KU-645-224

THE McDOUGALL PROGRAM FOR WOMEN

WHAT EVERY WOMAN NEEDS TO KNOW TO BE HEALTHY FOR LIFE

John A. McDougall, M.D.

RECIPES BY MARY McDOUGALL

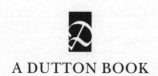

A DUTTON BOOK

A NOTE TO THE READER

The ideas, procedures, and suggestions contained in this book are not intended as a substitute for consulting with your physician. All matters regarding your health require medical supervision.

DUTTON
Published by the Penguin Group
Penguin Putnam Inc., 375 Hudson Street, New York, New York 10014, U.S.A.
Penguin Books Ltd, 27 Wrights Lane, London W8 5TZ, England
Penguin Books Australia Ltd, Ringwood, Victoria, Australia
Penguin Books Canada Ltd, 10 Alcorn Avenue, Toronto, Ontario, Canada M4V 3B2
Penguin Books (N.Z.) Ltd, 182–190 Wairau Road, Auckland 10, New Zealand

Penguin Books Ltd, Registered Offices: Harmondsworth, Middlesex, England

First published by Dutton, a member of Penguin Putnam Inc.

First Printing, January, 1999
10   9   8   7   6   5   4   3   2   1

Copyright © John A. McDougall, 1999
All rights reserved

 REGISTERED TRADEMARK — MARCA REGISTRADA

LIBRARY OF CONGRESS CATALOGING-IN-PUBLICATION DATA:
McDougall, John A.
    The McDougall program for women : what every woman needs to know to be healthy
    for life / John A. McDougall ; recipes by Mary McDougall.
        p.   cm.
    Includes bibliographical references.
    ISBN 0-525-94209-2 (alk. paper)
    1. Women—Health and hygiene.   I. McDougall, Mary A. (Mary Ann)   II. Title.
RA776.M4815   1999
613′.04244—dc21   96-34267
                                                                          CIP

Printed in the United States of America
Set in New Baskerville and Didot Roman
Designed by Eve L. Kirch

Without limiting the rights under copyright reserved above, no part of this publication may be reproduced, stored in or introduced into a retrieval system, or transmitted, in any form, or by any means (electronic, mechanical, photocopying, recording, or otherwise), without the prior written permission of both the copyright owner and the above publisher of this book.

This book is printed on acid-free paper.

THE McDOUGALL PROGRAM FOR WOMEN

Other Books by the Same Authors

The McDougall Quick & Easy Cookbook
The McDougall Program—Twelve Days to Dynamic Health
The McDougall Program for a Healthy Heart
The McDougall Program for Maximum Weight Loss
The New McDougall Cookbook
McDougall's Medicine—A Challenging Second Opinion
The McDougall Plan
The McDougall Health-Supporting Cookbooks—Volumes I and II

To Betty, Mary, and Heather—mother, wife, and daughter

Contents

ACKNOWLEDGMENTS

Our grateful appreciation to:

Tom Monte, for his excellent writing skills, which turned my serious scientific works into a book that personally touches the life of my readers; all of you who sent us your suggestions, recipes, and inspirational stories; and Patrick McDougall, for days spent in the medical library locating the research that supports the basic truths of the McDougall Program for Women. Many people work with us to help bring this vital message of health to you. Mary and I offer a special thanks to all of these dedicated people. They include the employees of:

- Dr. McDougall's Right Foods, the mission-oriented instant-food company that has made great health and weight loss effortless,
- The McDougall Program at St. Helena Hospital in the Napa Valley, a live-in experience that assures success with the McDougall Program (our professional staff locks you up for twelve days of summer camp), and
- The McDougall Health Clinic, where we make you feel like the most important person in the world when you call for help.

If you have any questions, or ideas you would like to share, please write or call.

The McDougall Health Clinic
PO Box 14039
Santa Rosa, CA 95403
Telephone: (707) 576-1654
FAX: (707) 576-3313
Book orders: (800) 570-1654
E-mail: drmcdougall@drmcdougall.com
On the web: http://www.drmcdougall.com

Dr. McDougall's Right Foods
101 Utah Avenue
San Francisco, CA 94080
Telephone: (650) 635-6000
FAX: (650) 635-6010
Food orders: (800) 367-3844
E-mail: drmcdougall@rightfoods.com
On the web: http://www.rightfoods.com

The McDougall Program/St. Helena Hospital
650 Sanitarium Drive
Deer Park, CA 94576
Telephone: (707) 963-6365
Reservations: (800) 358-9195

Reader's Note

This book offers you a real opportunity for rediscovering your health and appearance. However, diet is powerful medicine. Do not change your diet or start an intense exercise program if you are seriously ill or on medication unless you are under the care of a physician knowledgeable in nutrition and its effects on health. Do not change medications without professional advice. When appropriate, share this book with your doctor.

The people in this book are real. If you do as they have done, you should expect similar remarkable results. Although no treatment gives ideal outcomes for everyone, in most cases this approach offers you the best chance of rediscovering your health.

The McDougall Program for Women uses a pure vegetarian diet based around starchy vegetables with the addition of fruits and vegetables. If you follow the diet strictly for more than three years, or if you are pregnant or nursing, then take a minimum of 5 micrograms (mcg) of supplemental B_{12} each day.

Introduction

Imagine that you are a medical doctor and that six out of every ten patients you see are women, and imagine further that virtually all of these women suffer from illnesses that are preventable and very often treatable with the simplest of methods—a method that none of these women know about until they come to your office. When you, their doctor, apply your approach, the vast majority of these women are restored to good health. In fact, many undergo a remarkable transformation that is often described as "miraculous." As a scientist, you know that such "miraculous" recoveries are easily explained in medical terms. You also know that most of the women in the world today could experience similar healing miracles. Unfortunately, most women today are never told about this highly effective healing approach, and consequently they go on suffering until such disorders bring about an intense and terrifying health crisis that leaves them disfigured, or disabled, or dead.

Now imagine—as you look out your office window and consider the health crisis women face today—how you would feel if you were that doctor.

Now you've got a glimpse of how I feel.

I have been practicing medicine for more than twenty-six years, and I have watched a veritable parade of women come through my offices suffering from disorders that are very real and very dangerous, but all too often have been ineffectively treated or simply dismissed by other doctors. The consequence of inappropriate treatment is the inexorable progression of the illness until it explodes into one or another crisis. The array of possible outcomes are all too familiar: the diagnosis of cancer; the amputation of one or both breasts; a hysterectomy; a heart attack or stroke; the diagnosis of osteoporosis or of a serious fracture; hormonal imbalances, fluctuating menstrual periods, or an unstable and troubling menopause; and, finally, the presence of chronic pain.

Of course, this is to say nothing of the various stages of fear a woman passes through after she discovers a lump, or experiences abnormal periods or frightening discharges, or chest pain, or watches her skeleton shrink or her bones break.

Empowering Women to Make Choices About Their Health

The enormity of the women's health crisis is astounding. Although women live longer on the average than men, they often suffer more from chronic diseases. As the adage goes, "Women get sicker, men die quicker." By the first half of their ninth decade, about 50 percent of women will have died from heart disease, stroke, or cancer. Because the crisis is so great, many of us are led to believe that a solution doesn't exist. How could it? If there were an answer, it would be used—or so we are led to believe.

In fact, the answer to the women's health crisis does exist and is spelled out explicitly. Moreover, that answer is not hidden in some ancient and far-removed text, but is published in the most obvious place imaginable: the world's leading medical journals. It's right there for the whole world to see.

Unfortunately, most of the world's doctors have rejected the solution to the crisis, and instead have opted for non-solutions—a wide assortment of drugs and surgeries that palliate the symptoms of disease, at least temporarily, but fail to address their underlying causes. Which means that the illnesses only grow worse, until they bring about a crisis that requires even more extraordinary measures, or simply is too far advanced for anyone to do anything about.

It wouldn't bother me as much as it does if the women themselves decided to reject the solution to their disorders. Everyone should have that right. What disturbs me is the fact that women are not given the choice between the non-solutions and the real answer. All too often, they are led to believe that the prescribed drugs and surgery are the best available approaches. However, because these are not the best approaches, the modern epidemic of breast cancer, heart disease, osteoporosis, and so many other life-threatening disorders continues to afflict and kill millions of women prematurely.

You would think that the ineffectualness of the current approach would become obvious over time. Unfortunately, it hasn't. Each year, thousands of women undergo unnecessary mastectomies and hysterectomies; many more take hormones and pharmaceutical drugs that they do not need. In a state of fear, they undergo tests that are expensive and unrevealing. Women do all of this because they feel powerless to do anything else. Meanwhile, doctors remain silent about the fact that diet and lifestyle changes could prevent such diseases, and in many cases reverse them, even after they have reached a crisis point. Medicine has chosen to keep women ignorant of such facts. No wonder they feel helpless and hopeless.

Many of my readers are shaking their heads now and saying to themselves that such a statement is unbelievable. No doctor would deliberately keep important information from his or her patients.

Allow me to tell you a true story.

Fighting to Keep the Patient Ignorant

There are laws on the books in several states called informed consent laws, which are designed to tell women the likely results of various kinds of breast cancer treatments. These laws are also intended to inform women of their options and alternatives to the treatments. Such information is essential to anyone who wants to make a correct decision. You would think that, in a free society, doctors would insist upon such laws as the only ethical way they could conduct themselves for the benefit of their patients.

In 1981, I was living in Hawaii and in the fall of that year a group of concerned citizens approached me to help them establish an informed consent law for our state. At the time, only two other states, California and Massachusetts, had passed such legislation of informed consent for breast cancer treatment. Hawaii would be the third state, if we were successful.

My job in this effort was to inform members of the state senate subcommittee that aggressive surgical treatment, such as mastectomy, does not appear to prolong survival any longer than the non-deforming lumpectomy. The reason this is the case is because it takes eight to ten years, on average, for a cancer to grow large enough to be detected by mammography or palpation. If after eight to ten years the mass is indeed malignant, it will have spread beyond the breast to other parts of the body and consequently will be beyond the control of any kind of surgery, including a mastectomy. Given these medical facts (which I will present in great detail later in this book), it is obvious that many women are better off choosing a non-deforming lumpectomy over a mutilating operation, such as a mastectomy. However, because women are not informed of the medical facts they do not have a choice. Instead, they are often pressured into having a life-altering procedure that they do not need.

Our efforts to pass this essential and otherwise sane legislation were opposed by lobbyist Becky Kendro, assistant executive director of community affairs for the Hawaii Medical Association, the very powerful group that lobbied on behalf of the state's medical doctors. Despite her considerable efforts, Ms. Kendro was unable to refute the facts I presented, and as a result the bill for informed consent moved out of committee to be voted on by the state legislature.

About four months later I met one of the key advocates who was fighting for the informed consent law and asked why I had not heard about its passage. She explained that instead of offering women a full-fledged informed consent law, the Hawaii Medical Association had convinced legislators to allow physicians to place a general statement on the hospital surgical release form stating that a doctor had informed the patient of all risks and benefits of the proposed treatment. The informed consent bill never got out of committee.

I was outraged. How is a woman to know if she has been fully informed of all her options unless there is a specific law on breast cancer treatments requiring that she be told both the pros and cons of any such treatments. Moreover, by the time a woman finds herself in the hospital and ready to undergo surgery, she has already made her decision and is long past fighting for more information.

Thus, the Hawaii medical doctors had won the first round. The political activist I had been talking to vowed that we would do better next year.

On March 4, 1982, I went to the Hawaii State Capitol and testified before the Committee on Health, which was chaired by Senator Benjamin J. Cayetano (who would later be elected governor of the state). Once again, the business before the committee was Senate Bill No. 2636, the Hawaii law for informed consent for breast cancer treatment. As before, I presented the medical and scientific facts on the existing medical treatments. And as before, the same lobbyist for the state's doctors,

Becky Kendro, argued against me. Once again, she failed to prove her case to the committee members. This time, however, I was not nearly as naive about our chances of having the bill come before the full legislature. As I left the meeting, I asked Senator Cayetano if there was any chance this bill would fail to emerge from committee. He assured me the bill was on its way to the full Hawaii state legislature.

The next day I received a distress call. The bill was back in committee. The medical association's lobbyist, Ms. Kendro, had been replaced by a dozen physicians, some of whom were on the staff at the John Burns School of Medicine. They were there to stop the passage of the informed consent law. Upon being told of the full court press being put on by the doctors, I immediately closed my office for the day and hurried to the meeting, which was already in session.

Once again, I reported the scientific research demonstrating that women with breast cancer who underwent lumpectomy survived just as long as those who had undergone radical mastectomy. In other words, there was no survival benefit to those women who had undergone the more radical and disfiguring surgery.

After reading my testimony, I waited to be attacked by my colleagues. To my surprise they did not try to refute the science I had gathered. Instead, they argued that the medical community did not need to be told by the government how to inform women—they were already doing a good job of that, they said—and that the medical profession itself was capable of correcting any problems that might exist.

I asked the chief of surgery of the medical school, Dr. Thomas Whelan, how he informed a woman of the pros and cons of any treatment and her alternatives to such procedures.

"I tell her all of her options and then I give her a consensus paper that explains to her that mastectomy is the best way to go," he said. Hmm, I thought. No bias in that approach, doctor!

As to the claim that doctors can police their own house, I pointed out that in the previous year fewer than 8 percent of women with breast cancer had chosen a procedure other than breast amputation. And when we examined that 8 percent who did not have a mastectomy, we found that the majority of these women might have had the surgery were it not for the fact that they were too sick to withstand it. I then pointed out that the evidence supporting the comparable benefits of lumpectomy had been available for almost thirty years. Yet, the radical surgery still dominated. This fact could only mean that women were being encouraged—not to say pressured—into having the radical surgery, even when lumpectomy was just as good a choice for surviving. Obviously, doctors weren't keeping their house in order.

As the meeting ended, Representative Joan Hayes, who had undergone a bilateral mastectomy and whose daughter had already had a single mastectomy, took a copy of my testimony over to the group of medical school doctors and asked them why this document shouldn't be given to every woman who is diagnosed with breast cancer. They had no response.

The final act of this committee meeting was to instruct the Hawaii division of the American Cancer Society and the Hawaii Medical Association to write a brochure informing women of their choices and the pros and cons of the available treatments. After that order was passed, I stood up and said to the committee members that they should "expect an advertisement for a mastectomy." They all laughed. Little did they know.

From Bias to Informed Consent

On November 22, 1983, Representative Hayes sent a letter to the Hawaii Medical Association explaining to them that she was not satisfied with the brochure because it showed "a strong bias for the modified, or radical mastectomy." As I expected, it was essentially an advertisement for mastectomy. Was it a simple oversight that the committee designated to develop the brochure had failed to ask me to assist them? I called Reginold Ho, M.D., the head of the Hawaii division of the American Cancer Society. We agreed on a lunch meeting.

Dr. Ho did not come to lunch alone. With him was Ms. Kendro, the lobbyist for the state medical association, and about twenty other doctors. You might say that I didn't come alone either. With me was a stack of scientific articles two feet high, all supporting my position. I was not going to let any unscientific claims for radical mastectomy pass unchallenged.

After sparring over trivial matters for a while, I finally said, "We only have half an hour. It's time to address the issue at hand, which is to honestly inform women about results of various breast cancer treatments. The most important question every woman should ask when considering a specific breast cancer treatment is: 'How long can I expect to live after undergoing a specific therapy?' "

Then I pointed to the stack of articles I had brought with me and said, "I have here all the relevant scientific studies published on the subject. If anyone knows of a single reputable piece of research that supports a survival advantage of one treatment over another, please tell me." Dr. Ho and the others were silent. I continued, "Unless you tell women the simple fact that all surgical treatments result in equal chances of survival, I will not support any brochure you write and you will not get the legislature's approval."

A torrent of angry and meaningless protests followed from Dr. Ho, Ms. Kendro, and some of the others. Finally the lobbyist raised her voice well above the din of the meeting room and said, "If you think you're so smart, why don't you write it yourself."

"Okay, I will," I said. And in two weeks Dr. Ho, Ms. Kendro, and their colleagues had accepted my version of the brochure informing women of their treatment options—with a few politically correct modifications, of course. Still, the brochure was intact and effective. To my great surprise and pleasure, the medical association also asked me to write a few words telling women who had been diagnosed with breast cancer that they should also adopt a healthier diet in the hope of achieving a better outcome. These doctors knew me too well.

That year, the informed consent law for breast cancer treatment passed the Hawaii state legislature, and today Hawaii is among a handful of states that actually inform women of their treatment options and the likely outcomes from those treatments. One of the primary ways women were informed of their choices was through the brochure I had written.

Sadly, There Are Many Ways Around the Law

That brochure was not well received by most doctors and clinics who specialize in the diagnosis and treatment of cancer. Some chose not to give out the document; others offered patients their own substitutions for it. Both actions were breaking the law. As such deceptions became more widely known, the breach of a woman's right to full disclosure was addressed in the February 1988 issue of the *Hawaii Medical Association Newsletter.* The association reminded Hawaii doctors to follow the standards of informed consent. It also called the attention of doctors to the brochure, which should be handed out to patients, that "outlines the Breast Cancer Treatment Alternatives required by law."

Sadly, very little has changed in the years since we won that battle. Overaggressive treatment for breast cancer continues, with more than 65 percent of women still undergoing breast amputation. There are two reasons so few women choose the conservative therapy. First, surgeons still recommend mastectomies. Second, only a minority of women investigate their options.

One of the reasons women do not investigate their options is because they don't know where to look for answers. Their doctors are often powerful men or women who have strong opinions and seem to have the medical knowledge to back them up. The alternative to asking your doctor for the facts is to go directly to the medical literature, but many people are understandably intimidated by scientific journals. Not only is the language foreign to most lay readers, but people do not know how to evaluate the relative importance of an individual study. Finally, lay readers do not have any real experience with the most widely used treatments, or their alternatives, and therefore do not know how effective these approaches can be. In the absence of such knowledge and experience, people react from fear. The only thing they have to hold on to is their doctor's advice. Unfortunately, that advice is sometimes biased or ill-informed. The consequence is that a lot of women choose treatments that are ineffective at best, or harmful at worst.

Information That Empowers and Heals

That's the reason I wrote this book. In the pages that follow, I explain the causes of the leading health problems women face today, and how such disorders can be overcome. I describe the common current medical approaches to those disorders, and evaluate each therapy's benefits and risks. I then examine other options that are available. I offer many case histories of women who, when faced with these same disorders, chose to reclaim their power by using the program I offer in this book.

Once you understand the causes of a particular disorder, and how it can be overcome; once you fully understand the risks and benefits of any particular therapy; once you know very clearly all your options, you are in a position to make the best decision. You will feel in control and capable of managing your own way back to health.

Being in control is the first step in dealing effectively with fear, which is a big step toward gaining clarity and making appropriate medical decisions. Unfortunately, the current medical approach does not give women sufficient information to allow them to feel in control. All too often, women are made to feel dependent on the judgment of their doctors, which naturally engenders feelings of helplessness and fear.

Every adult patient should be treated with the respect and dignity adulthood warrants. In the patient-doctor relationship, that means that the doctor must fully disclose all the medical and scientific information available to him or her that is relevant to the patient's condition. That is not happening in medicine today. For a great may reasons, some of which I will discuss in this book, doctors often keep important information from patients. This practice is much more common in the relationship between male doctors and female patients. While there are many consequences to such behavior, the most fundamental one is that too many women take drugs they do not need, undergo an excessive amount of unnecessary surgery, and fail to experience the high quality of life they deserve.

As I will demonstrate, the effectiveness of my program has been proved in scientific and hospital settings, including the hospital where I practice medicine—and in the homes of hundreds of thousands of individual patients. In fact, the program I offer is not new. It is the oldest form of medicine in human history. It predates all the drugs you are taking, all the surgeries that you might be considering or have undergone. It is the foundation of medicine and the basis for true healing. Some 2,500 years ago, Hippocrates, the Father of Medicine, said, "Let thy food be thy medicine, and thy medicine be thy food." Twenty-five hundred years later, McDougall is saying, "Let thy food and thy exercise be thy medicine." I don't think Hippocrates would mind the slight addition.

In this way, I'm really an old-fashioned doctor, one who does not want people to take a lot of drugs and undergo operations they do not need—drugs and operations that very often do far more harm than good. Fortunately, I have the benefit of nearly a hundred years of science to back up my approach. In addition, I have the knowledge that, after more than two million years of life on this planet, humanity has come to depend on a certain way of eating and behaving in order to maintain its health. By combining science and traditional behavior, I have created a program that is as modern as the latest scientific discovery, and as old as humankind itself. On many occasions I have been told that my approach to medicine is ahead of its time. For example, in 1984 I published the first study on the use of a low-fat diet to treat women with breast cancer. A radical idea back then, but almost two decades later it is accepted as a commonsense recommendation, backed by solid scientific data, for this too often fatal disease. Now *The McDougall Program for Women* is a book whose time has come.

This book offers a program that can help you prevent serious disease. It can also help many women overcome illnesses that currently afflict them. If used correctly, it can boost your energy levels dramatically. Without counting calories or ever going hungry, you can achieve optimal weight and a much more youthful appearance. It will slow the aging process, improve your moods, and give you a much more positive view of life. The transformation that this program effects is not just the reduction or elimination of individual symptoms, but the enhancement of every aspect of your physical and emotional life. You're going to be amazed at what happens when you stop poisoning your body, and instead eat foods that strengthen your immune system, enhance your biochemistry, boost the health of your organs, and cause you to shed needless pounds.

This book contains vital information on health and medical issues for women of all ages and stages of life. It begins with a general understanding of why every woman should eat starchy foods, vegetables, and fruits. This is the basis for health, vitality, and an attractive appearance. Next I will provide you with guidance for experiencing a trouble-free pregnancy, giving birth to a healthy child, and how to nurture that child so that he or she has a strong foundation for life. Following this you will gain the information you need to protect yourself against cancer, and what to do if you have been diagnosed with some forms of cancer, particularly cancers of the breast. You will learn how to avoid having a hysterectomy. Then I will show you the way to achieve strong and healthy bones; how to reduce or eliminate menopausal symptoms naturally; and answer all the important questions regarding whether or not to take hormone replacement therapy. I'll also show you how you can avoid heart disease. Finally, we'll get down to the practical part with instruction on the complete McDougall Program, including practical alternatives to unhealthful foods and meals, and more than one hundred McDougall recipes for delicious and satisfying foods. In the appendix you will find information on major medical indications for the McDougall Program, the value of early detection tests, and why many manufactured low-fat foods are a health hazard. For those who are interested, I also provide a complete bibliography of scientific references that support my entire approach.

CHAPTER 1

Solving the Mystery of Women's Diseases

Ask any number of doctors why women suffer from such an array of physical disorders and they will tell you that nature somehow made mistakes in its design of a woman's body. The actual words may be, "They inherited their problems." After all, consider the plethora of chronic ailments women face, including numerous menstrual and reproductive disorders, diseased breasts, overfat bodies, hormonal imbalances, a troubling menopause, failing hearts, frail bones, and various forms of cancer. What other conclusion could you come to but that nature just didn't get it right? Something must be defective—in a word, a woman's genes. Because the genes fail, women must depend upon drugs and surgery to function and even to survive, or so the prevailing thinking goes.

But that's not the picture that emerges when we piece together the scientific evidence. On the contrary, we can draw no other conclusion but that after millions of years of adaptation, nature designed women perfectly—that is, to be healthy, vital, and fully alive, even after they are well into old age. Indeed, nature went so far as to give women an array of biological protections intended to help them thrive, even under the most demanding of circumstances, such as pregnancy, childbirth, and nourishing a baby.

Then what is going wrong? you may ask. Why do so many women spend their lives suffering from one health problem after another? If it is not some fundamental biological flaw, then what are women doing today that is so disabling and destructive to their health?

That's what this book is all about. In the chapters that follow, I will address the major health problems women face today and show you how they are caused, how they can be prevented, and how health can be restored by adopting a way of life that includes delicious and easy-to-prepare foods, along with a small amount of exercise. In the process, I am going to convince you that nature created women to be strong and healthy, and in fact gave each woman the physical foundation to achieve her full potential.

Everything I am going to say is based on scientific evidence that already has been published in the world's leading medical and scientific journals. For more than two decades, I have been converting the scientific and medical research into a practical and easy-to-follow program that hundreds of thousands have used to restore their good health. In the pages of this book, I will report my experience of treating women with my program, and I'll tell you about some of the remarkable recoveries of my female patients. I'll also show you in very explicit terms how you and your loved ones can do the same.

Why I Wrote This Book

Before we wade too far into the specific illnesses women must contend with, allow me to address a question that may arise in many of my readers' minds: Why is a male doctor writing a book about women's health? The answer is simple: I had to. No other medical authority is willing to tell you the things you need to know to preserve and regain your health—and the health of your loved ones. The fact is that all discussions about women's health today are founded upon a set of assumptions and biases that doctors refuse to acknowledge, but that women have come to accept. Unfortunately, the accepted way of performing medicine today is actually preventing women from getting the treatment they need to restore health.

The first of these assumptions is that the preeminent causes of disease are essentially genetic or unknown, and therefore beyond the control of women. Since the causes of their problems remain a mystery, women are left with no other choice but to believe that they are somehow defective and therefore condemned to a lifetime of medication and/or disease.

The reason this belief prevails is simply because *the vast majority of doctors will not tell you the extent to which your diet and lifestyle are the causes of your health problems.* Doctors fail to tell you that your behavior is hurting your body, mostly because physicians do not know any better; they are performing medicine in the way they were trained, with a total lack of a practical education on the importance of diet and lifestyle.

The second major assumption in medicine is that the only effective way to treat disease is through drugs, surgery, and/or radiation. All essential information about how diet and lifestyle can prevent or treat disease is avoided. Thus, when a doctor discusses reproductive, menstrual disorders, and PMS, he may recommend hormone therapy or even a hysterectomy, but he fails to tell you that appropriate diet and lifestyle often clear up the problems entirely, making drugs and surgery unnecessary. When discussing osteoporosis, or the loss of bone tissue, a doctor will inform a woman of the pros and cons of hormone replacement therapy (HRT), or the bone-sparing effects of a particular drug, such as Fosamax, but the physician does not tell her that a major way to prevent further bone loss is to avoid animal foods, including skim milk, even though it is well established that such foods increase bone loss. When women experience a difficult menopause, they are presented with the pros and cons of HRT, but they are not informed that their diets and lifestyles will dramatically reduce the symptoms of menopause; nor are they told that a healthy diet can actually decrease the toxic effects of HRT, making it far less likely that the drugs will cause cancer.

The current policy of avoiding the importance of diet and nutrition in women's health is most unfortunate for young women, who are in a position to prevent the tragic consequences that flow from a lifetime of unhealthy eating. In today's world, young women are not told that their diets and exercise habits will determine the strength of their bones, the kinds of periods they experience, the condition of their skin, the health of their breasts, their chances of contracting cancer, how rapidly they will appear to age, the kind of menopause they eventually will undergo, or whether or not they will need hormone replacement therapy. The only significance the word *diet* has for women is its effect on weight, a condition that itself has become so mysterious and intractable that many women now obsess about it. What doctors do not tell women is that the same diet that promotes health and prevents disease also controls weight—and it does it without your ever needing to count calories or go hungry.

There are so many people who lose weight effortlessly on the McDougall Program that it is impossible to give even a representative sampling. Jean Doyle, fifty-five, of California, wrote to me in 1996 to say, "I just want you to know that you literally saved my life. I was so sick of taking prescription pills that I was like a walking zombie. I had two heart attacks, two angioplasty surgeries, and nobody told me to change my diet. I just put my life into the doctor's hands. I finally got sick and tired of being sick. I started reading your books and heard your tapes. I threw all my pills down the toilet and adopted your program. I lost forty pounds in three months and have no more angina pain whatsoever." Jean went on to say that she had more energy than she had had in more than a decade.

Judy Cohen, of Florida, wrote to me in 1995 to say that "I saw you at the Orlando Health Expo and started following your diet after I listened to your talk. I have lost sixty-one pounds and stabilized." Judy stopped by to see me at my presentation at the 1996 Las Vegas Health Conference to show me photographs of her former self. I have been teaching this way of life for nearly two decades, but even I am still amazed by the miracle-like recoveries I see people make.

Linda Waller, forty-four, of Connecticut, wrote to me in 1998 to say that she had lost ninety pounds after reading my book *The McDougall Program for Maximum Weight Loss* (Dutton, 1994). "I have maintained this weight loss for more than four years," Linda wrote to me. "Your diet has become a part of my life. I don't even think of it as a diet anymore. It's just the way I eat."

In 1993, Patricia Paris, fifty-four, was suffering from severe sinus headaches, joint pain, stomach disorders, back pain, swelling in her knees, and chronic depression. She and her husband used to love to go dancing, but it had been many years since they had danced because Patricia's health had steadily deteriorated for more than the past decade. All that changed when she adopted the McDougall Program.

"Three and a half years ago, I saw your infomercial for Twelve Days to Dynamic Health," she wrote to me in 1996. "I could not believe all those claims could be true, but I thought to myself, 'What do I have to lose?' "

Indeed, as Patricia wrote, her life had hit bottom. "I would go through a bottle of pain pills a month . . . I used to be depressed all the time. I was in so much pain, I thought to myself, 'If I feel like this at fifty, what would it be like to be sixty?' I felt so lousy and tired and my stomach bothered me all the time."

She decided that a couple of weeks on the McDougall Program might be worth the effort. "After I had read your book and found out that I had to become a vegetarian, I didn't like the idea very much, but I thought I could last for twelve days. After the fourth day, the swelling I had in my knees disappeared and after the eighth day, all the pain was gone. I felt so good that to continue following your plan was easy. After a while, I didn't miss the meat and dairy. I actually prefer vegetables to my old way of eating, and everything you said was amazingly true . . . I haven't had a headache in over three years. . . .

"Now I have more energy than I had ten years ago, and I feel fantastic. . . . My depression is gone and my whole life has changed. . . . By the way, I also lost forty pounds, which isn't the reason I originally changed my diet."

Why Doctors Avoid the *D* and *E* Words

There are many reasons why your doctor doesn't counsel you on diet and exercise, but here are two of the most important: first, diet and exercise therapy are not as exciting to physicians and scientists as are the technical, pharmacological, virological, and surgical treatments available; and, second, there's too much greed in medicine today. In the time it takes a doctor to teach one person what to eat, what to buy in her grocery store, how to cook healthful foods, and what to eat in restaurants and while traveling, another doctor who relies on drugs can see a dozen or more patients. It's simple economics. But as I will show you, there's a big difference in the outcomes of patients who eat healthfully and walk regularly, versus those who rely on drug therapy. But drug therapy is only one way doctors can inflate the cost of treating their patients. Many tests and surgical procedures are widely accepted for women, even though science has proved they are not necessary in most cases.

Neither male nor female doctors are telling women these facts. And unless physicians start saying the kinds of things I am saying in this book, women are going to remain on a deadly treadmill: they will engage in behaviors that promote disease and, once they are ill, will gamble their lives on an array of treatments that all too often do not work.

In addition to these systemic problems within medicine is the thorny and much more nebulous issue of the relationship between the sexes. The problem of how male doctors treat women varies dramatically among physicians. There are a great many male doctors who have tremendous compassion and understanding for all their patients, but there are some who patronize women and dismiss their complaints with a proverbial pat on the head and a new prescription. When you add this rather amorphous but very real problem to an already one-sided relationship, you get the medical equivalent of a fast food restaurant. Women are often seen as the "soft" customers, the ones doctors can treat quickly, with maximum profit.

Underlying these issues is a larger problem we all must face today: a kind of cultural and historical denial of the real causes of disease. This denial allows us to continue consuming foods and living lifestyles that create illness. When such diseases arise, we turn to doctors for drugs and surgery that we hope will silence the symptoms. Nevertheless, both men and women have a limit to the quantity of poison they can take into their bodies. Once their tolerance levels are exceeded, they begin to manifest symptoms, and all the drugs and surgery in the world are not going to fully protect women from the ultimate consequences of those poisons.

Since I am among a handful of medical doctors who have the knowledge and the experience of using diet, exercise, and lifestyle to treat disease, I am one of the few people who can bring this message to women today. That's why I wrote this book.

Cataloging Women's Illnesses

In the course of telling you about my program and the many people who have overcome disease by using it, I am in no way making light of the problems that women face today. They are very real and extremely intractable, especially when treated with the current medical armamentarium. In fact, there has never been a time, I believe, that women experienced such a devastating health crisis as the one they face today. It seems that every single aspect of their physical health is under siege, beginning very early in life.

Consider a woman's life, beginning sometime between eight and sixteen, when most girls experience menarche, or the onset of their first menstrual cycle. For a modern girl, this initiation into womanhood, which in traditional cultures is often celebrated as one of life's great steps in maturity, is a major step into decades of pain and suffering. From very early on, many young girls experience irregular and painful periods; some have heavy blood flow that can last a week or more; others endure cycles of less than twenty-eight days; and still others suffer spotting or inadequate flow. Coupled with these problems is a list of discomforts collectively called premenstrual syndrome (PMS) that include headaches, cramps, water retention, anxiety, irritability, tension, and fatigue. As a girl develops further, she begins to experience tenderness in her breasts during the time of her period, a tenderness that, for many, becomes another source of monthly pain and worry.

Of course, this is to say nothing of the standard disorders that both boys and girls experience in early childhood, including colic, ear infections, stomachaches, constipation, inflammatory arthritis, tonsillitis, and appendicitis, that are also due to their diet.

From very early on, there is a growing awareness, even a fear, that the body is associated with all kinds of problems. And then the big issue arises: appearance.

Even before she enters womanhood, many young girls are already worrying about their weight, a problem that is created by a diet that almost guarantees weight gain, and by the excessive amount of pressure society, and very often family members, place on girls to be thin. The terrible trap women are caught in is that on the typical Western diet, girls can't help but gain excess weight. Nor can they lose it, which means the pressure only becomes more intense. By the fourth grade, 40 percent of girls have begun dieting. For most of these young girls, this will be the early start of a lifetime of dieting that will result in dozens and even hundreds of failures. Not only will such failures affect these women emotionally and psychologically, but many of the nutritionally imbalanced regimens they adopt will affect them physically, thus contributing to their health problems.

There are a lot of people looking at the social and family issues related to women and dieting today, and I applaud them all, but I cannot understand why more people don't stop to think about the kinds of foods young girls are eating now, and the relationship of those foods to overweight and obsessive dieting. The fact is that there are too many calories, especially fat calories, in the standard Western diet for a young girl or woman to burn as energy. Thus, weight accumulation is inevitable for many women, just as it is for men.

In addition to overweight are the many painful miseries of oily skin and acne, which are also directly related to the kinds of foods women eat. Appearance, a woman finds, is a constant source of frustration and emotional distress. By adolescence, a great many young girls have come to believe that their bodies are "the problem." Little wonder, therefore, that so many succumb to eating disorders, cosmetic surgery, or just plain self-hatred.

As they mature, "the problem" only gets worse. Many women suffer from an array of digestive disorders, abdominal pain, diarrhea, constipation (often referred to as spastic colon or irritable bowel syndrome), and gallstones. Again, all caused by their food choices. Overweight women suffer from higher levels of adult-onset diabetes, cardiovascular disease, and gallbladder disease. What women must realize is that the same diet that makes them overweight also makes them sick.

The senior years can be most unkind to women because that is when osteoporosis has caused a dangerous erosion of bone mass and makes a great many women vulnerable to fractures. A woman's skeleton reaches its peak strength sometime in her early to mid thirties, but from that point onward she begins to lose bone. Some women lose 50 to 70 percent of their bone tissue, causing many to suffer major fractures. For many, those fractures will be fatal.

In this, the most prosperous country in the world, old age has become synonymous with sickness and disability, especially for women. Far more women suffer from osteoporosis than do men, just as more women suffer from rheumatoid arthritis, lupus, scleroderma, multiple sclerosis, and Alzheimer's disease than do men.

BREASTS AND REPRODUCTIVE ORGANS

Throughout a woman's adulthood, her breasts are often her greatest source of worry. The tenderness she experienced in youth becomes outright pain in adulthood, often accompanied by the discovery of a lump or several lumps. The fear engendered from such a discovery is highly disruptive and, for many, often devastating. Yet, only half of the women who experience such problems actually consult a physician; when they do, they usually are told that they suffer from fibrocystic breast disease. However, all too often the doctor finds a malignant or cancerous growth. Breast cancer afflicts one in eight adult women. (In affluent communities, the illness attacks one in seven women.) More than 65 percent of these women will undergo mastectomies. Each year, nearly 200,000 women are diagnosed with breast cancer and approximately 46,000 die from the disease.

The reproductive organs are another site of trouble and worry. In addition to the list of menstrual disorders I mentioned, there are the problems of uterine fibroids, endometriosis, and cancer of the uterus. Fully one-quarter of women who become pregnant and give birth must undergo cesarean section. By the time they reach menopause, approximately one-third of women will have had their uteruses surgically removed. As with other problems, overweight only exacerbates these issues. Overweight women are more prone to polycystic ovary disease, breast cancer, and uterine cancer.

Women's health is in trouble from birth until death, and doctors are remaining silent about the causes of that trouble, as well as the most effective way of treating it.

To be fair, it is not just women who are in trouble. The November 13, 1996, issue of the *Journal of the American Medical Association* reported that one-third of Americans are affected by such chronic illnesses as arthritis, constipation, cancer, diabetes, heart disease, hypertension, various forms of indigestion, kidney disease, multiple sclerosis, and obesity. These problems are so widespread, in fact, that they account for three-quarters of U.S. health care bills. In 1990, the cost of treating chronic disease in the United States was $425.2 billion.

At some point, all of us have to take a good hard look in the mirror and ask: Why are we all suffering so?

Changing Your Lifestyle Is the Key to Healing

There's an old and rather tattered joke that provides perhaps the best advice medicine can give any patient when it comes to treating chronic disease. The joke goes like this: A patient goes to a doctor and says, "Doctor, I broke my arm in two different places. What should I do?"

The doctor replies, "Don't go into those places."

That's essentially the advice every woman should receive when she comes to a doctor and finds she suffers from one or another chronic illness. Doctors should be telling patients to avoid the causes of their problems. In effect, every doctor should be telling his or her patients, "Stop going into those places."

Stopping the causes of chronic disease requires the patient to change highly destructive behavior patterns. Let me give you an example. Coughing, wheezing, and shortness of breath are often due to chronic lung disease caused by cigarette smoking. The "acute care" solutions offered by doctors involve the use of cough syrups and bronchodilators, but these treatments cannot heal the injury caused by cigarettes. The solution is to stop inhaling cigarette smoke. As most former smokers know, the chronic coughing and wheezing usually stops within a week after they give up cigarettes. In time, the body heals itself of the damage done to the lungs by years and even decades of smoking. There's nothing a doctor can offer that's as powerful as the simple act of throwing away the cigarettes.

In the same way, most chronic diseases are caused by injuries to the body brought about by the foods people eat. It's that simple. The only way to solve the problem is to stop eating the foods that are causing the injuries. At the same time, we must eat foods that promote the healing mechanisms of the body. There is no doubt that the greatest abundance of healing nutrients and phytochemicals available in foods are concentrated in starchy grains, beans, vegetables, and fruit.

After reviewing the scientific literature related to the cause and prevention of chronic illness, former U.S. Surgeon General C. Everett Koop, M.D., put the matter plainly in *Nutrition and Health in the United*

States, the Surgeon General's report published in 1988. As the report stated, the "main conclusion is that overconsumption of certain dietary components is now a major concern for Americans. While many foods are involved, chief among them is the disproportionate consumption of foods high in fats, often at the expense of foods high in complex carbohydrates and fiber that may be more conducive to health."

Similar recommendations to eat fewer animal products and more plant foods have been made by *every other health organization*, including the American Heart Association, the American Cancer Society, the American Diabetes Association, and the American Dietetic Association.

Throughout this book, I'm going to show you how certain foods give rise to specific health problems that women face throughout their lives, but allow me to summarize very briefly ten ways harmful foods injure people every day.

Ten Disadvantages of an Unhealthful Diet

1. NUTRITIONAL DEFICIENCIES

When you hear the term *nutritional deficiencies*, you right away think of the old nutrition-related problems of beriberi (from insufficient vitamin B_1) or pellagra (from inadequate tryptophan), or scurvy (from insufficient C)—all due to inadequate intake of unrefined plant foods. Interestingly, today we face a new array of deficiency diseases, and these, too, stem from poor consumption of unprocessed plants.

Plant foods contain literally thousands of phytochemicals and antioxidants, powerful chemicals that are essential to the body's immune response and its capacity to repair damaged genes and cells. Without adequate consumption of plant foods, we are deprived of these chemicals that are essential to the prevention of disease and good health.

Plant foods are also the only source of fiber, which, though not a nutrient, is essential to good health. Just as it is deficient in other health-promoting substances, the standard Western diet is also deficient in fiber.

2. NUTRITIONAL EXCESS

It is said that we Westerners dig our graves with our teeth. No nutritional problem buries us deeper in disease than our reliance upon animal foods, such as red meat, poultry, dairy products, and eggs, all of which provide us with too much fat, cholesterol, animal protein, and calories. In addition to these are overconsumption of salt, vegetable oils, and refined foods.

You cannot regain your health if you eat excess amounts of fat and cholesterol, and, frankly, you cannot avoid excesses of both if you eat animal foods. The fastest way to optimal health is to eliminate all animal foods, vegetable oils, and refined foods, and rely exclusively on a starch-based diet that is rich in immune-boosting and cancer-fighting chemicals.

3. Hormone Imbalances

In several different ways, all of which I will discuss in detail later in this book, diet changes hormone levels—either for health or for illness. High-fat, low-fiber diets elevate estrogen and prolactin levels and keep estrogens circulating within the system, causing excessive stimulation of the reproductive organs and leading to unstable menstrual periods, PMS, fibrocystic breast disease, ovarian cysts, endometriosis, uterine fibroids, breast cancer, and endometrial (uterine) cancer.

Conversely, diets low in fat and high in fiber are associated with moderate to low levels of estrogen and prolactin, as well as with low incidences of these same diseases. The diet I recommend is one of the most powerful ways you can restore balance to your hormones and thus restore health to your reproductive organs and breasts.

4. Immune Reactions

Proteins found in milk and other animal foods can generate an immune reaction and cause your immune cells to attack your own tissues. For millions of people, such reactions cause mild aches, pains, stiffness in the joints, runny nose, fluid collections in the middle ear, postnasal drip, hoarseness, asthma, eczema, and bed-wetting. For millions more, however, the symptoms are far more severe. Immune cells can attack connective tissue, causing inflammatory (rheumatoid) arthritis and lupus. They can also attack the arteries, giving rise to atherosclerosis and heart disease, or the kidneys, causing severe kidney disorders (glomerulonephritis). Many scientists now believe that such immune reactions are from animal proteins, such as meat and milk proteins. Researchers also believe foreign proteins from cow's milk enter the bloodstream through the gut wall and stimulate immune cells to attack and destroy the insulin-producing cells of the pancreas. This food-caused reaction is the primary cause of juvenile, or type I, diabetes.

5. HAZARDOUS MICROBES

An increasing amount of our food supply is now tainted with harmful microorganisms, including E. coli, trichinella, and salmonella. Some of the beef herds in Europe now carry the organism that produces "mad cow disease," or Creutzfeldt-Jakob disease.

One of the least publicized but potentially dangerous sources of disease comes from cattle infected with bovine immunodeficiency viruses (BIV)—also known as bovine AIDS virus—and bovine leukemia viruses (BLV). On average, 40 percent of the beef herds and 64 percent of the dairy herds in the United States are known to be infected with BIV. Over 60 percent of dairy herds are infected with BLV. No one knows the extent to which these viruses affect human health, but common sense would dictate that it is not a wise choice to consume them ourselves, or feed them to our children.

Chemically, plants differ greatly from animals and therefore the diseases that affect plants—Dutch elm disease or aphids, for example—are never a threat to humans.

6. CHEMICAL CONTAMINANTS

Chemical pollutants from a variety of sources, including industrial waste and farming (such as pesticides, herbicides, and chemical fertilizers), are well known to cause diseases. Many scientists believe that such toxic chemicals play an important role in the initiation of breast cancer. These toxic chemicals are also believed to be involved in some allergic and autoimmune diseases. Because these chemicals are attracted to and stored in fat, their highest concentrations are usually found in animal-derived foods.

7. PHYSICAL INJURY

Many components of the rich Western diet harm the body by direct physical contact. Coffee and decaffeinated coffee, tea, and smoking have been shown to cause gastritis (heartburn) and lay the foundation for ulcers. Diets very high in salt cause chronic irritation of the stomach lining and contribute to stomach cancer. Hot spices can cause irritation and burn the intestinal tract from one end to the other.

In addition, many commonly consumed foods carry bacteria that can cause physical damage to the intestine, contributing to ulcers, colon cancer, and other diseases.

8. Free Radical Oxidation

Oxidation, or free radical production, causes the decay of cells, organs, and tissues within the human body. It contributes to more than sixty major illnesses, including heart disease, the common cancers, cataracts, disorders of the brain and nervous system, even simple aging. One of the primary causes of free radical creation is dietary fat. Other causes include cigarette smoke and chemical pollutants.

The antidote to oxidation and free radical production are *anti-oxidants*, which are found abundantly in plant foods. These chemical good guys restore health to cells and repair the damage to DNA done by free radicals. In the process, they protect us from the major causes of aging, disability, and death.

9. Acid-Base Imbalance

Your blood and much of your biochemistry is slightly alkaline on the acid-alkaline (pH) spectrum, a condition your body struggles to maintain. Plant foods are alkaline by nature and support the body's pH balance, while most animal foods are acidic and throw off the body's natural pH balance. In order to neutralize the acid that accumulates in the blood and tissues from an acidic diet, the body leaches its natural alkalizing buffers, the calcium and phosphates found in bones, into the bloodstream. The result is weaker, more porous bones, and the first step toward osteoporosis.

This leaching of calcium and phosphates into the bloodstream, followed by the excretion of this bone material through the kidneys into the urine, is also the beginning of calcium-based kidney stones.

10. Physical Straining from the Absence of Fiber

The fiber you consume from plants fills up with moisture, making bowel elimination regular, and stools soft and easy to pass. Heavy reliance upon fiber-free meat, poultry, dairy products and low-fiber refined grains results in tiny, rock-hard stools that are difficult to pass. The consequence is that many people struggle and strain to move their bowels, causing hemorrhoids, varicose veins, and hiatal hernia, which is often accompanied by symptoms of indigestion and chest pain.

If you currently eat the animal-based standard Western diet, you are injuring your body not once, but three or more times a day. When you think about it, you have to admit that it's a wonder you and every other person on this diet functions as well, and for as long, as you do. Still, we do not have to strain our minds to understand why women suffer from such a wide array of disorders. Women are not ill because of some flaw in nature's design, but because of the poisons on their plates.

Avoiding Hysterectomy

In 1987, Denise Sobel, a registered nurse from Sonoma, California, underwent surgery for the removal of an infected ovarian cyst that had ruptured. Her doctor wanted to do a complete hysterectomy, but after strong resistance from Denise, he promised to take out only the single ovary. When the doctor opened her up, he found that her entire abdominal cavity was covered with endometriosis, or the excessive growth of tissue that had spread from the endometrium. True to his word, the doctor took only the ruptured ovary, but when Denise came out of surgery, he told her that eventually she would have to have the hysterectomy.

In 1992, Denise began to experience severe pain and swelling of the remaining ovary. It had become so enlarged that two physicians in different parts of California insisted that she immediately have the ovary removed, along with her uterus. Both doctors told her that the ovary would never return to its normal size, and warned that if it continued to grow it would eventually hemorrhage, causing far more serious problems.

Denise knew of my programs at St. Helena Hospital, in the Napa Valley of California, where I run a twelve-day inpatient program that provides people with instruction in the full McDougall regimen. I also provide night classes for local people who want to learn what to eat, how to prepare the foods, and how to exercise.

As Denise wrote to me in 1995, "Eventually [I] signed up for one of your four-night classes. My life changed from the first class."

Within two months of taking the class and adopting the program—which she did after the very first night—Denise lost weight, no longer suffered any constipation, which "I had always had [thinking that this was normal]," and discovered that the pain in her ovary and uterus was gone. "I knew that my female parts felt better," she wrote to me.

However, she still believed that she needed a hysterectomy, based on her previous medical examinations and the insistence of her doctors. Convinced that she would be operated on, Denise wrote that, "I went for my preop examination with the M.D. in San Francisco. He examined me and told me that he did not feel justified doing the surgery as my ovary was normal, my uterus was freely movable—before, it was fixed—[the result of the excessive tissue that had become hardened], and sent me on my way!"

Needless to say, Denise has been practicing the McDougall Program ever since.

The current state of women's health does not have to persist. In fact, nature designed women so perfectly that they have the capability to overcome the disorders that may currently beset them. Women have the strength to regain their health and thrive.

To do that, they must first create the conditions that support the restoration of health. Those conditions are established by following the McDougall Program, which is what I want to describe to you next.

CHAPTER 2

Eating Your Way to Health

Just as it is for all other physicians, my daily medical practice is my greatest teacher. Every day I confront patients who come to me suffering from an incredible variety of disorders, and every day, I learn from these people. They reveal special insights about their illnesses, the mysterious associations between certain behaviors and the rise and fall of their symptoms, the therapies they have used, and the results they have experienced, Like other physicians, I have pored endlessly over medical journals in search of answers to the medical mysteries that people present me with each day. I have also used the best technology and most advanced therapies science can offer. And I can tell you that in all my experience, only one form of therapy prevents and effectively treats almost every chronic disease and disorder under the sun. It does it better than any other form of medicine I have used.

That singularly powerful form of medicine is this: a starch-based diet, composed chiefly of whole grains; whole-grain products, such as pasta, tortillas, and bread; beans and legumes; a wide assortment of vegetables; and fruits. In addition to this diet, I add a moderate amount of exercise, at least four days per week. The exercise need not be any more strenuous than a daily walk. I also strongly encourage people to eliminate the most toxic of their bad habits, especially smoking and excess consumption of coffee and alcohol.

I use this therapy every day, in both my professional and my personal life. In fact, I have used it to treat every member of my extended family when one or another of them faced an ordinary health problem or a life-threatening disease, and in every case this regimen succeeded far better than anything else that was attempted.

One of the most common experiences I have had in my medical practice is this: a woman comes to me with a disorder of some kind that has been treated by every known medication or surgery, only to see the symptoms persist or worsen. I listen to the description of her symptoms, assess her condition, and make a diagnosis. I then inform her of how food and lifestyle factors are causing her disorder, and how appropriate diet and exercise can restore her health.

Occasionally, I couple my diet and exercise regimen with drug therapy when I believe that a particular pharmaceutical can be effective in the short term, at least until she regains her health sufficiently to be freed from the drug. I then let the diet, exercise, and drug therapy do the rest. In a very short time, the woman is experiencing a dramatic improvement in health and I am gradually weaning her from the drug until she is entirely drug free.

I reach many more people through my books and media appearances. Each week, I get mail from people who have read one of my books or listened to my radio show or seen me on television. Rita Freeman, of California, is one such example.

In 1992, Rita was diagnosed with severe rheumatoid arthritis. As she said in her letter to me years later, "It came on slowly and sporadically, but by December 1992 the pain was excruciating and crippling. There were days that signing my name, getting up from a chair, or just shaking a hand were overwhelming tasks."

The pain Rita suffered would often keep her awake at night, or simply wake her in the middle of the night and prevent her from going back to bed. One morning, at three o'clock, she was awakened by the pain and could not return to sleep. As a way to distract herself from the pain, she turned on the television and, quite by coincidence, saw me explaining the relationship between diet and health. One of the people I had on the show was one of my former patients who reported her recovery from severe rheumatoid arthritis on my diet and exercise regimen. Seeing that patient and listening to my explanation piqued Rita's interest, and, as she later wrote, "I decided to give it a try. To say the least, I was cautiously optimistic. I had a hard time believing that a change in diet could improve my health so dramatically."

Rita bought one of my books and adopted the program. It wasn't long afterward that her skepticism vanished. "The results were gradual and subtle at first," she wrote to me. "My shoes started to fit very loosely, because the swelling in my joints had gone down. I could slide my wedding bands over my knuckle and started wearing them again.

"It wasn't until the day I ran down a flight of stairs that I realized something was really happening. I was halfway down the block before it dawned on me [that] 'I RAN.' I hadn't run in over a year. Walking was the best I could do, and some days I'd characterize it more like hobbling.

"But there was nothing quite as telling [as] when I *firmly* shook my doctor's hand. He was taken aback. The expression on his face will stay with me forever.

"After three months on the program, I was 85 percent back to my healthy self and off all the pills." Rita resolved to go that last 15 percent by adhering even more closely to the McDougall Program. At the time of her letter, Rita characterized herself and her recovery as a "walking miracle."

Introducing the McDougall Program

While the foods on the program are explained in much greater detail in chapter 16, I want to give you an idea here of what you should eat and what you should avoid in order to regain your health. As you read about food substitutions and practical steps for healthy meals and try the recipes, you will discover that there is endless variety in this diet, both in the foods and the herbs and spices you can use to make your meals delicious and completely satisfying.

The foods you should eat every day include

- Whole grains and whole-grain cereals, such as brown rice, barley, corn, millet, quinoa, oatmeal, bulgur wheat, and wheat berries
- Whole-grain products, such as pasta, breads, tortillas, cereals, and puffed grains
- Squashes, including acorn, buttercup, butternut, pumpkin, summer squash, and zucchini
- Roots and tubers, including potatoes, sweet potatoes, yams, carrots, rutabagas, and turnips
- Beans and other legumes, such as adzuki, black beans, black-eyed peas, chickpeas, kidney beans, lentils, navy beans, pinto beans, peas, split peas, and string beans
- Green and yellow vegetables, such as broccoli, cabbage, collard greens, kale, various kinds of lettuces, mustard greens, watercress; also celery, cauliflower, asparagus, and tomatoes
- Fruits, such as apples, bananas, berries, grapefruits, melons, oranges, peaches, and pears (limit servings to two to three per day)

In order to complement and enhance the flavor of these foods, the program allows most people to add small amounts of sugars, salt, and spices to the surface of their foods.

Once you learn to prepare these foods and allow your taste buds to adapt to the new flavors and textures, you will not feel any sense of deprivation. Nor will you feel any strong desire for the old high-fat, rich diet that you once barely subsisted on.

That old diet, of course, is the cause of so many of your problems. Like the cigarette smoker whose only real solution to her lung disease is to stop smoking, you must avoid all of the following foods if you are to restore your health.

- All forms of red meat, including beef, pork, and lamb. The human body simply cannot withstand all the fat, cholesterol, harmful bacteria, chemicals, and excess animal protein that these foods provide.
- Poultry and fish. Like all muscle foods, poultry and fish contain large amounts of cholesterol and significant amounts of fat.
- Dairy products, including milk, cheese, and yogurt, as well as the "low-fat" and "skim" versions of these foods. Whole-milk products are rich in fat and cholesterol, while both whole milk and the low-fat or skim varieties contain proteins and other potentially harmful constituents that trigger an immune reaction and cause allergies, joint and connective tissue disorders, heart disease, diabetes, and other serious illnesses.
- Oil, including olive, safflower, peanut, and corn oils. Oil is fat in its liquid form. All vegetable oils contribute to obesity, under the proper circumstances they all can promote cancer, and most of them are also involved in atherosclerosis of the arteries.
- Eggs. They are rich in fat, cholesterol, and animal protein, and deficient in dietary fiber and carbohydrate.

In addition, you should limit your intake of the following foods:

- Nuts, seeds, avocados, and olives—all are high in fat—as well as soybeans and soybean products, such as tofu, tempeh, and soy milk. Most soybean products are also high in fat; however, low-fat tofu and nonfat soy milk are used in some of our recipes. Some recipes also contain small amounts of nuts, seeds, avocadoes, and olives.
- Dried fruits. They are rich in concentrated calories.
- All fruits and other forms of simple sugars should be eliminated by people with high triglycerides and cholesterol.

- Legumes, such as beans, peas, lentils, and other high protein vegetable foods must be severely limited by people with liver or kidney failure and those with osteoporosis or kidney stones.
- Breads, bagels, and pastas. If you are concerned about your weight, these refined grains can slow your weight loss. They provide concentrated forms of calories that are quickly absorbed. Such rapidly absorbed calories raise insulin levels and cause the body to store more fat. Therefore, these foods should be eaten sparingly by people who want to lose weight. If you are thin and are not concerned about gaining weight, or you actually want to gain more weight, then you might add more of these to your diet.

DESIGNING A DIET AROUND BULKIER, STARCH-BASED PLANTS

Decades ago, people used to refer to plant foods—especially whole grains, pasta, beans, and the pulpier vegetables, such as squash—as starches. Rich in complex carbohydrates (long chains of sugar molecules that provide lasting energy and endurance), starches are also low in fat, low in calories, and high in fiber. They contain generous amounts of healthy plant proteins. They are also exceedingly rich in nutrition and contain no cholesterol. (Cholesterol is found only in animal foods.)

Many people who try to eat a more healthful diet fail to distinguish between the bulkier, starch-based plant foods, such as beans, grains and grain products, and the exceptionally low-calorie vegetables, such as leafy greens, broccoli, cauliflower, and sprouts. The starchy foods are luscious, filling, and create satisfaction. The yellow and green vegetables, while rich in nutrition and full of delicious flavor, especially when they are prepared properly, do not fill people up.

When people do not understand the difference between the two vegetable groups, they often make the mistake of subsisting entirely on the lowest-calorie vegetable foods. After a day or two on that extremely low-calorie diet, they complain that they're starving. "Nobody can eat this way," they say.

I agree completely—*nobody* can subsist on a diet composed mostly of these very low-calorie green and yellow vegetables. The secret to creating satisfying meals is to design your diet around delicious starches like beans, breads, corn, pastas, potatoes, sweet potatoes, and rice. People often think of these as the "comfort foods": oatmeal, pancakes, waffles, or hash brown potatoes for breakfast; bean and vegetable soups for lunch; and potatoes, spaghetti, or bean burritos for dinner.

These meals will fill you up, satisfy your taste buds, and still cause you to lose weight. In fact, because the foods on my program are so reasonable in calories, and especially low in fat calories, most people can eat as much as they want throughout the day and still lose weight while improving their health.

PUTTING THE McDOUGALL PROGRAM TO THE TEST

That's the experience people have who come to my center at St. Helena Hospital in the Napa Valley of California, or purchase one of my books and take up the McDougall Program. At St. Helena, we have collected the data from more than 1,500 patients who have participated in the twelve-day live-in program over twelve years. Over the course of those twelve days, people enjoy our "all you can eat" starch-based diet created by a talented chef, Carol Wallace. They also do some moderate exercise each day under the supervision of our exercise physiologist, Linda Schulz.

While our program is twelve days, we measure our participants' results after eleven days. After those eleven days, the average weight loss is four pounds for men and three pounds for women, even though people are encouraged to eat as much as they want, as frequently as they want, during the entire stay. Men starting out the program weighing more than 200 pounds experience an average weight loss of six pounds in eleven days, while women starting at over 175 pounds lose four pounds during the same period. For patients with high blood pressure (as defined as 150/90 mm Hg or greater), the average drop usually in twenty-four hours is 23/14 mm Hg. Most patients are taken off their antihypertensive medications on the first day of the program. The average drop in cholesterol in eleven days is 29 milligrams per deciliter of blood (mg/dl). If the cholesterol was 300 mg/dl or higher, then the average reduction is 65 mg/dl. Most medications are stopped during the twelve-day stay.

As remarkable as these numbers are, they do not begin to tell the story of the overall recovery people experience on the McDougall Program. When people eat this way consistently, and exercise moderately each week, the results are even more startling. Just ask Debra Miller, of Missouri.

In 1990, Deb was hospitalized with a pulmonary embolism and pneumonia for nine days. She was also obese. Once in the hospital, she was placed on the American Diabetes Association diet, which caused a small weight loss that was immediately replaced by even more weight once she resumed her normal diet a few weeks after she returned home. As Deb reported, she could not stay on the ADA diet.

Shortly after her weight returned, Deb's chiropractor gave her a copy of my book *The McDougall Program for Maximum Weight Loss.* Inspired by the information and especially by the recipes, Deb adopted the diet and exercise regimen and over the course of the next two years lost 113½ pounds. As Deb says, "I am a new person. I feel so good and am healthier today than I have been in years! I can't thank you enough for your advice, recipes, and encouragement."

BREAKING OLD HABITS AND GAINING NEW FREEDOMS

One of the experiences I find so encouraging is that so many people are able to stay on my diet. The difference between my recommendations and those of other respected authorities is a matter of degree. Since my only interest is the health of my patients, I can recommend what the scientific research clearly and consistently points to as the most health-promoting diet available, one made up of starchy grains and beans, green and yellow vegetables, and fruits. The diet contains *no* animal products and most of the plant foods are unrefined and unprocessed, or only minimally so. As you will see, this is actually the easiest program for most people to follow because the recommendations are so clear and the results so dramatic. More moderate or "watered-down" recommendations are often far more difficult to follow, because they offer equivocal recommendations—yes, you can have a little of this or that, but not too much. With ambiguous advice, it's hard to know when you've crossed the line and placed your health in jeopardy.

Another problem with such programs is that they do not bring about the kinds of dramatic results that would keep people inspired and on the program. Why struggle with a diet that will only give you small benefits? My program is designed to create maximum results, rapidly. And as my patients know, I am fond of saying that "big changes beget big results." The most effective and easiest way to change any habit is to make a clean break with it. Then your resolve is stronger and you have a greater buttress against the old temptations. Still, you will have to want to change; you will have to want to be healthy again. Anyone who is tired of being ill and living far below her potential is ready for the McDougall Program.

Having said all of that, I also want to say that if they are in relatively good health, most people can enjoy a refined flour product or a food that contains sugars occasionally or a holiday feast that includes animal foods without worry that they will harm their health or cause themselves to permanently go off the wagon. I have found that those who succeed on my program adhere to the McDougall diet every day and sustain it even when they travel or socialize, but their consistency gives them freedom so that at special family gatherings or holiday feasts they can enjoy the foods that their loved ones serve without doing any lasting harm to their health. (I like to refer to the short-term effects of going off the program as "McDougall's revenge." It doesn't last long, but it reminds people of the powerful effects of foods, both positive and negative.)

This is one of the larger truths that everyone who follows my program discovers: they have more freedom on the McDougall Program than they did before they adopted it. The reason, simply, is that feasting every day causes illness, which results in tremendous suffering and restriction. More people are prisoners of disease and obesity than any other form of confinement on earth. Health gives us the energy, the vitality, and the strength to enjoy life. Health is the basis for freedom. The McDougall Program is the basis for good health.

Finding All the Nutrients You Need in Plant Foods

One of the first questions people want answered when they change their diets is "Am I going to get all the nutrients I need to be healthy?" My unequivocal answer is yes. In fact, you will get an abundance of all the nutrients your body needs to restore and maintain health. Just as important, you will no longer be putting all that poison into your mouth, which means that the nutrients that have been supporting your body's efforts at combating all the fat, cholesterol, chemical toxins, and bacterial agents in your former diet will now go toward healing your chronic disorders.

But let's consider where nutrients come from and the amount of nutrition found in the McDougall diet.

ESSENTIAL NUTRIENTS

Nutrients are the raw materials found in food that enable our bodies to grow and function properly. These essential nutrients cannot be created by the body, but must be obtained through our daily food supply. That's why we call them essential.

Vitamins are essential nutrients. Of the thirteen essential vitamins, eleven are made by plants. One of the two remaining, vitamin D, is actually a hormone (not a vitamin) that is created by the body when plant sterols found in the skin interact with sunlight. It only requires about twenty minutes to an hour of sunshine daily on a patch of skin the size of your hand for light-skinned people to produce sufficient vitamin D.

And since vitamin D is fat soluble, it is stored in the tissues and therefore does not have to be replenished each day. Vitamin D is only considered an "essential nutrient" when there is not adequate exposure to sunlight.

The remaining essential vitamin not found in plants is vitamin B_{12}, which is made by bacteria and certain algae. Contrary to what most people believe, B_{12} is not produced by animals. Rather, it is contained in the flesh of animals after they consume B_{12}-producing bacteria and algae. B_{12} can be stored in your tissues for up to twenty to thirty years, which is why so few people today ever suffer from a deficiency of B_{12}. Still, I like to be cautious in all matters of health, so I tell my female patients, especially those who are pregnant, planning to become pregnant, or nursing a baby to take a B_{12} supplement. Also, if you are on the program strictly for more than three years, you should add a daily dose of B_{12}. You should take a minimum of 5 micrograms per day.

While plant foods are missing only two essential nutrients, they are bursting with vitamins, minerals, antioxidants, and compounds known as phytochemicals that are essential for health and boost immune function to fight off infections and cancer.

Animal foods, on the other hand, tend to be concentrated sources of individual nutrients, but overall do not provide a balanced range of vitamins and minerals. They are also low in or devoid of antioxidants— they contain insignificant quantities of vitamin C and beta carotene, for example—and contain no phytochemicals.

MINERALS

Minerals are tiny metals that make up the earth's crust, and the only source of minerals is the earth itself. Minerals make their way to the tissues of animals, including humans, after they dissolve in water and are absorbed by the roots of plants. Once absorbed, they are drawn into the roots, stems, leaves, flowers, and fruits of plants. Animals get their minerals either from eating plants or eating plant-eating animals. Minerals combine with proteins and other materials to build the underlying structure of all your bones, cells, organs, and nerve tissues. Minerals are also essential in maintaining all of these structures. Plants are the primary source of minerals for the animal kingdom, including humans, and thus are the most abundant sources of the myriad minerals the body needs.

As I will show in greater detail in chapter 11, all diets composed of whole, natural foods contain more than enough calcium to meet human needs. *In fact, a dietary origin of calcium deficiency is unknown in human beings.* No one who follows a largely unrefined plant-based diet (with no added milk products or calcium pills) has ever suffered from a disorder known as calcium-deficiency disease as a result of eating too little calcium. There is enough calcium in plants to grow elephants, horses, and hippos, which means that there's more than enough to grow human skeletons, frail by comparison.

Right about now, you're probably looking quizzically at this book and wondering, What about all of those health authorities urging me to guard against calcium deficiency and eat calcium-rich foods, especially milk, at every opportunity?

In chapter 11, I discuss the relationship between calcium intake and osteoporosis at length, but for now you should know that people who consume relatively high quantities of calcium by worldwide standards have *not* been found to develop stronger bones than those who have diets relatively low in calcium. Most of the world's population ingests 300 to 500 milligrams (mg) of calcium daily from plants, without consuming a drop of dairy products, yet these people are able to grow and maintain normal adult skeletons. Even the World Health Organization (WHO) recommends that people eat only 550 to 600 mg per day to get adequate calcium for good health and strong bones. Scientific research has shown that an intake of 150 to 200 mg of calcium per day is adequate to meet the needs of human beings, even during pregnancy and lactation.

I do not recommend that people consume such low levels of calcium, and on the McDougall diet you will take in as much calcium as many people do on the standard American diet. But as I will demonstrate in chapter 11, osteoporosis is *not due to dietary calcium deficiency* but instead is the result of ingesting too much animal protein and several other causes. As I mentioned in chapter 1, excess consumption of protein throws off the body's pH, making the blood and tissues too acidic for the body to maintain health. In order to alkalize this acid, and thereby reestablish a healthy pH, the body leaches calcium and phosphorous from bones. The result, moreover, is that the bones become porous, thus leading to osteoporosis.

PROTEIN

Interestingly, when people think about vegetable-based diets, they immediately ask whether or not they will obtain enough protein. Also, many who have read something about nutrition wonder if plants provide all the amino acids the body needs to make a "complete" protein. Not only do plants provide all the amino acids, but they also provide a balanced amount of protein—more than enough to maintain health, but not enough to cause disease. Let's look a little more closely at both of these issues, however.

All proteins are composed of amino acids, which are the chemical building blocks of proteins. There are twenty amino acids that make up all the proteins in the tissues of every living thing on earth: whales, viruses, plants, tigers, people. All of us are composed of the same twenty amino acids. However, each living thing's proteins are arranged in unique sequences of amino acids, just as all individual words are made up of the same twenty-six letters of the alphabet arranged in different sequences. Since humans can make twelve of the twenty amino acids, the eight we cannot produce are called *essential* amino acids, meaning that they must be obtained from our food supply. All eight are produced in abundance by plants. Nature designed her foods "complete" long before they arrived on the dinner table.

In the 1940s and early '50s, scientific studies demonstrated that people generally require about 2.5 percent of their calories from protein. In order to establish a recommended amount of protein that would be absolutely safe for everyone, including those who suffer from infectious diseases and injuries, the World Health Organization (WHO) doubled the amount that had been proved necessary, bringing the daily recommended amount of protein to 5 percent of total daily calories. This recommendation established in 1974 by the WHO scientists for men, women, and children still stands today, as well as a recommendation for pregnant women to eat 6 percent of their calories as protein, and lactating women 7 percent.

The period of human life when growth is most rapid is during infancy, when we double in size during the first two years. The food intended to nourish all of human development during infancy, including this rapid growth, is human breast milk, which derives only 5 percent of its calories from protein. This is a time in our lives when our protein needs are at their peak, yet nature meets those needs more than adequately with a food source that contains only 5 percent of its calories as protein.

Commonly consumed plant foods contain 6 to 45 percent of their calories as protein. In fact, protein is so abundant in plant foods that it is impossible for any dietitian or scientist to design a diet that is composed of unprocessed plant foods (starches and vegetables) and at the same time is deficient in protein. We would not have survived as a species if this were not true. Think about it. There were no RDAs throughout most of human history, and no one was thinking "Am I getting enough protein?" On the contrary, the only thing our ancestors were thinking when it came to food was "I'm hungry and is there enough food to satisfy me?" Plants provided that protein. In fact, there is enough protein in plants to grow elephants, horses, and hippos. Surely, there is enough to grow puny human beings, too.

If you look at the chart below, you will see that it is actually difficult, if not downright impossible, to meet the lowest minimum level established by WHO scientists—you're always above it.

PERCENT OF CALORIES DERIVED FROM PROTEIN

Beans (navy)	25	Potato	9
Broccoli	42	Rice (brown)	9
Cauliflower	31	Strawberries	8
Corn	13	Zucchini	17
Orange	9		

CARBOHYDRATES

Besides water, the essential nutrients that are consumed in the greatest abundance by people are carbohydrates. The reason, of course, is because one of our greatest nutritional needs is for energy, and carbohydrates serve as the primary source of energy for human cells.

Fats are a secondary source of energy. They can provide energy for some tissues, such as muscle, but only carbohydrates provide energy for red blood cells, some cells in the kidney, and the central nervous system, including the brain. When humans are deprived of carbohydrates by starvation or some forms of dieting, the body will convert proteins into carbohydrates, either by changing the proteins in your food to carbohydrates or by converting the proteins in your muscles. This is one reason why starving children look so emaciated: their bodies are converting their protein stores in their muscles into carbohydrates in order to sustain life. Carbohydrates are a universal source of energy for the body; every cell can use them. Fat is not.

We have been designed by evolution to crave carbohydrates. The tip of the tongue enjoys only one calorie-giving substance—carbohydrate—with our sweet-tasting taste buds. Our hunger drive is regulated primarily by carbohydrate consumption. If we do not get sufficient carbohydrates, we will continue to be hungry even after we have eaten great quantities of food. People who do not eat sufficient carbohydrates may become chronic overeaters, always searching their meals for adequate carbohydrates to satisfy their hunger and allow them to enjoy a relaxed sense of well-being.

We identify carbohydrates by their sweet flavor, which is the preferred taste above all others. We learned, through much trial, error, and suffering, that sweet-tasting foods were nutritious, while bitter-tasting ones were often poisonous. As a way to establish carbohydrate as the preeminent food for human consumption, nature designed us so that the taste buds that identify sweet taste are located on the tip of the tongue, thus allowing us to taste a little of the food without having to take it very far into our mouths before we knew if it was nutritious or poisonous.

Unlike carbohydrate, *fat provides very little satiety,* which is why you have to eat great quantities of it before you feel full, and you may never feel satisfied. This lack of satisfaction from low-carbohydrate, high-fat meals leads to a preoccupation with thoughts of food, and eventually many people become "compulsive overeaters" in their futile quest to become satisfied with the American diet.

Between 70 and 90 percent of the calories in a starch-based diet are derived from carbohydrates, which is why the McDougall diet is so filling and satisfying. There is no carbohydrate of any kind found in red meat, poultry, fish, shellfish, or eggs. Most dairy products are deficient in carbohydrate. Cheese, for example, contains only 2 percent carbohydrate. Lard and vegetable oils are all fat, with no carbohydrate. All of which helps explain why people who eat animal food–based diets overeat and are often overweight.

FIBER

The carbohydrates provided by nature are of two types: digestible and indigestible. Digestible carbohydrates are the source of most of our energy. The indigestible carbohydrates, commonly referred to as fiber, do not provide energy, but are essential for good health. They are synthesized only by plants. Animal foods contain no fiber.

Once inside the intestines, dietary fiber swells with water, giving stools bulk and making them soft and easily eliminated. Fiber binds with cholesterol, hormones, and environmental toxins, causing all three to be eliminated from the body before they can harm health.

Sugars that come in unprocessed plant foods, such as brown rice and vegetables, are bound up by the fiber in the plant. Once inside the intestines, these sugars have to be broken free from their fibrous matrix so that they can be used as energy. The work of extracting the sugars from the fiber takes time and effort. Consequently, the sugar molecules drip into the bloodstream at a slow, methodical rate. This is one of the reasons why people who eat a starch-based diet—one rich in whole grains, beans, and vegetables—have such abundant and long-lasting energy. The sugars are being absorbed into their intestines consistently throughout the day. This also prevents the extreme rising and falling of blood sugar levels, which, over time, can result in either a diabetic reaction or the opposite problem, hypoglycemia.

Boosting Energy with a Starch-based Diet

One of the most consistent changes people report after they adopt my program is the dramatic improvement in energy, usually after the first week on the diet.

That was one of the experiences that most gratified Sandy Sullivan, a reference librarian who lives in Indiana. In 1990, at the age of forty-eight, Sandy had entered perimenopause and suffered from severe hot flashes, migraine headaches, and chronic fatigue. "Most of the time, I just didn't feel good," she wrote to me later. "One or two days a month I had energy and everything was fine; the rest of the time I felt tired, spacey, and discouraged."

Sandy wanted to get her master's degree in library science, but "I just didn't have the energy to work eight hours a day in a busy job and then spend two evenings a week in class plus complete homework assignments and write papers." Limiting her life even further were the migraine headaches, which she often got on weekends. This, of course, was negatively affecting her marriage. Sandy tried many different diets, various forms of meditation, and bought a lot of self-help books, none of which helped to restore her health.

"Then I happened across your book *The McDougall Program—Twelve Days to Dynamic Health* at the library," Sandy wrote to me. "The fact that it only required a twelve-day commitment was what got me to try it. After only a couple of days I was feeling good, and after a week my energy was high and my headaches were gone. At the same time I got off coffee and Ativan which I had been using for insomnia . . . I couldn't believe the amount of energy I had. I felt better than at any time in my life." Other menopausal symptoms, such as hot flashes, were significantly reduced as well.

With her newfound energy and confidence, Sandy took on a challenge she had been afraid to face for years. Two years later, she had earned a master's in library science. "I completed my MLS at age fifty," Sandy wrote me, "and am now a reference librarian. I work eight hours a day and never feel tired. At the end of the day, I have energy to work at home, go out for a walk or whatever. I love my job."

Like so many people who have adopted this program, Sandy couldn't believe that a change in diet could help her so much. The reason, simply, is that most of us do not think of this relatively soft tool as medicine. But as I have learned over many years, through my own experience and that of tens of thousands of others, this rather humble and unceremonious approach to healing very often is the strongest medicine of all.

CHAPTER 3

Improving Your Chances for a Successful Pregnancy and a Safe Delivery

Every woman who has been pregnant, and every husband who has watched his wife during her childbearing months and delivery, knows that implicit in pregnancy is a wide array of emotions, including enormous joy and significant fear. In traditional cultures, people dealt with this spectrum of feelings by establishing all sorts of taboos and spiritual rituals designed to protect and celebrate women during this most delicate period of gestation and delivery. Even today, we are aware that the new life that is growing rapidly inside of your body is an awesome event. It is a mystery that none of us will ever fully understand. Becoming pregnant and giving birth is life's most affirming act, a statement of faith, even a defiance of death. While it is true that pregnancy is essentially a physical event, the experience extends beyond the physical, putting a woman in touch with her most primitive instincts, as well as her most lofty. All of us, women and men alike, experience a certain reverence about pregnancy and birth. More than at any other time in your life, you want to do everything right for your baby and yourself, because this experience, perhaps more than any other, puts us all in touch with life's terrible fragility, as well as its tremendous beauty.

In today's society, this pressure to do right by your child has given rise to all kinds of behaviors that we may believe to be healthful, but in fact may do more harm than good. This is especially true of a woman's diet during her pregnancy. Many women feel compelled to eat as much as they can, and to eat as wide a variety of foods as possible, believing that this will strengthen them and their developing babies during the demands of pregnancy and birth. We've all heard the clichés "Go ahead and have seconds; you're eating for two now," or "Eat a little bit of everything; it's not good to restrict your diet when you're pregnant." Behind such statements lie the beliefs that it's better to eat as varied a diet as possible to be certain that you're getting all the nutrition you need, and to gain a significant amount of weight during pregnancy.

Let me say at the outset that you should get all the nutrition your body—and your baby—needs. I'm all for maximizing the nutrient content of your diet. The question is, how can you get maximum nutrition rather than merely an overabundance of fat, cholesterol, calories, and protein, all of which can make your pregnancy difficult and, at the same time, place your unborn baby's health at risk?

In order to answer that question, we have to know the kinds of foods that offer an abundance of nutrition. Overall, animal foods offer a relatively narrow range of nutrients. They are often rich in protein; milk can provide significant amounts of calcium, and meat can provide significant amounts of iron. But animal foods are deficient in many vitamins and minerals, antioxidants, phytochemicals, and fiber. For example, milk has virtually no iron and meat has no calcium. Consequently, a diet based largely on animals foods, the standard Western diet, is low in many of the nutrients your body needs to maintain health.

In fact, the diet that is the richest in the widest possible array of nutrients is a plant-based diet. As I showed in the previous chapter, all the essential minerals, amino acids, and vitamins—save two—are found in abundance in plant foods. Plants are also the major sources of antioxidants, phytochemicals, and fiber. This is why nutritionists will tell you that if you are going to eat a balanced diet, one that contains all the nutrients your body needs, you have to eat vegetables, because that's where the nutrition is. Therefore, the best advice to a pregnant woman who wants to get the maximum nutrition for her baby is to eat a plant-based diet.

Unfortunately, many of the recommendations given to pregnant women have been wrong. There was a doctor in the late nineteenth century, Dr. Prowchownick of New England, who advised pregnant women to eat a diet rich in protein but low in fluids and calories so that the growth of the developing fetus would be stunted. Why would a doctor deliberately want to keep babies from growing to normal size? The recommendation was intended to compensate for the fact that many women developed abnormally small pelvises during the nineteenth century, because they worked in sweatshops and suffered from rickets due to an absence of sunlight. Since their pelvises were small, this doctor reasoned, they should eat a diet that would make their babies even smaller. Rather than deal with the cause of the problem, namely, the lack of sunshine, this doctor designed a program to shrink the babies to accommodate for a constricted birth canal caused by a serious, but easily correctable, disease.

Remarkably, this approach became very popular throughout the United States and remained so until after World War I. The practice stopped when scientists observed that during the war pregnant women living in Germany experienced low rates of preeclampsia, an illness characterized by high blood pressure, edema, and protein in the urine. Curiously, these low rates of preeclampsia appeared to be associated with low meat consumption. Once this was recognized, of course, doctors began to recommend that meat, and thus protein, be limited during pregnancy.

Still, the bad advice continued. During the early 1940s, doctors attempted to reduce the risk of preeclampsia by placing women on calorie- and sodium-restricted diets. Sometimes they would also prescribe appetite suppressants and diuretics to limit weight gain to fifteen to twenty pounds. Unfortunately, this regimen increased the rate of small babies and the infants' risk of death.

For most of this century, doctors recommended that women avoid excessive weight gain during pregnancy. That advice changed in the 1960s when doctors observed that small babies had a higher risk of death than larger ones. Physicians thus recommended that women gain significant amounts of weight during pregnancy. It naturally followed, therefore, that women should eat a great abundance of food— "you're eating for two now"—and that, in order to gain weight, they should eat lots of animal foods—meat, chicken, eggs, dairy products, and fish. The result, as you can see when you look around you, is oversized mothers and babies.

Only thirty-seven years ago a Joint Expert Group of the Food and Agriculture Organization of the World Health Organization pronounced that nutrition was of no great importance in pregnancy. Today, of course, we know differently. However, even to this day, experts in prenatal and infant nutrition disagree widely on such fundamental matters as how much weight a woman should gain and what her requirements are for energy, protein, and micronutrients. This confusion among the experts, of course, explains why so many women are bewildered about what to eat during pregnancy.

Gaining Excess Weight During Pregnancy

One of the most common responses to confusion about diet during pregnancy is for a woman to eat lots of high-fat animal foods in the hope that she will get all she needs to produce a healthy baby. Unfortunately, such a diet often makes both mother and baby too big to produce a normal delivery. Thus, an increasing number of women require cesarean sections. Fully one-fourth of pregnant women require surgical removal of their babies. In developed countries throughout the West, pregnant women usually gain between twenty-two and thirty-five pounds. Compare that to the fourteen pounds pregnant women on average gain in many traditional cultures and undeveloped countries. Many of these places, it should be pointed out, have better infant mortality rates than we do in the United States, and much lower cesarean section rates. (The U.S. cesarean section rate is the third highest in the world.)

Let's consider the effect of this weight gain on the mother. The more weight you gain during pregnancy, the more likely you will retain that weight. On average, women who gain less than 25 pounds during pregnancy are, six months after giving birth, about 2.6 pounds lighter than their prepregnancy weight. On the other hand, women who on average gained 36 pounds or more are 11 pounds heavier than their prepregnancy weight six months after delivery.

Overweight and obesity have a tremendous impact on a woman's health. Obese women are seven times more likely to have diabetes, four times more likely to suffer from high blood pressure, and twice as likely to develop pregnancy-induced hypertension than are lean women. Approximately 17 percent of obese pregnant women develop preeclampsia (or pregnancy-induced high blood pressure). Among moderately obese women, 6.5 percent suffer from diabetes during pregnancy, called gestational diabetes, and the diabetes risk may be as high as 20 percent in severely obese women.

Such acute disorders as diabetes and high blood pressure are not the only side effects of such a diet, however. Many women who follow the prevailing wisdom to gain weight during pregnancy suffer from chronic constipation, fatigue, and edema, all of which create tremendous discomfort. Little wonder, therefore, that many women associate pregnancy with being ill.

Fortunately, it now appears that doctors have begun to take notice of the fact that the more weight a woman gains during pregnancy, the more she and her baby suffer. A study published in the *Southern Medical Journal* found mothers living on a purely plant-based diet (vegans) were essentially free from preeclampsia. Out of 775 women on a vegan diet, only one had preeclampsia, when 10 percent, or about 77 women, would be expected to suffer from this condition under usual circumstances.

Other medical authorities are now attempting to encourage women to rely more on plant foods during pregnancy, especially for those who suffer from diseases caused by a high-fat diet and being overweight. A 1995 editorial in *The New England Journal of Medicine* stated, "The first-line treatment for women with gestational diabetes is diet, with reduction in fat intake and the substitution of complex carbohydrates for refined carbohydrates. In addition, moderate caloric restriction and exercise are recommended for obese women."

The best way to reduce calories is to eat vegetables. The reason, simply, is that vegetables are low in calories, yet they fill you up and they are extremely high in nutrients. You can achieve your optimal weight and never have to go hungry on a plant-based diet. (For more on weight loss, see my book *The McDougall Program for Maximum Weight Loss*.)

That's what Linda Foreman, of Nevada, discovered when she began the McDougall Program. Linda, who is 5 feet, 4 inches, followed the conventional wisdom while she was pregnant; she ate every kind of food available to her and found herself at a staggering 208 pounds after she gave birth. She tried various weight loss programs but couldn't maintain the diets and any weight she lost was quickly regained. Then she began the McDougall Program. As she wrote to me in 1996, "I began your program in September 1994 and have lost seventy-five pounds. My husband and I walk several times per week and recently took up bicycling, which has been so rewarding to both of us. We bicycle almost every weekend and many evenings."

Eating Less Can Be an Advantage

In chapter 1, I pointed out that nature so perfectly designed a woman's body that she and her unborn baby would be protected, even under severe dietary conditions. Let me give you a classic example of the toughness of women. During World War II, people in the Netherlands suffered from near-starvation conditions. At one point, the Dutch were forced to subsist for six months on 450 calories a day, a daily calorie consumption that was only one-sixth of what is generally believed to be adequate. Fortunately, the foods these women did eat were vegetables, mostly potatoes, some bread or grains, and whatever green or leafy vegetables could be found. Such foods are extremely low in calories, but high in nutrition. Even though a big potato contains only 109 calories, it's loaded with complex carbohydrates, protein, vitamin B_6, vitamin C, copper, iron, magnesium, manganese, niacin, potassium, and fiber.

Still, you would think that under such conditions, the most precious people in the population, pregnant women and their unborn babies, would suffer severe side effects from such a famine. But a comprehensive study of the effects of those six months of starvation on babies born during that period showed that the average birth weight was only eight ounces less than the weight of babies born during times of plenty. Infant death rates during the famine were the same as those during normal times, and there was no increase in the incidence of physical or mental disabilities of the children.

Why would pregnant women and unborn babies do so well under such harsh conditions? In fact, the human body adapts well to "undernutrition."

In the long history of human experience, famine has been much more common than abundance. Consequently, humans developed mechanisms to survive an inadequate food supply. We were even able to grow healthy babies during times when food was scarce. During such times, plant foods were the most plentiful. Animal food sources tended to be more unpredictable and seasonal. Our Paleolithic ancestors might have hunted for days and weeks before making a kill, and even when they did, the animal may have been small, and there was no refrigeration to preserve the remains. The foods they subsisted on in the meantime were plant foods, which were far more constant and abundant throughout nature.

This dependence on plant foods continued with the birth of civilization and persisted even up to relatively modern times. When you examine the cultures of Japan, China, India, Africa, the Caribbean, Mexico, and many of the native American peoples, you find an overwhelming dependence upon starches, such as rice, corn, potatoes, and beans, and a vast variety of green, yellow, and orange vegetables. Our Paleolithic ancestors subsisted on vegetables largely because that was what was most available in nature. Our more recent ancestors depended on plant foods because animal foods were extremely expensive and most of our ancestors were poor, farmers or craftspeople. This is true even for most Western Europeans.

The one thing the human body did not experience commonly, at least not until the twentieth century, was a sudden overabundance of fat, cholesterol, and protein. Consequently, we never developed adaptive mechanisms to cope with the rich diet that most of us eat today. That's one reason why we become ill when we eat such foods.

Still, the question remains: What do mother and child need to experience a healthy pregnancy and birth?

Good Nutrition for a Healthy Pregnancy and Birth

ENERGY REQUIREMENTS

The first thing you need to grow a healthy baby is energy, which comes from food in the form of calories.

Between 60,000 and 80,000 extra calories are needed to grow a healthy baby. That averages out as 250 to 300 additional calories a day during the second and third trimesters, an additional amount that you can easily meet by eating only plant foods. Overall, calorie consumption for pregnant women has been estimated to increase from 2,200 kilocalories (kcal) to 2,500 kcal a day.

Glucose, the carbohydrate derived originally from plant foods, is the primary metabolic fuel your baby needs most when it is an embryo, a fetus, and a newborn immediately after delivery. To ensure that they get adequate calories, pregnant women naturally become hungrier as the pregnancy develops; this is especially true during the last two trimesters of pregnancy. If they are eating a lot of plant foods, they will be getting not only additional calories but also lots of additional nutrition.

In many parts of the world, women do not eat more food in order to meet their caloric needs. Rather, their bodies obtain the extra calories by increasing their efficiency. In other words, they are able to derive more of the calories available in food and use them more efficiently as fuel. Pregnant women from the Philippines and rural Africa who do hard physical labor take in no more food during pregnancy, and sometimes eat even fewer calories when they are pregnant. Yet, they thrive and give birth to healthy babies, because the foods they eat are primarily nutrient-dense plants that easily provide the raw materials needed to grow a healthy baby.

PROTEIN REQUIREMENTS

A pregnant woman and developing child need the most amount of protein during the last six months of pregnancy. During that time, between 5 and 6 grams of protein are needed per day, or a total over the entire six months of about two pounds. A starch-based diet provides between 44 and 130 grams of protein per day for a woman consuming 2,200 kcal of food. The World Health Organization recommends that a pregnant woman consume 6 percent of her calories from protein; a lactating woman should derive 7 percent of her calories from protein, according to WHO scientists. This amount is easily supplied by plant sources. Rice alone contains 8 percent of its calories in protein; corn, 12 percent; potato, 11 percent; and beans, 28 percent.

Of all the nutrients in the food supply, pregnant women tend to consider protein one of the most important for themselves and their developing babies. Therefore, they often emphasize protein-rich foods, such as meat, eggs, dairy products, and fish. Despite claims that pregnancy-induced hypertension can be prevented with a high-protein diet, there is no evidence that a high-protein intake during pregnancy is beneficial, and in some cases, it may actually be harmful.

One important study suggests caution when it comes to adding more protein to a pregnant woman's diet. In Guatemala, pregnant women in two villages were given a high-protein calorie supplement; pregnant women in two other villages subsisted on their normal plant-based diet to which a high-calorie supplement with no additional protein was added. Researchers found that birth weights were influenced more by the number of calories consumed than by the protein content of the diets. Unfortunately, the women who had received the extra protein actually had far worse outcomes. They gave birth to a greater number of babies who were underweight, suffered a greater number of premature deliveries, and had higher rates of infant mortality than the women in the two villages who ate their usual plant-based diets with no additional protein.

MINERAL REQUIREMENTS

Minerals are essential for the health and development of your unborn child; fortunately, they are abundant in almost all diets, and are particularly plentiful in diets based on plant foods. As I said in chapter 2, all minerals originate in the earth. Plants draw up the calcium, copper, iodine, iron, zinc, and other minerals from the soil and incorporate them into their tissues. The plants are then eaten by animals, which incorporate the plant's wealth of nutrition, including its minerals, into their tissues. Thus, plants are the primary source of minerals in the food supply. A plant-based diet provides all the minerals a pregnant woman and her unborn child need.

Calcium

A developing fetus requires approximately 30 grams (one ounce) of calcium to develop healthfully, which he derives from his mother's blood. That 30 grams represents about 2.5 percent of a woman's overall calcium supply. In a wondrous feat of increased efficiency, a woman's body during pregnancy actually increases its ability to absorb calcium from her food and retain it in her body. This accomplishment is facilitated by a woman's small intestine, which increases its absorption of calcium, and her kidneys, which decrease their excretion of calcium into the urine. Thus, the woman's calcium supply internally increases to meet her own needs and those of her baby.

Although calcium intake varies widely around the world, no specific problems associated with dietary calcium deficiency have been identified. Studies worldwide on various populations of people show no need for extra calcium during pregnancy. Neither the number of children nor the duration of breast feeding are a risk for loss of bone or fractures later in life. As a result of recent studies on calcium needs during pregnancy the U.S.-Canadian guidelines have been revised in 1998 to recommend that no increase in calcium intake is required during pregnancy or lactation.

When a pregnant American woman thinks about adding calcium to her body, she automatically thinks she needs to drink more milk. Yet after they are weaned from their mothers, billions of women worldwide consume no milk and produce perfectly healthy and strong children. The fact is that dairy products are truly unnecessary for good health.

Iron

Iron is a constituent of hemoglobin (blood), myoglobin (muscle), and numerous enzymes. Iron deficiency during pregnancy can elevate the risk of premature birth, lower birth weight, and infant mortality.

A woman's body contains about 2.2 grams of iron, which is equal to the weight of a dime. New tissues of the fetus and mother require a total of about 1 gram of extra iron. Once again, a woman's body performs a feat of magic during pregnancy by increasing its absorption of iron to gain additional amounts of the mineral. This occurs at the end of her first trimester, or sometime in her second, between twelve and thirty-six weeks into her pregnancy. At this point, the ability of the small intestine to absorb iron increases to 9.1 times its normal capacity.

A pregnant woman requires approximately 5 mg of additional iron per day, especially in the latter half of her pregnancy; plant foods meet and exceed this need (see the chart below). However, many women immediately think of animal foods, especially beef, when they think of sources of iron. In fact, research has shown that vegetarians have a higher iron intake and higher blood levels of iron than nonvegetarians. One of the reasons may be that people who eat a plant-based diet take in more vitamin C, or ascorbic acid, which enhances iron absorption. Just as important, those who follow a healthy diet tend to avoid milk products, tea, and coffee, all of which inhibit iron absorption and lead to iron deficiency.

SOURCES OF IRON (Plant Foods vs. Animal Foods)
(mg iron for 100 calories of the specified food)

Asparagus	2.7	Beef	0.8
Cherries	0.8	Chicken	0.6
Beans (white)	1.8	Fish (salmon)	0.7
Broccoli	3.4	Eggs	1.3
Carrots	1.2	Milk	0.0
Rice (brown)	0.4	Cheese	0.0

Because iron is so important to pregnant women, many are convinced that they need iron supplements; however, clinical studies do not demonstrate that iron pills offer any clinical benefit to a woman's health or that of her baby. Supplementation may even harm some women.

Research has shown that iron supplementation can inhibit the absorption of zinc from the intestines. Iron supplements can also irritate the gastrointestinal tract, causing nausea, vomiting, or constipation, and may overstimulate the production of blood. Elevated blood or hemoglobin levels are associated with an increase in the same side effects that iron deficiency creates, perhaps because high hemoglobin is associated with preeclampsia.

Incidentally, some children who ingest their mother's iron supplements die as a result of overdosing on iron. I doubt that nature intended women to take pills in order to remain healthy during pregnancy.

VITAMIN REQUIREMENTS

As I explained in chapter 2, plant foods provide all but two vitamins, D and B_{12}, in abundant supply. Vitamin D is easily obtained from sunlight (twenty minutes to an hour of light, per day, on the face of light-skinned people provides all the vitamin D they need) and is stored in the body. B_{12} is obtained through bacteria, algae, and animal food sources.

In fact, the actual risk of experiencing a B_{12} deficiency is extremely small, since it is stored in the body for years. However, B_{12} deficiency has been reported in infants born to mothers who have been longtime vegans and to macrobiotic mothers who have avoided all animal foods for many years. No significant neurological disorders or symptoms were reported in either case. However, to avoid any risks, vegetarian women who scrupulously avoid animal foods and who are pregnant or breast-feeding *must* add a nonanimal source of B_{12}, such as a vitamin supplement, to their daily diet (approximately 5 micrograms per day).

Toxic Effects of Vitamin A Supplementation

Vitamin supplementation can be dangerous, especially the addition of vitamin A. The adverse effects of vitamin A supplementation—the type found in animal products and referred to as retinol—have been known for more than forty years. The risk of birth defects is 480 percent greater for women taking more than 10,000 international units (IU) of vitamin A per day than for those taking 5,000 IU.

Pregnant women who take vitamin A supplements have a one in fifty-seven chance of having a child who suffers from a deformity of the head and face, nervous system, thymus, and/or heart. Pregnant women should also avoid liver and liver products because they frequently contain high amounts of vitamin A or retinol. Dairy products and some vitamin-fortified foods can also provide a significant amount of this toxic, or teratogenic, form of vitamin A.

On the other hand, no risk has been found with the intake of beta carotene, a plant-based chemical that the body uses to synthesize vitamin A.

Folic Acid Deficiency

The most frequently encountered vitamin deficiency in the Western industrialized world, particularly in the United States, is an insufficiency of folic acid, one of several compounds referred to as folates. While it can cause significant harm to pregnant women—folic acid deficiency commonly causes megaloblastic anemia during pregnancy, which is characterized by very large blood cells—it is much more harmful to unborn babies.

Conclusive evidence has shown that folic acid deficiency in the developing fetus causes incomplete development of the spine, skull, spinal cord, and brain. Such deformities, known as neural tube defects, are the second most common major birth defect in children in the United States. Surpassed only by congenital heart defects, neural tube malformations occur in approximately one out of every thousand births. Each year 2,500 children are born in the United States with neural tube defects.

The severity of deformity caused by folic acid deficiency can be as minor as a missing patch of skin at the base of the spine or scalp, or the complete opening of the backbone (referred to as spina bifida occulta). More severe manifestations include the failure to develop the lower spinal cord (referred to as spina bifida), which is accompanied by paralysis. In its most severe manifestations, some children are born without a brain or skull development (a condition called anecephaly).

Other potential birth defects that can be caused by folic acid deficiency include hydrocephalus, cleft palate, serious heart defects, limb abnormalities, narrowing of the intestines, and failure of proper kidney development.

The best way for a woman to ensure that she has sufficient folic acid in her body is to eat a plant-based diet. Folic acid was named because it was found originally in leafy vegetables. Plants make the folates and therefore contain large amounts of this essential nutrient. Unfortunately, 50 to 95 percent of the folate is destroyed by prolonged cooking and processing such as canning. Therefore, it's essential to eat fresh or lightly cooked vegetables: try steaming them or boiling them for a few minutes. Think foliage! Some of the best sources of folic acid include legumes, whole grains, and fresh green vegetables (see the chart on page 53).

On the other hand, all forms of meat, except liver, and all dairy foods are low in folic acid. Concentrated fats and oils are devoid of the vitamin. The typical daily American diet contains less than 200 micrograms of folates. Ideally, well over 400 micrograms should be consumed each day.

The absence of adequate folate in the typical American diet is particularly threatening because most pregnancies are unplanned and neural tube deformities tend to occur in the first two weeks of pregnancy. Thus, the quantity of vitamins you have in your blood and tissues at the time of conception is very often what determines a child's neurological health.

Moreover, the entire diet plays a pivotal role in proper development. Obese women are two to four times as likely as trim women to have babies with debilitating birth defects. Even adequate folic acid intake does not reduce the risk for the heaviest women. The point is that every woman, no matter whether she is pregnant or not, should eat a diet rich in plant foods to eliminate the threat of nutrient deficiencies or excesses and their terrible side effects.

In Mexico, mothers who consume a diet high in beans and rice and low in meat and dairy foods consume far more vitamins A and C, folate, iron, and vegetable protein. These women have fewer low-birthweight infants, less intrauterine growth retardation, and fewer infant deaths than white Americans or Mexican-Americans.

SOURCES OF FOLIC ACID
(micrograms of folic acid in 1 cup cooked food)

Asparagus	176	Corn	76
Barley	128	Fish	10
Beef	12	Garbanzo beans	282
Beef liver	420	Green cabbage	40
Black beans	256	Margarine	0
Broccoli	104	Milk	12
Butter	0	Olive oil	0
Cheese	36	Oranges	60
Chicken	16	Peas	127

Many health authorities have suggested fortifying the national food supply with folic acid to protect against deficiencies at the time of conception. Unfortunately, folic acid supplementation will not prevent about 30 percent of birth defects, because other components in the diet are also important for proper fetal development. That's the blessing of a nutritionally rich plant-based diet: you don't have to worry about whether you're getting enough of a particular nutrient; they're all included.

Keep in mind that your entire diet plays a pivotal role in the healthy development of your unborn child. Developmental abnormalities of the fetus are too complex to ascribe to a single vitamin deficiency; the whole diet must be taken into account.

Combating Birth Defects

Many environmental poisons threaten the developing fetus, and they tend to be much more concentrated in animal foods than plant foods. Once ingested by the mother, environmental pollutants can damage the genetic material, or DNA, in the cells of the developing child, which causes a wide assortment of birth defects. Scientists know that such defects account for much of the disability in children throughout the world and are the leading causes of infant mortality in developed countries.

Although there are several ways that such toxic chemicals can enter a woman's body, including through the lungs, skin, and mouth, the foods we eat provide by far the greatest chemical assault on the fetus. The primary carrier of such toxic chemicals is dietary fat, especially the fat that comes in meat, dairy products, eggs, and fish. Grazing animals eat plants and drink water that have been tainted by industrial poisons. Usually such toxins originate in polluted rivers, soil, rainfall, or farm runoff. Once the animals eat the grass and other plants that have been contaminated, these poisons accumulate in their fat cells—the same fat cells that are later consumed by humans either as meat or milk products. A similar series of events occurs in fish that swim in polluted lakes, rivers, and poisonous parts of the oceans. Fish that swim in poisoned waters ingest the toxins, which accumulate in their fat.

A recent study found that school-age children in Michigan who were exposed to low levels of polychlorinated biphenyls (PCBs) while in the uterus had an average decrease in IQ scores of 6.2 points. Women who ate at least twenty-six pounds of Lake Michigan salmon or lake trout over a six-year period had children with reduced IQs and associated deficits in general intellectual ability, short- and long-term memory, and the ability to focus and sustain attention. Such chemicals damage the nervous system of the developing child. PCBs have been banned in the United States since the 1970s, but their residues persist in the environment and find their way into our food supply. Fatty fish are a major source of human exposure to PCBs. Other important sources of these highly toxic chemicals are dairy products and meats.

CHEMICAL DANGERS

Environmental chemicals may be responsible for developmental abnormalities in the sexual characteristics of young boys. According to an article published in the May 1993 issue of the *Lancet*, "The incidence of disorders of development of the male reproductive tract has more than doubled in the past 30 [to] 50 years, while the sperm counts have declined by half."

Both the volume of semen and the sperm count have fallen, while such disorders as testicular cancer, urethral abnormalities, and failure of the testes to descend (cryptorchidism) are statistically on the rise.

Scientists believe that estrogen-like compounds found in the environment are among the causes of such abnormalities. They base their opinions on the fact that similar abnormalities have been seen in sons born to women who were once treated with the estrogen compound DES during pregnancy. There are ample sources of environmental estrogens, including cows that continue to give milk even after they are pregnant. The pregnancy results in high levels of estrogen (estrone sulfate) that are excreted into their milk.

Moreover, DES and other synthetic estrogens have been used widely throughout the livestock industry to promote cattle growth for more than thirty years. In fact, during the first twenty years of their use they were not recognized as a risk to humans. Many estrogen-like chemicals, such as dioxins, are found in the environment, where they make their way to humans through the food chain.

HARMFUL FOOD ADDITIVES

Substances intentionally put into our foods also pose a significant risk to unborn children. The most common kind of brain cancer in young children, known as astrocytoma, has been linked to the consumption of nitrosamine-containing cured meats by their mothers. Brain cancers account for about one in five childhood cancers. Research has found that consuming vegetables, fruits, and fruit juices protects against the development of brain cancers.

ALCOHOL

Alcohol consumption during pregnancy has been shown to increase the risk of spontaneous abortion; growth retardation; low birth weight; congenital anomalies; emotional, behavioral, and mental disorders; and death. Fetal alcohol syndrome is a specific pattern of malformations that occurs in the children of alcoholic mothers; this condition inhibits normal growth and development and is characterized by structural defects such as a smooth upper lip, joint abnormalities, and disorders of the heart. One study of pregnant women who were heavy drinkers found that one-third of their children had the syndrome and another third suffered from its milder effects. Only one-third were judged to be normal. With even moderate drinking—one to three drinks a day in the first trimester—abnormalities can be found. The effects of binge drinking are not known.

Pregnant women who drink are far more common than you might

think. One study reported that 38 percent of women consume some alcohol during pregnancy.

CAFFEINE

A study at Johns Hopkins University found that women who consumed more than 300 mg of caffeine a day (more than three cups of regular coffee or eight sodas) reduced their chances of conception by 26 percent. On average, a couple maintains a 20 percent chance of conceiving each month; with extra caffeine consumption by women those chances are reduced to 15 percent.

Caffeine intake before and during pregnancy has been found to double the risk of spontaneous abortions in women; this finding is consistent with animal studies. The risks are greater when caffeine is consumed during pregnancy rather than before. Currently there is little research to implicate caffeine consumption with congenital malformations, but there is some association with intrauterine growth retardation.

CIGARETTES

Researchers found that smokers were 15 to 20 percent less likely to become pregnant, no matter how much caffeine they drank. Another study of four thousand couples that compared smokers to nonsmokers found the average amount of time it took nonsmokers to conceive was 2.6 months. Those who smoked more than ten cigarettes a day required four months to conceive. The effects of cigarette smoking are seen in every trimester of pregnancy, from increased spontaneous abortions in the first trimester to increased premature delivery rates and decreased birth weights in the last trimester. Nicotine causes constriction of blood vessels to the uterus, and possibly the umbilical cord, and smoking produces carbon monoxide. These effects combine to retard the growth of the fetus.

Throughout history, and even today, babies have been born to women who followed diets based on a variety of starchy vegetables, with no dairy products and very little meat. Rich foods, including meats, poultry, fish, and refined and processed foods, have always been eaten as condiments or limited to special occasions. Such a diet provides both baby and mother with an abundance of nutrition, which is the basis for good health.

Pregnancy is a normal state of health, not a time of illness. A pregnant woman's body undergoes many natural adjustments to nourish and support fetal growth and development and, at the same time, prepare her for nursing. On a starch-based diet your body takes in a far richer supply of carbohydrates, vitamins, minerals, phytochemicals, and fiber. You will also get plenty of plant-based protein, while consuming small amounts of fat and no cholesterol. You will gain an optimal amount of weight, without becoming overweight or obese, and you will lose that additional weight quickly. You will feel good throughout your pregnancy, without suffering the standard array of chronic illnesses, including high blood pressure, diabetes, fatigue, and constipation.

Enjoying a Healthy Pregnancy

At thirty-seven years of age, Gloria Tanner, of New York, had had trouble getting pregnant for her entire adult life and even believed that her chances of conceiving had been lost. In January 1987, she adopted my program for an onset of adult acne, which the program quickly cleared up. After following the program faithfully for eleven months, Gloria found herself unexpectedly and joyfully pregnant.

After reading more about my program, Gloria, a registered nurse, decided to remain on the McDougall diet after she became pregnant. Her energy levels were so high during her pregnancy that she was able to walk three miles a day for three days each week and swim laps at her local health club.

"It was a wonderful time," Gloria wrote to me. "I could advise and encourage my patients who were sharing my experience to follow a low-fat, nonanimal-product eating plan, as well.

"My total weight gain was twenty-two pounds. I exercised and worked up to delivery," Gloria reported. "I felt great—almost superior to my ordinary unpregnant state!" When her big day came, Gloria experienced some "mild backache all afternoon, which I had no idea was actually back labor until a friend had me time my backache!" Gloria went to the hospital at 7:30 P.M. and gave birth to a "gorgeous six-pound, fifteen-ounce baby boy at 8:30, without any drugs. Pretty good for an 'older' mother's first delivery."

As a postscript, Gloria told me that she remains on the McDougall Program, and her son, who has developed into a strong and smart boy of normal height, has tested in the gifted range in IQ. Said Gloria, "So you can tell people that having a vegan pregnancy and infancy can turn out just fine."

Why Is Change So Slow?

Even with the overwhelming scientific data showing the benefits of a starch-based diet, change is imperceptibly slow. At the bottom of this stagnation is fear. Mothers- and fathers-to-be are afraid that if the woman does not eat all of the high-calorie, high-fat, high-protein foods most other women eat, their baby somehow will be deprived of what he or she needs to develop normally. Virtually every mother and father confronts this fear. I know: Mary and I faced it, too.

We had just made the final modifications on our strict vegetarian diet shortly after the birth of our second child in 1975. Five years later, Mary became pregnant with our third. Much to my astonishment, Mary was soon buying cheese, fish, and eggs—the high-protein, high-calcium fare—fearing that such foods might be essential for a pregnant woman and her baby. I knew that Mary knew better, but we were pioneers of sorts—at least in our families and among those we knew—so there was no one to turn to for reassurance that our principles were both true and safe. Three months later, Mary suffered a miscarriage. I would never say that these foods caused her miscarriage, but they certainly did not guarantee a full-term and healthy pregnancy, either.

Still, the miscarriage was traumatic and caused Mary to think about her diet and pregnancy. We both learned a lot from that experience. Two years later, Mary was pregnant again. I waited for the cheese, or at least some fish, to steal its way back into our house, but none of those foods darkened our refrigerator. Experience had cured Mary of her fears. During her entire pregnancy, she ate no meat, foul, fish, or dairy products. She also reports that this was a wonderful time of her life. She was full of energy and did not suffer the customary bloating and edema that is so common during pregnancy. (She could easily slip her rings on and off her fingers each day.)

By the time she gave birth to our son, Craig, she had gained only 15 pounds and after delivery she was only one pound heavier than her prepregnancy weight. She lost that one pound and two more in a week. Over the next three years, Mary kept her weight five pounds below her prepregnancy, thanks to the fact that she was nursing and eating a starch-based diet. She tells me today that her pregnancy with Craig was one of the happiest and healthiest periods of her life.

CHAPTER 4

Giving Your Child a Healthful Head Start

When I ask my female patients to describe their experience of breast-feeding, they offer a wide variety of answers, but virtually all of them say that nursing connects them to their babies, to motherhood, and even to nature as no other experience ever has. One woman I know put it this way: "When I breast-feed my baby, everything in my life slows down. I experience life in a new way. I'm in my body—not in the car or at the office thinking about something else I have to do. I'm right here in this moment, doing something that is so right. I see my baby nursing and I know that I am giving him something that will affect his entire life. I also feel connected to that long line of women who were mothers who did the same thing I am doing, going all the way back to the beginning. This is what mothers do in nature."

Breast-feeding affects our lives in so many ways that it's actually impossible to write about it without realizing that we are able to express only a small fraction of its meaning and importance. The more science discovers, the more awe-inspiring this living, liquid tissue becomes.

Protecting Infants Against Disease

Breast milk contains water, carbohydrates, fats, proteins, vitamins, minerals, and many other substances that are precisely engineered to promote the growth and development of a human infant. It is a complete food, providing all the nutrients a baby needs to develop healthfully for at least the first six months of life. Unlike infant formulas, which are a relatively recent phenomenon, breast milk is the proven substance, having been the foundation for infant health for millions of years. Not only does it offer infants the perfect nutrition, but breast milk helps to protect and develop infants in countless other ways.

Long before a baby's immune system becomes strong enough to ward off diseases by itself, mother's milk provides babies with an incredible abundance of immune cells and antibodies designed to protect an infant against all kinds of pathogens. In fact, it is a mother's immune system that guards her baby. Within hours of being exposed to a bacteria or virus, a mother begins producing immune cells, antibodies, and immunoglobulins, all specifically designed to eradicate the pathogen to which she and her baby were exposed. All of these immune constituents flow to her baby through her breast milk. No matter whether the source of the illness is airborne or blood-borne, whether it infects the intestines, chest, ears, urinary tract, nervous system, or brain, mother's milk provides an army of immune cells all designed to wipe out the potential disease, usually before it takes root in the infant's system.

Breast milk promotes the growth of friendly bacteria in the baby's intestinal tract, such as *Lactobacillus bifidus*, that inhibit the spread of disease-causing bacteria, including *Staphylococcus aureus*, which can cause a variety of illnesses in the throat, sinuses, lungs, and skin. Breast milk forms the basis for healthy intestinal flora for the rest of the child's life. Human milk is also anti-inflammatory, which means it suppresses the swelling that often accompanies illness and injury, which can also cause pain.

In yet another way of protecting infants against bacterial and viral infection, breast milk contains sugars that block harmful bacteria from attaching to the baby's cells and tissues. Breast-feeding protects babies from the harmful microbes that cause influenza, ear and throat infections, pneumonia, severe diarrhea, bacterial meningitis, botulism, urinary tract infection, and necrotizing enterocolitis. This is only one of several reasons why breast-fed babies experience fewer ear infections than bottle-fed children.

In fact, research has demonstrated that breast-fed infants have one-fourth the risk of developing serious respiratory and intestinal diseases, and one-tenth the risk of being hospitalized with a life-threatening bacterial infection. Breast-feeding also appears to protect children from serious inflammatory bowel diseases, including ulcerative colitis and Crohn's disease. In developing countries where children are most challenged by poor sanitation and bacterial and viral infections, bottle-fed infants are at least fourteen times more likely to die of diarrhea, and four times more likely to die of pneumonia than breast-fed infants.

Such protection may even extend to adults who were breast-fed as infants; they have a significantly lower risk of contracting allergic diseases like eczema, asthma, and food allergies. Some studies suggest that breast-feeding also reduces the risk of contracting cancer, especially lymphomas and acute leukemia. The 1997 position statement on breast-feeding from the American Academy of Pediatrics states, "There are a number of studies that show a possible protective effect of human milk feeding against sudden infant death syndrome, insulin-dependent diabetes mellitus, Crohn's disease, ulcerative colitis, lymphoma, allergic diseases, and other chronic digestive diseases."

Breast-feeding Promotes a Healthier Nervous System

Remarkably, studies have shown that children who were breast-fed consistently produce higher scores on intelligence tests than those who were bottle-fed. This capacity to promote the healthy development of the nervous system and brain extends even to babies who were born prematurely and thus did not have the full nine months in the womb to develop their nervous systems. Studies have shown that when seven-year-old children who were prematurely born but were breast-fed are tested for intelligence, they score 8.3 points higher, on average, than children who were prematurely born but were bottle-fed. Additional research has shown that, in effect, the more breast-milk a child consumes, the higher that child's IQ will be later in life.

These higher IQ scores may be a consequence of breast-feeding's ability to protect and enhance the development of the nervous system. Breast milk provides a rich supply of essential fats and sugars that may make the nervous system more resistant to injuries from viruses or to autoimmune diseases later in life, including such illnesses as multiple sclerosis. But there may be even more dramatic reasons why breast-feeding enhances human intelligence.

More than just a source of nutrition, breast milk is now recognized as a powerful cocktail of hormones, neuropeptides, and substances with an opium-like effect called natural opioids that not only promote healthy maturation of the nervous system, but may actually shape a newborn's brain and behavior. Scientific study is focusing not only on breast milk but also on the human breast, because this is where some essential hormones are thought to be developed.

At the Weizmann Institute of Science in Rehovot, Israel, Dr. Yitzhak

Koch and his colleagues have shown in animal studies that hormones essential for healthy development of the nervous system are produced by breast tissues. While the discovery was made in animal research, the scientists are certain that similar events take place in the human breast, making breast-feeding essential to the full development of the human nervous system.

The breast "is a unique gland, an underestimated gland," Dr. Koch told the *New York Times*. "Its activity is much more complex than people had thought."

Because certain systems, most notably the nervous system and the digestive tract, are not fully developed at the time of birth, scientists now recognize breast-feeding as an essential step in the process of bringing a human infant into full development.

Scientists suggest that the human breast may be an external counterpart to the placenta, the organ of metabolic interchange between the fetus and mother during pregnancy. The breast may be essential to completing the job of human physical development that was begun in the womb.

"They may be complementary organs," Dr. Koch said. "The placenta is responsible for regulating the growth and differentiation of an embryo. But after birth, not all the organs of the infant are fully developed. The brain is still growing. The breast could be doing a similar job [for the brain that the placenta did for the embryo]."

Certainly, the abundance of hormones that flood breast milk seem to support such speculation. Included among the hormones in breast milk are:

- Melatonin, which may help the body keep time and regulate certain circadian rhythms, such as appetite and the wake-sleep cycle
- Oxytocin, which may help the baby develop his ability to make affirmative responses; it may also be needed to establish a loving bond between mother and child
- Thyroid hormones, which may help ward off symptoms of congenital hypothyroidism
- Bradykinin, which is needed to recognize pain
- Endorphins, natural opiate-like compounds that enhance mood and act as natural painkillers
- An insulin-like growth factor, which is needed to produce healthy skin and nerve development

Many more hormones found in breast milk are now being identified and studied. In addition, scientists assert that the importance of these hormones lies not only in what they do independently, but also in how they work synergistically to promote the healthy development of the brain, liver, pancreas, intestines, and other organs.

At the Oregon Health Sciences University in Portland, researcher Dr. Martha Neuringer says that we've just scratched the surface of what may be present in breast milk. "Human milk is an incredibly complicated substance," she told the *New York Times*. "It contains proteins we haven't even identified yet, much less know the function of."

Much about breast milk and breast-feeding remains a mystery to doctors and scientists. But based on what we do know, every doctor, nurse, and health professional should be promoting breast-feeding without reservation or compromise.

Other Advantages of Breast-feeding for Baby—and for Mother

If there is anything in human nutrition that is greater than the sum of its parts, it is breast milk, which is so much more than all its nutrients and hormones, simply because it comes with a mother's love. Dr. Grantly Dick-Read, now seen as the father of the natural-birth movement, says a newborn baby has three primary needs: the food from his mother's breasts, the warmth of her arms, and the security of her presence. Breast-feeding provides all three.

A full-term baby spends nine months in the warmth of her mother's womb. Since her mother's blood is her blood and her mother's body is her body, she and her mother are one. The experience of birth, however, is the sudden separation from the larger world the infant has occupied. No matter how loving and wonderful that birth may be, it is, on some level, a shock. Suddenly, the baby is thrust into the world of air, bright lights, changes in temperature, new sounds, clothing on her skin, and lifeless surfaces on which she often rests. To be taken into her mother's arms and held close to her mother's body, to suckle and be nourished by her mother's breast, is to be reunited in some way with the physical source of her life. It's no wonder that scientists make the analogy between the breast and the placenta, because there is nothing closer to the womb in an infant's life than her mother's breast.

Breast-feeding is a tactile experience—one might even call it the unity of touch, nourishment, and love. But there are many other sensorial experiences that go with it, including sounds, smells, and visual interchanges that reinforce bonding and love. The longer the duration of breast-feeding, the more measurable the quality of mother-child bonding. All of this had been shown to produce significantly lower incidences of child abuse and of those conditions collectively termed failure to thrive.

There are many benefits for the mother as well. Breast-feeding right after birth releases the hormone prolactin, which in turn shrinks the mother's uterus, preventing bleeding and hastening recovery. Breast-feeding also limits fertility and thereby provides effective birth control. A 1996 study published in the *British Medical Journal* found that when practiced correctly, lactation was 99 percent effective in preventing pregnancy for up to six months in women who breast-fed consistently.

By breast-feeding, a woman provides 700 to 1,000 calories to her infant each day. That is a significant number of calories—women usually consume between 2,000 and 2,800 calories a day—which can result in equally significant weight loss and/or a lot more pleasurable eating. As long as an overweight woman eats a starch-based diet, she will lose that extra weight effortlessly after pregnancy and will do it without ever having to go hungry. You may not need any additional exercise to lose weight, either. As every mother knows, tending to a baby is a workout in anyone's book. Of course, a little exercise would be a nice addition for better fitness.

New research has shown a clear correlation between breast-feeding and a significant reduction in the risk of ovarian cancer and in the risk of breast cancer for premenopausal women. And women who breast-feed have a lower risk of suffering from osteoporosis.

Risks Associated with Bottle-feeding

Nothing in infant formula or cow's milk compares favorably to human breast milk in any of the areas discussed above. There is none of breast milk's immune-enhancing elements in either infant formula or cow's milk, and none of the hormones needed for proper growth and development of organs and systems. In addition, research has shown that bottle-feeding is associated with a wide array of common physical problems, ranging from stomach and intestinal disorders to an increase in the risk of sudden infant death syndrome (SIDS).

One reason why formula and cow's milk may be associated with an increased risk of disease is that both actually promote the attachment of disease-causing bacteria to an infant's cells. Since there are no immune cells being pumped into the baby's blood from the mother, the child is even more susceptible to such bacteria and the illnesses they cause.

The list of ailments commonly associated with bottle-feeding is long. Research has shown that bottle-feeding contributes to digestive disorders, including inflammatory bowel disease, celiac disease (associated with intestinal disorders, anemia, and malfunction of the pancreas), obstruction of the stomach outlet (or hypertrophic pyloric stenosis); acute appendicitis; tonsillitis; and tooth decay and crooked alignment of teeth (malocclusion). Unlike bottle-feeding, breast-feeding appears to enhance proper development of the jaws and teeth, causing teeth to come in straight and aligned.

Bottle-feeding is also associated with higher rates of obesity in both children and adults. More bottle-fed children also suffer from an inability to grow normally and, later in life, tend to have higher rates of coronary heart disease and multiple sclerosis.

In addition to being devoid of so many essential components, formulas have also been found to contain a high degree of aluminum, which research has shown may cause disorders of the bone, brain, and nervous systems of infants. The aluminum in formulas probably comes from several sources, including the soybeans used to make the formulas, the formula's additives, the manufacturer's processing, and the storage containers that hold the liquid, often for extended periods of time. (It should be noted that soy products also contain an abundance of phytoestrogens, which are discussed in chapter 6.) The chart that follows shows the relative amounts of aluminum in various substances to which infants are exposed.

ALUMINUM CONCENTRATIONS IN MILKS
(measured in micrograms of aluminum found in a liter of liquid)

Breast milk	9	Preterm	300
Whey-based	165	Soy	534
Fortified	161	Casein hydrolysate	773

Studies have shown that infants are at risk of experiencing aluminum poisoning when they consume aluminum in amounts that are greater than 300 micrograms per liter of the "milk" substance. As the chart shows, the risk is especially frightening for infants fed soy- and casein-based formulas. According to a study by the formula manufacturer, Mead Johnson Nutritionals, in the United States approximately 50 percent of all newborns and 87 percent of 3-month-old infants are fed a commercial formula either as their sole source of nutrition or as a supplement to breast milk.

JUVENILE DIABETES

Among the most disturbing findings is that bottle-fed babies have higher rates of type I or juvenile diabetes. One study showed that children who are breast-fed for more than twelve months have only half the risk of developing diabetes as bottle-fed babies. In fact, the longer an infant is breast-fed, the lower his or her risk of developing diabetes.

The rates of juvenile diabetes are especially high among children who drink cow's milk. In some susceptible children, cow's milk protein passes intact through the wall of the intestine into the bloodstream. The body reacts to the cow's milk protein in the same way it would to foreign protein from a virus or bacteria. Antibodies are made to defend the body against these foreign proteins. Unfortunately, the antibodies do more than attack the cow's milk proteins; they also attach themselves to human tissues that contain sequences of amino acids that are also found in the cow's milk protein. In the case of juvenile diabetes, they attack the insulin-producing cells of the pancreas and destroy these tissues over a period of five to seven years. Once these cells are destroyed, the body loses its ability to produce insulin; the child develops type I diabetes and will need insulin shots for the rest of his or her life. Having diabetes makes a person susceptible to a host of other serious disorders, including coronary heart disease, blindness, kidney failure, and gangrene and the consequent amputation of limbs. And milk proteins can trigger the immune system to attack other tissues.

The American Academy of Pediatrics Work Group on Cow's Milk Protein and Diabetes Mellitus in 1994 concluded: "Early exposure of infants to cow's milk protein may be an important factor in the initiation of the β [beta] cell destructive process in some individuals," and "The avoidance of cow's milk protein for the first several months of life may reduce the later development of IDDM or delay its onset in susceptible people."

Dairy foods, including cow's milk, are the leading causes of food allergy in children and adults. Some experts estimate that more than 60 percent of people are allergic to cow's milk protein. Common symptoms include runny nose, fluid collections in the middle ear, postnasal drip, hoarseness, asthma, eczema, and bed-wetting. Chapter 11 examines osteoporosis, just one of the many other serious disorders associated with drinking milk and eating other dairy foods.

In addition to these problems, cow's milk has too little iron and too much protein (breast milk contains only 1.3 percent protein, while cow's milk contains 3.3 percent or more). High-protein diets are associated with a wide assortment of diseases, including osteoporosis. Cow's milk is the perfect food for supporting the life of a baby cow, but it's not suited to nourishing a human infant.

SUDDEN INFANT DEATH SYNDROME

Over the past twenty-five years at least nineteen studies have analyzed the relationship between bottle-feeding and sudden infant death syndrome, also known as crib death or SIDS. Twelve of those studies found an increased risk for SIDS with bottle-feeding; seven showed no effect. Overall, the evidence indicates that if you choose to bottle-feed your baby, your child's risk of SIDS will be two to four times greater than if you breast-feed your child.

The reason why bottle-feeding increases the risk of SIDS remains unknown. There may not be a single answer. Certain children may be more in need of the wealth of nutrients and hormones breast milk provides. Another theory proposes that while asleep, bottle-fed infants regurgitate their stomach contents and inhale the cow's milk (or soy) protein into their lungs, causing an anaphylactic reaction to these foreign proteins that can lead to death.

Changing Attitudes About Breast-feeding

Professional health organizations, including the American Academy of Pediatrics, the American College of Obstetrics and Gynecology, and the American Dietetic Association, have developed position statements declaring breast milk superior, and ideal, for infants. You would think that if all of these organizations were endorsing breast-feeding then most everyone else would be doing so, too. Unfortunately, that is not the case. Part of the problem is that these endorsements are not translated into the practices and policies of doctors, nurses, and hospitals.

Pediatricians who encourage women to breast-feed, such as Dr. Carole A. Stashwick of the Dartmouth Medical School, point out that doctors and nurses in hospitals often do not encourage mothers to start nursing their infants immediately after birth. Hospitals generally separate mother and child after birth, and place restrictions on the duration and frequency of breast-feeding, making the process difficult. Unless the baby is fed on demand he is likely to cry, giving the impression that he is not getting enough to eat. The automatic reaction at many hospitals is to give the infant supplements of water and formula. Infants should be placed on the breast immediately after being born, and breast-feeding should begin within an hour of birth.

Many hospitals further undermine women and breast-feeding by sending new mothers home with free samples of formulas. This unconscionable act is often cited as the most detrimental of all practices that keep women from breast-feeding, because it puts the hospital's credibility and authority behind the practice of bottle-feeding.

Meanwhile, drug companies promote bottle-feeding through advertisements and pamphlets that are sent directly to doctors. Such companies are aided in their attempts to undermine breast-feeding by willing physicians and nurses who either fail to educate women on the importance of breast-feeding or subtly encourage women to use infant formula.

Health workers defend their failure to encourage breast-feeding on the grounds that they do not want to make mothers feel guilty. Given the importance of breast-feeding to the health of every child—indeed, to the health of our entire society—medical professionals and government officials should be acting in exactly the opposite way. We must educate the public so thoroughly that everyone recognizes that breast-feeding is essential to human health. Health and government officials must encourage employers to allow more women to work at home, without the threat of losing their jobs or their career opportunities; they must also allow women to work shorter shifts, at least while they are nursing their babies. More women should be educated on how to express breast milk and provide it for their children while they are at work. We should make it easier for women to breast-feed in public places. Government officials should also enact legislation giving women more maternity leave from work.

Meanwhile, more mothers and grandmothers should encourage their grown daughters to breast-feed their children. This is no longer happening today. Breast-feeding, once considered normal motherly behavior, is now considered by many women as optional or even extraordinary.

The Department of Health and Human Services has announced the goal that by the year 2000, 75 percent of American women would breast-feed their infants for at least the first three months of life, and that 50 percent of mothers would breast-feed for the first six months. A study conducted by Ross Laboratories, a baby formula company, reported in 1992 that 53.9 percent of women nurse their babies in the hospital, and 20 percent were still breast-feeding six months later. Experts predict that those numbers will not increase—many think they will fall—unless our society provides more encouragement and support for women to breast-feed.

SUPPORTING WOMEN WHO WANT TO BREAST-FEED

Mothers who are uncertain about breast-feeding, or whether or not they can make it work with their schedules, need clear and complete information on the importance of breast milk and ways in which they can establish a routine to feed their infants.

There is so much disinformation in our society concerning breast-feeding that it's a wonder that so many women do breast-feed their children today. Many people tell pregnant women that it's painful to breast-feed, that they will have to restrict their diets to protect their children from the effects of certain foods, or that many women simply do not produce enough milk to adequately nourish their infants.

New mothers should know that it is extremely rare that a mother cannot produce an adequate supply of milk to nourish her baby. Breast-feeding should begin as soon as possible after birth, and the newborn infant should remain with the mother. Newborns should be nursed whenever they show signs of hunger, such as increased alertness or activity, mouthing, or rooting (crying is a late indication), and nursed eight to twelve times every twenty-four hours until satiety, usually ten to fifteen minutes on each breast. No supplements (water, glucose water, formula, and so forth) should be given to breast-feeding newborns. Nursing, as a rule, should not be painful. Moreover, the healthiest diet for you, the mother, is also the healthiest one you can be eating for your nursing infant: a starch-based diet with the addition of fruits and vegetables (supplemented with 5 micrograms of B_{12} daily). The addition of animal products, refined foods, and fats and oils slightly decreases the nutritional quality of the breast milk, but greatly increases the risk of contamination with environmental chemicals like pesticides and herbicides. Adding dairy products to a mother's diet will result in dairy proteins in her milk, which will eventually be absorbed by her infant, who could develop allergic reactions such as colic. Furthermore, no increase in calcium intake from any source (neither milk nor supplements) is required by the nursing mother.

Every pregnant woman should consult a lactation counselor during pregnancy, and again at the first sign of any trouble during nursing. These helpful women are found in the phone book, or through La Leche League. Or contact them on the Internet at www.lalecheleague.org. They can answer any and all questions you may have about breast-feeding.

Stopping Breast-feeding

Closely observing your baby's development will give you clues as to when to introduce solid foods. At about six months of age babies develop teeth for chewing. Their hands become sufficiently coordinated to grab solid foods and put them into their mouths. The American Academy of Pediatrics recommends that a baby be breast-fed exclusively for the first six months of life. The addition of any other liquids to a child's diet should be given by cup, not by bottle, in order to help maintain breast-feeding. Solid food should be introduced slowly, one item at a time, during the next six months of life. By solid, I mean soft vegetables, like potatoes, sweet potatoes, and squash; and grains, or soupy vegetables and grain broth. Vegetables and grains should be thoroughly mashed with a fork or by putting them through a baby food mill.

Once a child starts eating solid foods it's natural to reduce somewhat the amount of breast milk provided, but every mother should be cautious at this point. Introducing solid foods too early, or relying upon them too heavily, will deprive your child of essential nutrition from breast milk. As the child ages, the mother can breast-feed less frequently, while the child relies increasingly on solid foods. The foods fed to children at six or eight months still tend to have a low nutrient density, especially if they are still provided in soupy broth. This means that breast milk will still be needed during this transition to solid foods, and ideally should continue for at least two years.

What would medical authorities and government officials do if a new, nontoxic drug became available that could save the lives of more than a million babies worldwide each year? Think about how they would react if that remedy could reduce the risk of multiple diseases throughout life, improve intelligence, and foster social well-being. And consider further what would happen if that potion cost nothing to produce and could be taken by mouth. I can assure you that it would be prescribed universally. Breast-feeding can do all this and much more. Let breast milk do all of this for your child.

CHAPTER 5

Preventing Premature Sexual Development in Children

Parents of young children today will tell you that they are concerned about their children "growing up too soon," by which they mean being forced to deal with issues of sexual desire and relationships long before they have the mental and emotional maturity to deal with such issues. Most adults point to the media—television, films, and print—as the primary sources of concern. By exposing children to adult images and passions, parents argue, the media force our children to deal with sexual issues and desires long before they are ready. What people do not realize is that the primary cause of premature sexual development in children is the food they eat.

What effect does food have on the sexual natures of our children? The modern Western diet, rich in fat and low in fiber, is causing dramatic changes in human development and triggering the onset of puberty long before nature ever intended. The diet does this by altering hormone levels, which causes adult physical characteristics, reproductive functions, and sexual desires to emerge in people who, chronologically, are still children. As a result, puberty is occurring in children at younger and younger ages. By eating this high-fat diet ourselves, and encouraging youngsters to eat such foods, we are thrusting our children into the adult world long before they have the life experience and emotional and intellectual maturity to deal with that world.

Some of the sexual changes are truly startling because of the fact that they are occurring in very young children. A recent study from the

University of North Carolina at Chapel Hill, published in the medical journal *Pediatrics*, reported that "girls seen in a sample of pediatric practices from across the United States are developing pubertal characteristics at younger ages than currently used norms. . . . At age 3 years, 3 percent of African-American and 1 percent of white girls showed breast and/or pubic hair development, with proportions increasing to 27.2 percent and 6.7 percent, respectively, at 7 years of age. At age 8, 48.3 percent of African-American girls and 14.7 percent of white girls had begun development."

Here are the average ages for the onset of key sexual characteristics in girls.

	African-American	White
Breast development	8.87	9.96
Pubic hair	8.78	10.51
Menses	12.16	12.88

Boys are maturing much earlier as well. However, there have not been as many studies of boys' sexual development, perhaps because their secondary sexual characteristics are not as evident, or the overt physical changes as dramatic, so early in life.

As a result of this accelerated rate of development, girls are entering puberty at younger and younger ages. Scientists have calculated that every ten years, the age at which girls experience puberty drops two to six months.

This is happening in developed countries throughout the world. In Norway, the age of menarche, or the first menses, has dropped steadily during the past 160 years. In 1830, girls experienced their first period—and thus were capable of bearing children—at the age of 17.2 years. In 1950, girls began menstruating at the age of 13.2 years. Similar changes have been seen in other western European countries during the same period.

- In Britain, the average age of menarche has fallen from 16.5 years to 12.8 years during the past 150 years.
- In the United States, girls started their first periods at age 14 years in 1900; by 1960 they were menstruating by an average age of 12.7.
- In Japan, in 1875 girls became women at 16.5 years of age. In 1950, they started their first periods at age 15.2. By 1960, the age of menarche was 13.9; by 1970, it fell to 12.5. With the steady adoption

of the Western diet since World War II, Japanese girls now experience sexual maturity at the same age as American girls.

Interestingly, the oldest onset of sexual maturity was observed among native women of Papua New Guinea in the 1960s, who did not get their periods until sometime between 18 and 19 years of age. These native people ate a diet that was nearly vegetarian, with only very small amounts of animal foods. Needless to say, the diet was exceedingly low in fat and cholesterol, but rich in fiber and plant nutrients.

Causes of Early Maturation

During the past two hundred years—and especially during this century—humans have moved away from the diet that we as a species evolved on. Instead of relying on unrefined plant foods, as our ancestors did, we have shifted to animal foods and highly processed foods as the primary sources of nutrition. With that change has come the dramatic rise in fat and cholesterol consumption, along with the equally dramatic reduction in fiber and plant nutrition. The steady increase in our consumption of beef, other red meats, dairy products, eggs, poultry, and fish has caused sexual maturity to occur at younger and younger ages.

Scientists have long observed the connection between changes in diet and early sexual maturation. Several studies have shown a correlation between diets high in fat, protein, and processed foods with early onset of menstruation. Indeed, researchers have observed that vegetarian women experience their first menstruation later in life than nonvegetarians.

Another factor affecting menarche is vigorous exercise, which has been shown to delay the onset of puberty. Of course, girls today eat a high-fat diet and do not exercise; today's lifestyles are more sedentary for both men and women.

Diet and exercise affect hormone levels, and the most important hormone for sexual development in young girls is estrogen. Estrogen promotes the development of secondary sex characteristics. It causes the uterus to grow, the vaginal tissues to become thicker, and the breasts to develop. Estrogen combines with other hormones to cause the tissues lining the inside of the uterus to grow and, if pregnancy has not occurred, these tissues are shed as menstruation.

The relationship between estrogen and health does not stop with the early onset of puberty. Estrogen levels play a key role in the onset of other diseases, especially breast cancer. Young girls who experience early puberty are many times more vulnerable to this terrible disease than girls who enter puberty later in their teens.

Controlling Estrogen Levels

Diet controls estrogen levels in several ways: by controlling body weight and in particular by increasing body weight; by determining the kind of bacterial environment in the intestines; and by introducing environmental chemicals into our systems.

CONVERTING FAT TO ESTROGEN

We all know that a high-fat diet is the primary cause of weight gain. As more fat is consumed, fat cells in the adipose tissues expand. These fat cells become factories for estrogen production.

The process begins with the creation of male hormones, called androstenediones, which are produced by the adrenal gland and ovaries. In the fat cells, these male hormones are converted into estrogen. The fatter a person is, the more hormone he or she produces. Young girls who are most at risk for having high estrogen levels are those who are obese. As fat consumption and weight increase, estrogen levels rise, causing accelerated physical and sexual maturity in young girls.

CONVERTING BILE ACIDS INTO SEX HORMONES

Fat cells are not the only source of higher estrogen levels in children. Another is the kind of bacteria that populates a young girl's large intestine. A high-fat, low-fiber diet promotes the production of a type of bacteria in the intestinal tract that has the ability to convert bile acids into sex hormones, including estrogen. These hormones are then absorbed through the intestinal wall into the bloodstream.

Not only do people on high-fat diets have more of these bacteria, but their bodies also produce more bile acids, which the bacteria use to convert into hormones. The reason for this is that bile acids are produced by the liver in order to digest fat. If your child eats a high-fat diet, she has more bile acids in her intestines and therefore converts more of these into sex hormones.

RECIRCULATING ESTROGENS

Estrogen circulates through a healthy body only once. The hormone is produced by the ovaries and fat cells and secreted into the bloodstream, where it travels throughout the body and affects the hormone-sensitive organs, including the breasts, uterus, ovaries, skin, and other tissues. After one complete passage, all of the estrogen is removed from the body by the liver, which excretes the hormone into the intestinal tract, where it is eventually eliminated with the feces.

To prevent estrogen from being reabsorbed by the body, the liver attaches a nonabsorbable substance to the hormone. A high-fat, low-fiber diet, especially one high in meats, encourages the growth of intestinal bacteria that are capable of breaking apart these nonabsorbable compounds, thus allowing the estrogen to be absorbed into the bloodstream over and over again. Once in the bloodstream, these freed estrogens merely add to the overall estrogen load, repeatedly stimulating the hormone-sensitive tissues. The net effect is to increase the overall estrogen levels in a woman's body.

THE ESTROGENIC EFFECTS OF ENVIRONMENTAL POISONS

The higher up you go in the food chain, the greater the concentrations of environmental chemicals in the tissues and fat cells of the animals. The way it works is simple enough: plants containing toxic residues are consumed by animals. Over time, those toxins accumulate and become concentrated in the fat cells of the animals; they enter your body whenever you consume animal foods. Thus, red meat, dairy products, poultry, and fish are the primary sources of environmental chemicals in the American food supply.

Once inside your body, these chemicals migrate to the fat cells, where they interact and combine. Many of these chemicals, especially pesticides such as atrazine, DDT, dieldrin, endosulfan, and toxaphene, have an estrogenic effect. Individually, their effects are weak, but when these chemicals are combined in your tissues, they can become exceptionally powerful estrogens, increasing their impact by 160- to 1,600-fold.

It should be noted that Americans used record quantities of pesticides, insecticides, and herbicides in 1995, despite claims by the chemical industry and farmers that they are cutting pesticide use.

ESTROGENS IN MILK

What most of the people who smile when they see a milk mustache on their favorite celebrity don't realize is that the glass of milk they're drinking is loaded with hormones. Most milk-producing cows today are pregnant. Unlike most humans, pregnant cows continue to lactate. The pregnancy causes high levels of estrogen (estrone) to circulate in the animal's body. And, not surprisingly, the milk produced by these pregnant cows also contains high levels of estrogen.

The Disadvantages of Early Sexual Development

The consequences of premature sexual development permeate our society. Instead of concentrating on school and their long-term career goals, children are forced to deal with adult sexuality, which encourages them to make unwise sexual choices that very often lead to disease. Three million teenagers suffer from sexually transmitted diseases annually, including herpes and HIV infection that eventually leads to AIDS.

Early sexual development prevents young people from developing the skills needed to maintain relationships; it leads to premature marriage and divorce. More than 90 percent of teenage marriages end in divorce. The logical consequence of young people having sex is an increase in teenage pregnancies. One million teenagers become pregnant each year and nearly half of them give birth. The birth rate for young teens between the ages of fifteen and seventeen is steadily rising: it rose 27 percent between 1985 and 1991. In 1991, nearly four in one hundred girls between the ages of fifteen and seventeen gave birth.

Children having children results in high rates of single motherhood, a disruption or discontinuation of the mother's education, and poverty. A teenage mother has a far greater risk than older women of experiencing complications in pregnancy and childbirth, including premature and prolonged labor and preeclampsia.

Infants of young mothers are also in danger: they have a 9 percent chance of suffering from low birth weights (under 5.5 pounds)—the average in the United States is a 7 percent chance. These babies have a greater risk of complications such as respiratory distress syndrome and bleeding. They are also forty times more likely to die during their first month of life than normal-weight infants.

The age at which children mature sexually also affects their adult height and health. Interestingly, children who reach sexual maturity later in life eventually grow taller, on average, as adults. The reason for this is that sex hormones close the growth (epiphysial) plates of bones, halting further longitudinal growth. Early menarche is also associated with a much higher risk of breast cancer and heart disease in women.

As a nation, we must create social policies that implement the dietary goals and recommendations that so many government agencies recommend. We must begin by feeding our children a starch-based diet that allows them to develop naturally and will give them the stability to think, feel, and act as children—right through most of their teenage years. This will give them the time to develop intellectually, emotionally, and psychologically, so that their sexual development can be influenced by the maturity of their character. Only then will we have the basis for a stable and clear-thinking society.

CHAPTER 6

Protecting Yourself Against Breast Cancer

Breast cancer is perhaps the most frightening of all diseases facing women today, and the one around which there is the most confusion. If you were to listen only to the prevailing medical voices, you would have good reason to be scared and bewildered. The incidence of breast cancer began climbing steadily in the early 1970s and only recently started to level off at its current rate, which very likely is the highest ever seen in human history. Meanwhile, despite billions of dollars spent on cancer research in general, and on breast cancer in particular, science has yet to provide a clear set of recommendations designed to prevent the illness. The only consistent recommendation offered today is for women to have regular mammograms, which, as we will see in the next chapter, is a dubious recommendation at best. The fact is that women seeking ways to avoid breast cancer and gain control over their health have been abandoned by many doctors and the leading health agencies.

Breast cancer presents every woman with a life-altering choice: she can either wait for the National Cancer Institute to offer a clearly defined preventive program (which, it must be admitted, is still a very long way off, especially when you consider that the war on cancer began in 1972 and we are still waiting) or take matters into her own hands and protect herself from the disease. This chapter offers you the clearest set of guidelines yet devised to prevent an illness that, many scientists believe, is largely caused by environmental factors, most of which are under your control.

What Causes Breast Cancer?

A woman's chances of contracting breast cancer in 1960 were 1 in 20. In the 1970s, they jumped to 1 in 14, and as of this writing, in 1997, the American Cancer Society tells us that a woman's chances of getting breast cancer are 1 in 8. Approximately 184,300 women will be diagnosed with breast cancer this year, and about 44,300 will die of the disease. This is occurring in the face of enormous publicity and consequent increase in public awareness.

But what effect is that awareness having on women? Does the increased publicity, which lately has risen to a crescendo, offer women an action plan or some tools for prevention? Unfortunately, the answer is no. The media's reporting on breast cancer research, which is where most women get their information, is often muddled and contradictory. For years, we read that a high-fat diet was believed by many scientists to be a leading risk factor in the onset of the disease, but later evidence offered conflicting findings and since then many scientists have equivocated on fat's role in the onset of the illness. Meanwhile, scattered reports turn up about exercise, DDT, and the increased risk facing obese women. Without a larger context and a specific set of recommendations attached to such reports, this information has little impact on women's lives.

The topic getting much of the attention these days is genetics. Yet, scientists admit that the presence of the BRCA-1 gene, now identified as the breast cancer susceptibility gene, only accounts for at most 5 percent of all breast cancers.

The combination of a heightened awareness and the absence of any clear guidelines has caused women to react in a variety of ways. Many have become politically active; others are understandably angry and afraid; and still others have simply surrendered, frozen with the anticipation of the disease. But what else can women do? The answers may surprise you.

RISK FACTORS

We have known for a very long time that most cancers are triggered by environmental sources. At the turn of the century, pioneering cancer researcher Rolo Russell recognized that death rates from cancer were highest among those "countries that eat more flesh." The American Cancer Society took nearly a century (September 16, 1996) to recommend that Americans reduce their consumption of red meat because of its link to the cause of colon and prostate cancer. Research has consistently found a close association between the intake of meat specifically, and high-fat foods in general, to other forms of cancer, including those of the rectum, endometrium (uterus), kidney, and breast.

After distilling virtually all of the relevant cancer research, the Harvard School of Public Health concluded in 1996 that nearly 70 percent of all cancers today can be attributed to smoking, diet, drinking habits, and a sedentary lifestyle. Only 2 percent of the modern cancers appear traceable to environmental pollution, and only 10 percent of all cancers to a person's genes.

Though genetic research is getting a lot of publicity today, the subject is murky at best, because cancer-promoting genes still need the right environmental conditions in order to be expressed. Just because your mother may have developed breast cancer does not necessarily mean that you will, especially if you eat a diet and live a lifestyle that is very different from your mother's. The opposite is also true: just because your mother didn't develop breast cancer doesn't mean that you won't, especially if you eat a diet that supports the growth of cancer.

A perfect illustration of this point is the Japanese experience. For decades, Japanese women were thought to be genetically protected from breast cancer because their rate of developing the disease was only one-sixth that of American women. As long as Japanese women remained on their traditional diet of rice and vegetables, their apparent "immunity" remained intact. However, when they migrated to the United States and adopted more American eating habits, their protection vanished. Within a single generation, their rates of breast cancer jumped to nearly those of American women.

The Japanese cancer rates, which correlated so accurately with their dietary habits, led many scientists to believe that fat alone might be the cause of breast cancer. Other research, including human epidemiology, laboratory, and animal studies, supported this conclusion. But then two studies conducted by scientists at Harvard University found no relationship between fat and breast cancer, which had a devastating effect on women who thought that they could prevent breast cancer by eating a healthier diet. Reports of these studies also reinforced unhealthy behaviors among women who wanted to hear good news about their own bad habits. As a result, many people believed that those studies exonerated not only fat but also a lot of other unhealthy dietary habits.

One of the big mistakes that scientists made initially when examining the research on Japanese women was to overlook the fact that the Japanese diet is loaded with plant foods which, in addition to being low in fat, are also rich in all the immune-boosting and cancer-fighting chemicals that our bodies need to be healthy. By focusing exclusively on fat, they singled out a powerful poison, but neglected all the health-promoting compounds that are missing in the standard American diet. In the process, they allowed a dangerous misconception to settle on our society, which was that fat alone was the source of disease. When fat was proved to be a contributing, but not independent, cause of cancer, many people simply threw up their hands and decided to go back to indulging their tastes for animal and processed foods, fat, and sugar. This misconception no doubt contributed to the unprecedented rates of breast cancer in our society.

Dietary Risks

The first thing you must understand is that it is highly unlikely that breast cancer has a single cause—even a single dietary cause. No individual risk factor, not even fat or chemical pollution, is as potent alone as it is when combined with other environmental poisons. Together, these agents combine to form a massive assault on the human cell, like a barrage of arrows hitting a target at once. Focusing on any one risk factor, even fat, to the exclusion of the others is a mistake.

Allow me to describe for you a low-fat diet that passes for a healthy regimen in our society, but in fact is a cancer-promoting diet. This menu of breakfast, lunch, and dinner, plus snacks, is sure to cause disease.

- *Breakfast:* Egg white omelet; sugar-coated cereal with skim milk; white bread and jelly; coffee with sugar and low-fat creamer
- *Lunch:* Turkey sandwich on white bread; a scoop of low-fat cottage cheese; Jell-O; skim milk
- *Dinner:* White-flour quesadilla made with low-fat cheese; charcoal-broiled swordfish; white rice cooked in chicken broth; cola; angel-food cake with low-fat frosting
- *Snacks:* Have any of the following on a regular basis: SnackWells cookies, licorice, soda crackers, reduced-fat Entenmann's cakes, low-fat potato chips, hard candies

This diet derives less than 10 percent of all its calories from fat, yet it is a prescription for disease. Here are just a handful of its problems:

- The diet is rich in protein, especially animal protein, which is associated with higher rates of cancer as well as osteoporosis.
- It is devoid of fiber, which leads to constipation, hemorrhoids,

polyps, diverticulosis, and colon cancer; the absence of fiber also promotes the growth of harmful intestinal bacteria that result in higher blood levels of estrogen, the female hormone that promotes breast cancer.

• It is rich in milk proteins, which trigger destructive immune reactions and may contain cancer-causing viruses.

• It is deficient in antioxidants and other immune-boosting and cancer-fighting substances.

• The sugar, refined foods, and white flour products are loaded with calories that promote overweight and obesity, which, as I will show, are an independent risk factor for breast cancer.

• The diet promotes high insulin levels, which cause fat to be stored in tissues and contribute to weight gain.

• The charbroiled fish contains nitrosamines, a known carcinogen.

• The cola beverages contain substances that deprive the bones of calcium and contribute to osteoporosis.

• The diet is devoid of the innumerable vitamins, minerals, antioxidants, and phytochemicals that the body needs to support its immune system and protect itself against a wide array of illnesses, including breast cancer.

Now, think of the woman who eats this 10 percent fat diet, perhaps for years, and then gets breast or colon cancer, or suffers from osteoporosis later in life. She has gone to great lengths to follow the recommendations of the leading health authorities by avoiding fat and cholesterol. Yet, she has contracted a life-threatening disease. What other reaction could she possibly have except frustration, anger, and an overwhelming feeling of defeat?

Each day, we take in between one and five pounds of food. For a great many of us, that daily food allotment is five pounds worth of poison, and only one of those poisons is fat.

The Cancer Cycle

Cancer is thought to begin when the cell's command center, its genetic code or DNA, is damaged. Once the DNA is injured, cells either die or are stimulated to replicate relentlessly until they engulf the human organism.

These mutant cells can be created by a variety of insults, but most of them are caused by oxidants, or free radicals, which are highly reactive oxygen molecules that break down cells and deform DNA. Free radicals cause the atoms in your body to lose electrons. In order to maintain balance and stability, an atom must have as many protons (positively charged particles) as it does electrons (negatively charged particles). When an atom loses or gains one or more electrons, it will attempt to restore balance by stealing the electrons it needs from a neighboring atom or donating an electron. This results in destabilization of nearby atoms, triggering a cascade of chemical reactions that result in the breakdown of cells. If this breakdown occurs in the cell's nucleus, the DNA can mutate and trigger the creation of a malignant cancer cell.

Unfortunately, some degree of oxidation cannot be avoided because it occurs as a normal by-product of cellular metabolism and immune function. Your cells give off oxidants simply by burning oxygen, consuming nutrients, and replacing dead cells, such as when your body rebuilds its bones or restores the tissue in your eyes or your liver. Thus, oxidant formation is part of life. In fact, the rate at which we create oxidants determines how fast we age and whether or not we contract a serious illness.

Mammals, including humans, produce oxidants at very different rates, depending on how fast their metabolisms work. Since smaller animals, such as mice, have much faster metabolisms than humans, they produce a lot more oxidants. At the University of California at Berkeley, cancer researcher Bruce N. Ames, Ph.D., and his colleagues have estimated that rats experience 100,000 oxidant hits to every cell in their bodies each day. Most of those hits strike directly at the cells' DNA.

Since human metabolism is much slower than a rat's, each of your cells receives only about 10,000 oxidant hits a day, say Ames and his coworkers. Still, that's a lot of injuries to your cells and your DNA. Fortunately, your cells contain enzymes that repair damaged DNA and heal most of the injuries caused by oxidation.

However, you can expose yourself to additional oxidants through your diet and lifestyle. There is a point, unique to all of us, at which overexposure outstrips our ability to repair damaged cells and DNA, thus making us vulnerable to disease, including cancer.

There are many sources of oxidants and free radicals, but among the most common and powerful are dietary fat; cigarette smoke; pollutants in the air, water, and soil; radiation and radioactive particles in the environment; and the intake of certain pharmaceutical drugs. All of these sources of free radicals are therefore also causes of degenerative illnesses, such as heart disease, cancer, and other potentially lethal disorders.

FIGHTING CANCER

Just as oxidants cause the breakdown of cells and DNA, antioxidants restore cellular and DNA health. They do this by donating electrons to unstable atoms, or those that are in decay. In the process, antioxidants restore health to cells and tissues. In this way, antioxidants slow the aging process and prevent disease. Antioxidants also boost your immune system and help you fight cancer.

There are many antioxidants, but the three that people are most familiar with are vitamins C, E, and beta carotene, the vegetable source of vitamin A. In addition to these are vitamin B_6; glutathione; bioflavonoids (a group of compounds found in vegetable foods); several minerals, including selenium, zinc, copper, and manganese; and an amino acid called L-cysteine. These antioxidants are concentrated in plant foods, such as vegetables, whole grains, beans, and fruit.

Scientists now recommend that everyone eat at least five servings of these plant foods per day, in almost any combination, in order to get an adequate supply of antioxidants. Without these five servings, your immune system and cancer-fighting mechanisms can become depressed, which means that when a cancer cell manifests, your body will not be able to destroy it.

Dr. Ames and his colleagues have calculated that those who fail to eat the recommended five servings of antioxidant-rich foods have twice the risk of developing cancer of those who do not eat them each day. That may explain in part why breast cancer rates have reached such unprecedented levels.

Of course, in addition to the antioxidants are the innumerable phytochemicals found in plant foods, which are chemicals that directly inhibit cancer formation and promote cellular health. When you eat plant foods, you are getting an abundance of both the antioxidants and the phytochemicals.

STIMULATING TUMOR DEVELOPMENT

Scientists have long recognized that breast cancer is a hormone-dependent disease, meaning that it needs the female hormone estrogen to encourage rapid growth. Among the evidence supporting the link between estrogen and breast cancer is the fact that breast cancer is one hundred times more common in women. Also, women who have lost their ovaries early in life have far lower rates of breast cancer than those who have not lost these hormone-producing organs. Likewise, women who have taken estrogen pills appear to experience higher rates of breast cancer than those who do not take therapeutic estrogens either as birth control pills or hormone replacement therapy (HRT).

Not only has the scientific research shown that breast tumors grow more rapidly with estrogen stimulation, but when estrogen levels are dramatically reduced, tumors shrink. All this knowledge about hormones and breast cancer has led to the use of a synthetic anti-estrogen drug, such as tamoxifen, for the prevention of breast cancer. Unfortunately, there are potentially serious side effects from this medical treatment, including cancer of the uterus and blood clots. Besides, a healthy diet that reduces estrogen stimulation of the breasts is a safer, cheaper, and more effective approach.

A FORMULA FOR DISEASE

The fact is that many people on the rich Western diet consume the perfect formula for cancer every day. They expose themselves to high levels of oxidants and free radicals, which in turn damage cells and DNA. At the same time, they deprive themselves of plant sources of antioxidants and phytochemicals, which means that when a cancer is triggered, their bodies lack the resources they need to destroy the proliferating cells. Once the cancer cells have a foothold in their system, their bodies provide the chemical support needed to nourish the cancer, namely high levels of female hormones.

Another chemical substance that acts like a fuel for cancer cells is cholesterol. Research has shown that cancer cells require high levels of cholesterol to proliferate. Interestingly, the same foods that promote high estrogen levels also contribute to high blood cholesterol. Those dangerous foods are animal products, such as red meat, poultry, dairy foods, eggs, and fish.

Ten Changes You Can Make to Save Your Life

If we are to stop breast cancer in its tracks, we must address all its causes and the many elements that support the proliferation of the disease. Here are ten changes you can make that can do just that.

1. ELIMINATE THE PARTS OF YOUR DIET THAT ARE HARMING YOU

Many aspects of the typical Western diet encourage the creation of breast cancer, and support its growth. The first of these is fat.

Eliminate All Animal Fats and Extracted Vegetable Oils

Research from around the world has shown a strong correlation between the consumption of both animal and vegetable fats and breast cancer mortality rates. Excess consumption of fats, including those extracted from vegetable sources, promotes the growth of cancer in several ways. The first and perhaps most important is by creating free radicals that trigger the cancer process. One study showed that after consuming canola oil, blood levels of beta carotene and vitamin E dropped significantly in all twelve study participants. This reveals that oxidation levels increased dramatically, requiring reserves of antioxidants to be expended in order to maintain cellular and genetic health.

Fats Promote the Production of Hormones: The second way fat encourages breast cancer is by promoting high levels of female hormones. As most people know, women's ovaries and adrenal glands produce estrogen. However, most people do not realize that estrogen is also produced in significant quantities by fat cells. In fact, the more fat you consume, the higher your estrogen levels will be.

Young girls who eat a high-fat diet typically experience their first periods sooner than those who eat a low-fat diet. For example, the British diet derives 43 percent of its calories from fat, the Chinese diet, 15 percent. The average British girl experiences her first period at the age of thirteen, while a Chinese girl starts having her periods at seventeen.

Research has confirmed that women who experience their first period early in life, such as those in England, have higher rates of breast cancer than those who start their periods later in their teenage years. The reason for both earlier menses and higher rates of breast cancer is higher estrogen levels.

At the opposite end of a woman's childbearing years, menopause occurs later in life in women with high estrogen levels. And not surprisingly, late menopause is associated with higher rates of breast cancer. On average, Chinese women experience menopause at about the age of forty-eight, while British women undergo menopause at about the age of fifty. British women who are fifty-five to sixty-four years old have levels of the powerful female hormone estradiol 171 percent higher than those of Chinese women of the same age.

Why do high estrogen levels lead to breast disease? Scientists do not fully understand the mechanisms by which higher-than-normal levels of estrogen cause breast cancer, but they do know that estrogen overstimulates both breast and uterine tissues, which causes significant changes in both areas of the body. For example, women with high estrogen levels experience swollen and tender breasts around their menstrual cycle, when estrogen levels are peaking. For some, the pain is considered severe. When these tissues are consistently overstimulated and inflamed, scar tissue can form within the breasts, causing milk ducts to become blocked and clogged. These areas become sites for cysts. Similarly, high estrogen levels trigger muscle cells within the uterus to proliferate, causing cell clusters to form, some of which can grow into fibroid tumors. While most of these breast and uterine tumors are benign, a minority of the growths emerging in the breast especially can be cancerous. Because higher estrogen levels are involved in both diseases, it follows that women with fibrocystic breast disease are at greater risk of developing breast cancer.

Some studies have shown that women with breast cancer also have higher-than-normal levels of prolactin, a hormone that stimulates changes in breast tissue and prepares the breast for milk production. Not by coincidence, research has shown that dietary fat promotes higher levels of prolactin.

Fats Encourage the Reabsorption of Estrogens: In order to limit the potentially harmful effects of estrogen, the body normally allows the hormone to circulate through the system only once. Once estrogen passes through the liver, it is combined with a chemical substance that prevents the hormone from being reabsorbed by the small intestine. Instead, it is eliminated through the feces. By preventing estrogen from making its way back into the bloodstream, the body keeps estrogen levels from becoming too high.

Unfortunately, a high-fat diet promotes the growth of bacteria in the colon that produce enzymes capable of uncoupling the estrogen from the nonabsorbable chemical substances. Once free of these estrogen complexes, the estrogen can be reabsorbed into the bloodstream, thus allowing it to recirculate through the system. The result is higher estrogen levels in a woman's body. This is yet another way that fats boost estrogen levels and promote disease.

Fats Depress Immune Response: Both animal and vegetable fats depress immune response and promote metastasis, the ability of cancer cells to invade tissues and spread throughout the body. Animal studies have shown that certain types of fats have greater cancer-promoting capacities. Polyunsaturated vegetable fats that are high in *linoleic* acid (n-6), which is normally found in corn, sunflower, and safflower oils, appear to increase the incidence of breast cancer in animals.

On the other hand, polyunsaturated oils that are high in *linolenic* acid (n-3), which is found in canola and linseed (flaxseed) oils, seem to inhibit cancer growth. (Soybeans are high in both types of polyunsaturated fat.) Omega-3 oils found in fish also inhibit cancer growth.

However, after the addition of small amounts of linoleic acid (like corn oil), n-3 fats lose some or all of their ability to block tumor growth. Therefore, it appears that a small amount of linoleic acid must be present for a fat to be cancer promoting. Of course, this small amount of linoleic acid is found in all natural human diets. The reason why some studies have shown olive oil to be cancer promoting and others have not is probably because of the varying amounts of linoleic acid in commercially available olive oils. There appears to be some balance between n-3 and n-6 fatty acids that is ideal for tumor inhibition; unfortunately, that ratio varies with different experimental models. Because all of the types of fatty acids have been found to be cancer promoting under some circumstances, prudence would dictate that all fats, regardless of who labels them "good fats," be kept to a minimum in your diet.

There are other ways in which fats depress the immune system. Immune cells, especially the macrophages, identify disease-causing agents, such as bacteria, viruses, and cancer cells, by touching them with their sensitive cell membrane. Once they identify a threat to your health, macrophages are capable of creating a variety of lethal responses that can neutralize the potential threat. They also mobilize other immune cells, including CD4 cells that direct the overall immune response and beta cells that produce antibodies that attack the invader.

Unfortunately, all fats, including polyunsaturated essential fats, have the ability to coat the macrophage cell membrane and thus prevent it from recognizing pathogens and cancer cells. This, of course, allows the cancer cells and disease-causing agents to proliferate unchallenged.

McDougall's Recommendation: To win your battle against cancer, avoid all animal food sources of fat—including meat, poultry, dairy foods, eggs, and fish—and eat vegetable fats only in their original state, which is as whole grains, vegetables, beans, and fruits.

Eliminate Cholesterol

Cancer cells appear to require a high concentration of cholesterol to grow. Moreover, a cholesterol-lowering diet and drugs have been shown to inhibit the growth of tumors in animal studies. Interestingly, chemical by-products of cholesterol, called cholesterol epoxides, have been shown to be carcinogenic in animal studies. Not surprisingly, the higher the blood cholesterol level in women, the higher the concentration of these cancer-causing cholesterol epoxides in a woman's breast fluids.

The sole sources of cholesterol are animal products, which become even more carcinogenic when they are prepared in certain ways. Grilling or frying all forms of meat, including beef, pork, lamb, poultry, and fish, releases at least ten known cancer-causing substances. Among these cancer-causing substances is a group of compounds called heterocyclic amines, which are also present in cigarette smoke. What's more, the concentrations of these carcinogens go up as the cooking temperatures get higher, and the longer the meat is cooked.

McDougall's Recommendation: To win your battle against cancer, eliminate all animal foods, which will remove all cholesterol from your diet. Plant foods contain no cholesterol.

Avoid Chemical Toxins in Your Food

The highest concentrations of toxic chemicals are found in the fat cells of animal flesh, including the flesh of fish, poultry, and meat, and in eggs and dairy products. These are the primary sources of cancer-causing chemicals affecting Americans and much of the Western world.

Once inside the body, these chemicals migrate to and become concentrated in the fatty tissues of a woman's breasts. Some of the chemicals associated with breast cancer include pesticides, herbicides, industrial chemicals (such as the plastic compound bisphenol-A), and some polychlorinated biphenyls (PCBs).

Widespread use of DDT (a pesticide) began in the United States in 1946 and ended in 1972 because of its sustained toxic effects on the environment. However, U.S. produce imports from other countries have pesticide residues 5,000 percent higher than current U.S. standards of DDT. Some studies show as much as a fourfold increase in relative risk of breast cancer with high DDT exposure. Women with breast cancer have also been found to have a 50 percent to 60 percent higher concentration of the main metabolite of DDT (DDE) in breast specimens compared with women without cancer. DDT chemically mimics estrogens. When studied singly, these chemicals may have only a weak estrogenic effect. However, when the chemicals were tested in combination, estrogenic activity shot up 160- to 1,600-fold. Americans used a record amount of pesticides, insecticides, and herbicides in 1995 despite claims by the chemical industry and farmers that they are cutting pesticide use.

Recently, one large study examining the relationship between DDT and breast cancer cast doubt upon the pesticide as an independent risk factor in the creation of the disease. Scientists acknowledged, however, that no one knows what the synergistic effects of these chemicals are when they are combined inside the human body.

The exact mechanisms by which these compounds might cause cancer are unknown and their relative importance is debated. The National Research Council, an arm of the National Academy of Sciences, confirmed in 1996 that many natural and synthetic chemicals cause cancer, but that their importance was minimal compared with the effects of overconsumption of calories and fats.

Chlorine is added to drinking water to kill bacteria. Chlorine will react with organic material found in water to form compounds (trihalomethanes) that are known to cause an increase in cancers in humans. The compounds act by promoting tumor growth through direct contact with the tissues.

McDougall's Recommendation: To win your battle against cancer, avoid all chemical pollutants whenever possible by eating a diet low on the food chain, which is made up primarily of plant foods. Also, whenever possible, buy organically grown produce and drink only clean (unchlorinated) water.

Limit Iron Intake

Excess iron increases production of free radicals and appears to stimulate growth and proliferation of cancer cells. Research has shown that the rapid growth of cancer cells seems to require additional iron in the blood and tissues. A big source of iron, especially the type that is most readily absorbed by the body, is red meat. Conversely, many plant foods contain substances such as phytates that bind with iron and prevent it from producing free radicals.

McDougall's Recommendation: To win your battle against cancer, avoid excess iron and its harmful effects by eliminating all meat.

2. CONSUME FOODS AND NUTRIENTS THAT PROMOTE HEALTH

It isn't enough to eliminate the disease-causing parts of your diet; you must also consume nutrients and chemicals that boost your immune system and fight cancer.

It is no coincidence that animal foods and processed fare are also conspicuously lacking in the health-promoting substances. Fortunately, by the divine plan of mother nature, plant foods offer all the good things your body needs, while leaving out the bad.

Eat Foods Rich in Fiber

The fiber in plant foods binds with estrogens in the intestines and causes them to be eliminated through the feces. *The New England Journal of Medicine* reported that vegetarian women on high-fiber diets eliminate two to three times more estrogen in their feces than nonvegetarians. As I said earlier, one of the keys to protecting yourself against breast cancer is to keep your estrogen levels low, and one of the most powerful ways of doing that is by eating a high-fiber diet.

Fiber's ability to lower estrogen levels is truly amazing. One study showed that a group of postmenopausal women who adopted a high-fiber, low-fat diet experienced an average drop in their estrogen levels of 50 percent. Scientists have reported that a 17 percent reduction of estrogen can reduce the risk of breast cancer fourfold to fivefold.

McDougall's Recommendation: To win your battle against cancer, eat a fiber-rich plant-based diet. Remember, only plant foods contain fiber.

Eat an Abundance of Plant Foods to Get Adequate Amounts of Antioxidants

Two of the three most powerful known antioxidants, beta carotene and vitamin C, are only found in plants, and most of our vitamin E also comes from plants, such as whole grains. As I mentioned earlier, antioxidants remove free radicals and restore health to atoms, molecules, cells, and DNA. Antioxidants have also been shown to boost immune response and to help prevent all forms of the major degenerative diseases. A large population study of 6,500 Chinese done by Cornell researchers found that daily consumption of foods high in antioxidants was associated with lower rates of cancer.

It is important that we obtain these immune-boosting and cancer-fighting substances in their natural state, as plant foods, where they act in combination with other natural chemicals. When given in supplements of a single nutrient, antioxidants may cause unhealthy reactions. Pharmacological doses of beta carotene can result in competition with the other 50 naturally occurring dietary carotenoids, inhibiting their protective effect against cancer. Two recent studies have shown an increase in the risk of developing lung cancer when smokers were given supplemental beta carotene.

McDougall's Recommendation: To win your battle against cancer, consume antioxidants as part of a diet of vegetables, whole grains, beans, and fruits, while avoiding supplements of these important immune boosters and cancer fighters.

Eat an Abundance of Plant Foods to Get Adequate Amounts of Phytochemicals

Plants produce chemical compounds that have powerful anticancer effects. Among these are a group of chemicals collectively referred to as phytoestrogens (*phyto* means plant). These are weak estrogens that compete with the cancer-promoting estrogens in a woman's body for the estrogen receptor sites in the cells of her breasts, uterus, ovaries, and other tissues. By occupying these estrogen receptor sites, these safe phytoestrogens decrease hormone stimulation of tissues and thus inhibit the growth of cancer.

A plant-based diet results in a very large intake of phytoestrogens. In the average Japanese woman, these substances are found to be one hundred to one thousand times higher than the estrogens made by the woman's own body. More than fifteen phytoestrogens have so far been identified in human urine. They are found in edible plants and are divided into two main groups called isoflavonoids and lignans. Isoflavonoids are found mostly in unfermented soy products. The lignans are found in the dietary fiber of many plant foods, including whole grains, berries, fruits, and vegetables; they are especially high in flaxseed.

Scientists have admitted that we have only scratched the surface of such knowledge about the anticancer effects of plants. There is a huge army of unknown and still to be discovered phytochemicals in plants that protect us. Here is a summary of some of the ones we do know about.

Plant Foods That Fight Cancer

• Cruciferous vegetables (broccoli, cabbage, kale, Brussels sprouts, collard and mustard greens) contain numerous cancer-fighting compounds, including a substance called sulforanphane, which scientists have labeled a "major and very potent" trigger for detoxifying tissues and blood and for promoting production of cancer-preventive enzymes.

Cruciferous vegetables, especially watercress, also contain a substance known as phenethyl isothiocyanate (PEITC), which has been shown in animal studies to inhibit the creation of lung tumors after the animals have been injected with a powerful tobacco-specific carcinogen.

• Soybeans and soybean products. The April 1993 *Proceedings of the National Academy of Sciences* stated that soybeans and soybean products contain a substance called "genistein," which blocks blood vessels from growing to tumors. Like all other tissues, tumors require blood and oxygen to survive. By preventing blood vessels from attaching to these clusters of cancer cells, genistein literally suffocates and starves the tumor to death.

Scientists who have studied how blood vessels support the growth of cancerous tumors now believe that genistein may turn out to be an important adjunct in cancer therapy because it attacks the cancer cells without affecting normal cells.

• Beans. The American Health Foundation reported that beans contain high quantities of phytoestrogens, which may protect breast tissue and other organs from cancer-causing estrogens. It has been shown that Hispanic women who eat their traditional diet rich in grains and beans have lower rates of breast cancer than women who consume the standard American regimen.

• Shiitake mushrooms. Research at the U.S. National Cancer Institute and the Japanese National Cancer Institute have reported that shiitake mushrooms may boost immune response and promote the body's cancer-fighting mechanisms. Shiitake have also been shown to lower cholesterol.

McDougall's Recommendation: To win your battle against cancer, eat a diet based on starchy vegetables along with a wide variety of legumes; mushrooms; green, leafy, yellow, and orange vegetables; along with small amounts of fruits, all of which provide a rich supply of immune-boosting and cancer-fighting chemicals.

3. LOSE WEIGHT

Women who are overweight or obese have significantly higher rates of breast cancer than those who are lean. The likely reason is that overweight women produce far more estrogen than lean women. Being overweight is especially dangerous for young women. A thirty-year-old woman who is ten pounds overweight faces a 23 percent higher risk of developing breast cancer than a woman of normal weight, while a woman of the same age who is twenty pounds overweight faces a 52 percent higher risk of breast cancer than women the same age who are lean.

Because their ovaries have stopped producing estrogen, postmeno-pausal women who are obese derive the greatest amounts of estrogen from their fat cells. Moreover, the type of estrogen these fat cells pro-duce has been shown to increase the risk of breast cancer.

In order to reduce calories, you must drastically reduce fat. Fat is the most concentrated source of calories in the food supply. A gram of fat contains nine calories, while a gram of carbohydrate contains only four. Processed foods, including those made up of refined grains and sugar, have been stripped of their fiber and water and had their calories con-centrated, which means that the more processed foods you eat, the more calories you will consume. Also, processed foods often combine sugar, refined flour products, and fat, making the food all the more calorically dense.

Most animal studies show that a diet high in calories, independent of the amount of fat, promotes cancer growth.

McDougall's Recommendation: To win your battle against cancer, re-strict your diet exclusively to unprocessed whole grains, fresh vegetables, beans, and fruits. It's virtually impossible to eat too many calories from a diet based on whole grains and other starches, coupled with an abundant supply of green and yellow vegetables, and some fresh fruits. Such a diet will allow you to eat as much as you want, without being hungry. At the same time, you will achieve your optimal weight effortlessly.

4. EXERCISE

Regular exercise tends to lower estrogen and progesterone levels in-dependent of any weight loss that may result from exercise. With lower hormone levels comes a reduced risk of contracting breast cancer.

After studying twenty-five thousand women who exercised regularly—that is, at least four hours per week—scientists found that those who exercised had a 37 percent lower risk of contracting breast cancer than those women who were sedentary, according to a 1997 report pub-lished in *The New England Journal of Medicine*. The researchers found that reduction in risk was independent of the women's diets, body weights, or number of children they had borne. Animal research con-firms this finding. Animals made to exercise regularly have far lower rates of breast tumors than sedentary animals.

On the other hand, animals that are forced to exercise excessively have higher rates of breast cancer. The cancer-promoting effects of ex-cessive exercise were found to be directly related to the intensity of exercise being forced on the animals. Researchers speculated that one of the mechanisms for the promotion of cancer may be stress, which may increase the secretion of prolactin, a breast-stimulating hormone. Excessive amounts of exercise have been shown to suppress the immune system of humans as well.

McDougall's Recommendation: To win your battle against cancer, exercise daily as an enjoyable pastime. Do not overstress yourself. Rather, take brisk walks. If you are physically able, walk at least two miles per day.

5. Avoid Alcohol

Alcohol raises a woman's estrogen levels; it weakens the immune system's ability to repair damaged DNA; and it damages the liver's ability to detoxify cancer-causing substances in the blood. Research has shown that the consumption of just two drinks a day, regardless of the type of alcoholic beverage, increases your risk of breast cancer by 25 percent.

While it is true that some research indicates that alcohol may reduce the risk of heart disease, its tendency to raise your risk of breast cancer makes it a dangerous substance that should ideally be avoided or at least minimized.

McDougall's Recommendation: To win your battle against cancer, avoid all alcoholic beverages. When the pros and cons are weighed against each other, there are good reasons to see alcohol as a bad habit.

6. Stop Smoking

The more a woman smokes, the greater her risk of contracting breast cancer, according to a study conducted in Switzerland and reported in the May 5, 1996, issue of *American Journal of Epidemiology*. Women who smoke less than half a pack of cigarettes a day still experienced double the risk of contracting breast cancer as compared with nonsmokers. For those who smoke more than a pack a day, the risk was 4.6 times greater than for nonsmokers. Also, the younger a woman is when she starts smoking, the greater her risk of contracting cancer. Cancer-causing substances from cigarette smoke are found in breast fluids, where they may have a direct carcinogenic effect.

Passive smoke inhalation is also a very significant problem. Research has found a threefold increase in the risk of breast cancer among nonsmoking women who are regularly exposed to tobacco smoke at home or at work. To date, the effect of smoking has only been measured in postmenopausal women with breast cancer.

McDougall's Recommendation: To win your battle against cancer, do not smoke, and avoid secondary smoke whenever possible.

7. ELIMINATE MEDICATIONS

Among the chemicals considered to cause cancer, nearly one-half are medications. Women exposed to DES (diethylstilbestrol, once used in hopes of preventing miscarriages) have a 35 percent higher risk of breast cancer than those who were not exposed. Women who have used hormone replacement therapy for more than five years to prevent osteoporosis have a 50 percent higher risk of contracting breast cancer than those who never adopted HRT. Both therapeutic estrogen and synthetic progestins appear to promote cancer. Women who started taking the birth control pill before they were thirty-six, and used the pill for four years or more, have more than twice the breast cancer risk than those who never used the pill.

The good news is that there is no evidence of an increased risk ten years after cessation of the therapy. That means that the longer you are off the pill and disease free, the greater your chances of avoiding breast cancer entirely.

Immune-suppressing drugs, such as prednisone and azathioprine, along with cancer chemotherapy drugs (the alkylating agents), also cause breast cancer. Other commonly prescribed drugs, including blood pressure medication (such as the calcium channel blockers), increase breast cancer risk by as much as 65 percent. Cholesterol-lowering medications are suspected of increasing cancer risk as well. (See chapter 14 for more information about drugs used to treat heart disease.)

McDougall's Recommendation: To win your battle against cancer, reduce or eliminate all medications. Pharmaceutical drugs have adverse side effects. Breast cancer may be one of them.

8. AVOID RADIATION

The risk of contracting cancer increases in direct proportion to the amount of radiation dose one is exposed to. Radiation damages DNA, transforming healthy cells into cancerous ones. High-dose ionizing radiation exposure to the chest, such as that seen with strong X-ray examinations (fluoroscope for TB victims) and radiotherapy, is known to cause breast cancer. Even airline flying may present a danger to some women. A study of 1,577 female flight attendants who were followed for

13.9 years found an excess of breast cancer that may have been caused by the high exposure to solar radiation while flying at high altitudes.

Exposure to electromagnetic radiation from video monitors, electric blankets, and power lines has also been suspected of causing breast cancer. Women whose primary lifetime occupation exposed them to high levels of magnetic fields had a 43 percent increase in risk of breast cancer. An interesting theory as to how such radiation may harm the body is that radiation exposure during the day may reduce melatonin secretion at night. Melatonin, a hormone produced by the pituitary gland, has been shown to have anticancer effects. The reduction in melatonin may allow tumors to progress.

Still, the research examining the effects of magnetic fields is in its infancy and there is much controversy in this area. A recent study of 383,700 people in Finland found no association between electromagnetic radiation and breast cancer. Even so, it's best to be on the safe side, especially since there is enough evidence to warrant caution.

McDougall's Recommendation: To win your battle against cancer, avoid exposure to radiation. There is no safe threshold below which an increase in cancer risk does not occur.

9. BREAST-FEED YOUR BABIES

One of the benefits of a full-term pregnancy is a reduction in your risk of breast cancer. Added benefit is gained from breast-feeding. The possibility that breast-feeding might reduce the risk of breast cancer was raised seventy years ago, when the inability to lactate was commonly reported in women with breast cancer. Women with breast cancer show a history of low secretion of milk from the same breast, and women who breast-feed from only one breast have an increased risk of breast cancer in the unsuckled breast.

Breast-feeding also reduces the number of ovulations, which means that breast tissue is not exposed to as many estrogen and progesterone surges from the ovaries, thus reducing the number of times breast tissue has been stimulated and inflamed by estrogen. This also keeps the overall estrogen levels lower.

Breast-feeding may also reduce or eliminate carcinogens from the breast. Worldwide research has shown that in countries where breast-feeding is popular, people also consume a plant-based diet. Unfortunately, research has also shown that as people become more affluent, they tend to give up a healthier diet for themselves as well as their newborns.

McDougall's Recommendation: To win your battle against cancer, become pregnant and breast-feed.

10. CONTROL STRESS

Adverse life events seem to affect the development of breast cancer by possibly depressing the immune system through the production of adrenal hormones (glucocorticoids). A review of eighteen studies found that the suppression of strong emotions was a risk factor associated with the onset of breast cancer. A great deal of evidence has accumulated showing that stress can suppress your immune response and lead to a wide array of diseases. For some people, that may include cancer.

Research has shown that one of the best ways to handle stress is through regular exercise. Another way is to write down your thoughts and feelings in a journal or diary. At Southern Methodist University (SMU), professor of psychology James W. Pennebaker, Ph.D., found that writing about stressful and even traumatic events for twenty minutes a day, for four consecutive days, had a dramatic effect on the immune system. Immunologists Janice Kecolt-Glaser and Ronald Glaser measured the immune responses in study participants before and after they did their confessional writing and compared the results to a control group that did no such writing. The researchers found that the people who wrote in their journals about some emotionally stressful events had dramatically improved immune responses. Other research has shown that immune response is stronger in people who meditate or pray regularly.

On the other hand, studies looking at two of life's most traumatic events—divorce and widowhood—found no correlation between such stressful experiences and breast cancer.

McDougall's Recommendation: To win your battle against cancer, do your best to live a balanced life and engage in emotionally nurturing activities, including exercise, meditation, prayer, or journal writing. Such activities may have a salutary effect on your immune system, and in any case will contribute to the quality of your life.

The Role of Genetics and Aging

There is much talk these days about genes and the influence of aging on breast cancer rates, but these factors have been grossly overrated. Most people with breast cancer today do not have the BRCA-1 gene, yet they have the disease. Rather than having the breast cancer susceptibility gene, they had the breast cancer susceptibility diet and lifestyle. That is the far more likely danger facing women today—and one that they can control!

The strongest indicator of genetic susceptibility is contracting the disease early in life. The BRCA-1 is carried by one in three hundred women and is implicated in at most 5 percent of cancers in all age groups. However, approximately 25 percent of women who contract breast cancer before the age of forty have the BRCA-1 gene. Women carrying BRCA-1 have an 85 percent chance of developing breast cancer by the age of eighty; half of those cases will have occurred before age fifty. Testing for BRCA-1 is not readily available and is, unfortunately, expensive. Furthermore, doctors do not know if mammography, breast self-examination, and/or prophylactic bilateral mastectomy will reduce the chances of a woman carrying this gene from dying.

That said, we must acknowledge that breast cancer does run in families and the chances of contracting the disease increase with age. About 80 percent of cases occur in postmenopausal years. Also, women who have a first-degree relative (sister, mother, or daughter) with breast cancer have two to three times the normal risk of contracting the disease. However, many of the families who experience breast cancer in successive generations encounter the disease because toxic dietary and lifestyle patterns are often handed down from one generation to the next. If your mother or one of your sisters got breast cancer, the thing to do is to immediately change your way of life, starting with the adoption of the McDougall Program.

McDougall's Recommendation: *Ignore the things you cannot change and instead adopt a healthy diet and lifestyle today. That's all you can do. Most of the risk that is passed down through families lies in the dietary and lifestyle habits that we learn from our parents. You can change these.*

There will always be scientists and doctors who will tell you that we don't know enough yet to recommend changes in diet and lifestyle as a way of combating breast cancer and other serious diseases. Don't listen to them. Instead, remember your history. Thirty-five years ago, some scientists argued that lung cancer could not possibly be caused by cigarette smoking because no direct, proven mechanism could be found that related the two. Interestingly, some of these same scientists also argued that the association people were seeing between cigarette smoking and high rates of lung cancer was actually due to improved reporting. Today scientists are using the same arguments with breast cancer.

Take the advice of the old aphorism that says that if something looks like a gun, feels like a gun, and kills like a gun, it's probably a gun. You don't need a team of scientists to confirm what you already know.

The same is true for breast cancer and the many factors that "appear" to cause the disease. If it looks like a cause of illness, treat it like one. All of the details concerning the mechanisms of breast cancer do not have to be known before you take action. Adopt the McDougall Program and make these ten changes today. They could save your life, and the lives of those you love.

CHAPTER 7

Evaluating the Benefits of Mammography

Perhaps you are a woman in your forties who is concerned about breast cancer and wondering if you should have regular mammograms, as you are advised to do by the National Cancer Institute and the American Cancer Society. You want to act responsibly and if you were ever diagnosed with breast cancer you would hate to think that an early mammogram might have helped you. Reinforcing your own doubts and fears are the many images you are regularly exposed to by the media that show women of your own age having mammograms. This, of course, increases the pressure on you to fall into line and have the test done. But before you have the test, ask yourself a few basic questions: "Should I be getting a mammogram now, at my age?" "Will the test improve the quality of my life?" "Will it save my life?" "Is this the best breast cancer prevention?"

The answer to all four of these questions, unfortunately, is no, especially if you are under fifty or over sixty-nine years of age. In between these ages the benefits are far fewer than you now believe.

There is no better illustration of the public relations success achieved by the reigning cancer authorities than the image of so many thousands of women each year running to their doctors for mammograms. Unfortunately, that's what all of these images amount to: a public relations extravaganza. For the vast majority of these women, mammography is a waste of time, money, and the emotional distress associated with the test and its results. It may even be dangerous to your health.

When considering whether or not to have a mammogram, there are six essential points you need to know, all of which you will learn from this chapter:

1. Mammography is a blunt instrument, incapable of precise detection of the presence of cancer, especially for women in their forties, whose breast tissue tends to be more dense and therefore even more difficult to assess. In addition, there are a great many "false positives," especially for women in their forties, meaning that many of the women who are diagnosed by mammography as having cancer do not actually have the illness.

2. Most studies have found that having a mammogram in your forties will not extend your life if you get cancer, no matter when that cancer is detected. Women in their forties who avoid mammograms and who contract breast cancer live just as long as those who contract cancer but do have mammograms. As Dr. Barbara Rimer, director of cancer prevention and research at the Duke University School of Medicine, told the *New York Times*, routine mammography before the age of fifty does not save lives.

3. Though it will not save your life, a mammogram before you are fifty will dramatically increase your risk of undergoing needless tests and surgical procedures, even though the odds are that no cancer will be found.

4. As yet, there is no such thing as "early detection." Medical science has yet to develop the technology or diagnostic means for determining the presence of cancer at its early stages. By the time a malignant tumor is spotted by a mammogram, the cancer has already spread to other parts of the body in almost all cases. Instead of an increase in survival for many women, all early detection will mean is an increase in the time they will have to worry about dying from their disease.

5. Labeling someone as a cancer patient has severe individual and social consequences. People who have been diagnosed with cancer will find it difficult or impossible to get health or life insurance; many have difficulty getting jobs or are discriminated against by employers. Cancer patients suffer profound fears, as do their loved ones. And all of these problems arise after having a test that provides little or no survival benefit and does not improve the quality of one's life. Does the treatment of breast cancer detected by mammography prolong life, or does detection only increase the costs and prolong the burden of living with the disease?

6. The primary problem of cancer screening with mammographies is the waste of health care dollars and well-intentioned efforts by

caring health care providers. Our precious resources would be better spent teaching women how to prevent cancer by diet and lifestyle changes.

By reading this chapter, you will learn the relative advantages and disadvantages of this test, which I hope will lead you to make the right choice.

What Is Mammography?

Mammograms are X rays taken of the breast to determine the presence of cancer. Currently, many cancer authorities and some cancer organizations, such as the American Cancer Society and the National Cancer Institute, recommend that every woman over the age of forty undergo regular mammograms. Women older than fifty should have them annually, say the experts, while women under fifty should have the test at least once every two years.

Mammography came into general use as a screening test in the early 1960s and then dramatically increased during the 1980s when recorded cancer rates skyrocketed due to more diagnoses, not more cancer. Today, the great majority of women forty years of age and older undergo regular mammograms. According to the National Cancer Institute, 60 percent of women between the ages of forty and forty-nine had at least one mammogram during any two-year period in the 1990s. Sixty-five percent of women between the ages of fifty and sixty-four had at least one mammogram during that time, and 54 percent of women sixty-four years of age and older had mammograms during those years. These percentages indicate that many millions of women in all three age groups are having mammograms.

Women hold two basic and persuasive assumptions that encourage them to have the test. The first is that the test is an accurate assessment of the health of their breasts; the second is that it is likely to detect cancer early enough to save their lives. Unfortunately, neither of these assumptions is true.

The Accuracy of Mammography

Breast cancer is so emotionally charged, so fraught with fear, that when a woman is told that she may have the illness the psychological impact on her can be devastating—even when later she is informed that she doesn't have it. According to Dr. Barbara Rimer, women who have been told that they have breast cancer suffer for months with symptoms very much like those of posttraumatic stress syndrome, even when they later discovered that they did not have the disease. "It's not a benign experience," she said. The distress caused by a suspicious mammogram has been so overwhelming that women have been known to commit suicide.

If that's the case, there must be a lot of women walking around who are shell-shocked. Consider the facts. After undergoing a mammogram, about one woman in ten is told to come back for further analysis, usually because the mammogram has proved "inconclusive." About one in twenty is told that the test revealed an "abnormality," which requires more tests. These facts reflect the experience of women in all age groups, but younger women, those between forty and fifty years of age, are particularly at risk of having false positives, or suspicious-looking abnormalities.

Dr. Edward Sondik, the deputy director of the Division of Cancer Prevention and Control at the National Cancer Institute, told the *New York Times* that a suspicious lesion will eventually be found in about *half* of all women between forty and fifty who have annual mammograms—lesions that later are discovered not to be cancer. A recent study in the April 1998 issue of *The New England Journal of Medicine* found the risk of having a false positive test is over 56 percent for women having a mammogram every other year after the age of fifty (a total of ten mammograms). Furthermore, 26 percent of women report worry and anxiety three months after they have been told they don't really have breast cancer.

These are just the "abnormalities" and the "inconclusive" conditions within the breast that doctors find. In addition to these are the thousands of women who are informed that the findings of a mammogram suggest the possibility of cancer. Of these women who then undergo a biopsy, 80 percent are later told that they have no cancer at all. Unfortunately, they had to undergo surgery to discover that fact.

The point is that mammography is highly suspect, especially in women in their forties. Consequently, if you decide to have a mammogram, don't be surprised if you enter into a long and emotionally stressful period. The chances are very good that all that emotion will be for nothing.

Sadly, the inaccuracy of the test works in both directions. Researchers have found that mammograms miss as many as 44 percent of cancers in women in their forties, which means that nearly half of all women in their forties who do have cancer are told that they are healthy. One reason is that women in their forties typically have denser breast tissue, which makes it more difficult for a mammogram to read accurately. In women fifty and older who have cancer, between 10 and 15 percent are given clean bills of health by the mammograms. Both groups of women are usually diagnosed with cancer a year after these inaccurate mammograms are performed.

NONINVASIVE CANCER

Between the obvious inaccuracies lie the gray areas that present medicine with another set of challenges, particularly the condition known as *carcinoma in situ*, which is the presence of noninvasive cancer cells that do not spread in the vast majority of cases. Many doctors do not consider this condition "real" cancer because it is very unlikely to threaten a woman's life. The cells *look* like cancer, but in most cases do not behave like cancer; that is, they do not spread and result in sickness or death. Carcinoma in situ is far more common than many people realize. Forty percent of women in their forties who died of causes other than cancer and who later underwent autopsy and had their breasts removed were found to have these microscopic lesions in their milk ducts. Had those same women survived the accidents or the illnesses that killed them, the vast majority of them would not have developed breast cancer. Yet, because carcinoma in situ is so widespread, it quite naturally turns up sometimes on mammograms.

Researchers have found that between 10 and 17 percent of all cancers discovered on mammograms will be noninvasive carcinoma in situ. Even though this condition is unlikely to threaten a woman's life, the vast majority of these women will undergo mastectomy, radiation, and/ or even chemotherapy after being diagnosed by mammogram.

Before the general introduction of mammography, ductile carcinoma in situ of the breast accounted for less than 1 percent of breast cancers, which means that the rest of the women who had the condition were not treated; most of them lived their entire lives without ever realizing they had it. These days, this condition accounts for half or more of newly diagnosed breast cancers in women under fifty in the United States, and most cases were treated.

AVOIDING MASTECTOMY

In 1989, Sheila Anderson, then thirty-seven years old, of San Francisco, had a biopsy of her left breast after a physical examination and a mammogram detected a suspicious lump. Sheila's doctors diagnosed her as having intraductal carcinoma in situ, and a surgeon told her that the treatment of choice was mastectomy. Sheila questioned the diagnosis, which precipitated another examination, this one not unlike an inquisition.

"I had to go into this large conference room, where there were these thirty doctors all sitting around a long conference table," Sheila recalled recently. "There was a section of the room that was curtained off where I was examined again. After looking at my charts and going over my examination again, they told me that they concurred with the surgeon and the recommended treatment. I should have a mastectomy."

Sheila's medical group "was afraid of being sued, that was the reason they got me to have another examination in this room," she said. "They all seemed blasé about the whole thing. They just put the little breast tissue slide on the little screen and two or three looked at it and then reviewed my examination and then said, 'We concur with the diagnosis. You should have a mastectomy.' Then they all started to talk about where they were going for lunch, as if I wasn't even there.

"I was dying in the corner of the room, watching my whole life go forth in front of me," Sheila said. "It felt like I was in the midst of this assembly-line thing, with these doctors only half-interested in the process.

"It just didn't feel right to me, so I did a lot of research in the area and then I went to Dr. McDougall, who suggested that I consider not having the surgery. He also recommended that I see another physician at Seaton Medical Center, in Daly City, California, who was an expert in the treatment of cancer, including the treatment of carcinoma in situ. Dr. McDougall told me that this doctor at Seaton didn't like to operate on carcinoma in situ and that he could examine me and tell me whether I needed the mastectomy.

"Right away, I adopted the McDougall Program and became a complete vegan. Before that, I ate a lot of fatty foods, especially a lot of sweet fatty foods, like sweetened dairy products and pastries. I also ate a lot of animal protein—meat and chicken. But I eliminated all of that stuff and ate a strictly plant-based diet.

"I started to feel better on the McDougall diet pretty much right away. I decided I was not going to have the surgery. That was nine years ago. I have regular blood work done and I'm monitored by my doctors and I'm fine. I feel great. I'm forty-six years old and I never had the surgery."

Do Mammograms Save Lives?

Given all the encouragement women get to have mammograms performed, you would think that there is an enormous body of scientific evidence demonstrating that women who have the test done actually live longer than those who do not. That is, after all, the point to all this testing, isn't it? The assumption is that the test allows doctors to catch the cancer at an early stage, when it is more responsive to treatment, and by treating the cancer early you will be able to live longer. If you do not live longer by having a mammogram and undergoing treatment then what's the point of the test and the treatment?

Unfortunately, there is no great body of scientific evidence showing a survival benefit from mammograms. So far, there have been eight randomized studies examining the question of whether women who undergo mammograms live longer than those who do not. Of the seven experiments so far published, only two have shown a survival benefit, while the other five have shown no statistically significant survival benefit at all, even for women fifty years of age and older. (One study is still waiting publication, but preliminary results do not suggest overall benefit.)

The two studies that did show a benefit engendered great enthusiasm for mammography among doctors and other health professionals because it apparently showed about a 30 percent reduction in death rates among women who had mammography. However, when these two studies were analyzed carefully, scientists realized that mammograms would show a very small survival benefit only after many thousands of women had the test done.

For example, of the two studies showing a survival benefit, the most encouraging experiment is the one referred to as the Health Insurance Plan of New York, which found only one less death per year is achieved when a total of 7,086 women undergo a mammogram. In other words, you'd better be feeling really lucky if you expect to be that one woman in seven thousand who will derive a survival benefit from a mammogram. In any case, these numbers may represent a statistical truth, but they are not a practical one for most women. Even when we apply the only two studies to show a survival benefit, the odds are very small that your life will be extended because you had a mammogram. A 1997 review in the *Lancet* of the combined experiences of screening programs in Finland found that 200,000 women were screened to prevent twenty deaths from breast cancer. This benefit must be balanced against the anxiety, trauma, health care costs, and potential operative complications encountered by 28,000 women (14 percent) who had false positive tests.

The latest research on mammograms showed no benefit from the test. The Canadian National Breast Cancer Study found absolutely *no* survival benefit, regardless of the number of mammograms performed on women or the age of the woman screened. Here is a summary of the research and its conclusions.

Study	Location (Years)	Age at Entry	Significant Benefits?
Shapiro (HIP)	United States (1963–1969)	40–64	Yes—29% reduction in deaths
Anderson	Malmo, Sweden (1976–1986)	45–69	No
Tabar	Two County (1977–1983)	40–74	Yes—30% reduction in deaths
	Kopparberg, Sweden	40–74	Yes
	Ostergotland, Sweden	40–74	No
Bjurstam	Gothenburg, Sweden (1982–Present)	40–59	No (unpublished)
	Women under 50 (1983–1994)	39–49	Yes—45% reduction in deaths
UK	United Kingdom (1977–1981)	45–64	No
Roberts	Edinburgh (1979–1988)	45–64	No
Rutqvist	Stockholm (1981–1985)	40–64	No
Miller	Canada (1980–1987)		
	NBSS1 Women Under 50	40–49	No—36% increase in deaths
	NBSS2	50–59	No

Significant reductions for women over the age of 50 were only found in the HIP and the Swedish Two County Studies.

After reviewing and weighing all the evidence on mammography, two eminent scientists concluded that the benefits from mammography are so small that health agencies should no longer encourage them, and public funding for mammograms should be stopped. Publishing their conclusions in the British medical journal *Lancet* (July 1, 1995), Dr. Charles Wright, clinical professor at the Department of Health Care and Epidemiology at the University of British Columbia, and Dr. C. Barber Mueller, one of the world's most famous breast cancer surgeons, concluded: "Since the benefit achieved is marginal, the harm caused is substantial, and the costs incurred are enormous, we suggest that public funding for breast cancer screening in any age group is not justifiable."

It's also very important to note that *only one study on its original analysis has shown a significant survival benefit for women under the age of fifty.*

Writing in a 1989 edition of the *British Medical Journal*, M. Maureen

Roberts, clinical director of the Edinburgh Breast Cancer Screening Project since 1979, stated, "We can no longer ignore the possibility that screening may not reduce the mortality in women of any age, however disappointing this may be. . . . I believe that a rethink is required before the programme goes much further. I feel sad to be writing this; sad because naturally after so many years I am sorry that breast cancer screening may not be beneficial. I am also sad to seem to be critical of the many dear and valued colleagues I've worked with over the years, particularly those who have made such a magnificent contribution to the care and welfare of women with breast cancer. But they will recognize that I am telling the truth." Ms. Roberts's article was published posthumously after her death from breast cancer.

EVALUATING THE RISKS FOR YOUNGER WOMEN

Most countries throughout the world do not recommend mammograms for women under fifty. The United States, Australia, Iceland, and the Canadian province of British Columbia are the exceptions. Among the reasons most of the world does not encourage the tests for women under fifty is because mammograms simply yield too many errors and too few benefits for the cost.

On the other hand, there are a plethora of good reasons why women in this age group should stay away from them. Among the most important is that women in their forties who undergo mammograms are subject to more tests and treatment, much of it unwarranted and sometimes even dangerous.

For every single cancer discovered in their respective age groups, women in their forties will have 2.5 times more biopsies than women over fifty, and three times more surgical procedures. Thus, women in their forties undergo a lot more procedures than women older than fifty, yet they have far fewer cancers.

Ironically, doctors already know that women in their forties are at a far lower risk of having cancer than women in their fifties, because only about 20 percent of all cancers occur in the younger group. A thorough review of the research by the National Institutes of Health Consensus Development Conference held on January 21–23, 1997, produced a *Statement: Breast Cancer Screening for Women Ages 40–49*. "The Panel concludes that the data currently available do not warrant a universal recommendation for mammography for all women in their forties." The report went on to say, "About 2,500 women would have to be screened regularly in order to extend one life. For those women whose survival is extended, the length of life extension is not known."

SHOULD WOMEN IN THEIR FORTIES HAVE MAMMOGRAMS?

Recommend Routine Screening	Do Not Recommend Routine Screening
American College of Radiology	U.S. Preventive Services Task Force
American College of	American College of Physicians
Obstetricians and Gynecology	American Academy of Family Practice
American Cancer Society	Canadian Task Force on Periodic
American Medical Association	Health Examination
National Cancer Institute	National Institutes of Health

The Dangers of Unnecessary Treatment

In February 1993, an international workshop on mammograms found that for every one thousand women under fifty who had mammograms, no fewer than seven hundred would require further testing. Of those seven hundred, only fifteen tumors would be found. Remarkably, despite all of this overtesting, seven cancers would be *missed*.

Overall, nine out of every ten biopsies done on women in their forties find no cancer. That statistic alone should tell you how imprecise mammograms are at finding cancer in women in their forties. Among the cancers that are found, many are actually carcinoma in situ. In one study, ductile carcinoma in situ accounted for 63 percent of cancers diagnosed in women under fifty. Unfortunately, a great many women will get the full treatment after their carcinoma in situ is discovered, meaning they will undergo mastectomy, radiation, and chemotherapy.

All those mammograms, extra biopsies, and surgical procedures come with a price. One recent study referred to as the Canadian trial showed that women younger than fifty who underwent mammograms have a 36 percent higher risk of dying from breast cancer than those who do not undergo a mammogram. The risk of dying increased for women who had mammography because of the treatments that followed.

According to an editorial in a 1991 issue of the *Lancet*, "one explanation may be the type of treatment offered to women with mammographically detected breast cancers—usually a combination of surgery and radiotherapy." Treatment sometimes kills—and if there is little or no survival benefit to offset these deaths, then the overall risk of dying is increased. There is also the small possibility that the radiation from the mammogram will cause breast cancer. This may be particularly dangerous to younger women, whose breast tissue is more sensitive to radiation than that of older women.

An editorial in the 1994 issue of the *Journal of the American Medical Association* contradicted the publication's long-held position on mammography in younger women: "But wistful wishing cannot alter the fact that mammographic screening in women under the age of 50 does not reduce deaths, while for those over the age of 50 years it saves lives. The reasons for these results are unknown and need to be resolved."

The Dangers of Breast Compression and Radiation

It may seem trivial to some people, but I want to point out that during a mammogram, the breast is compressed by the X-ray machine in order to provide a better X-ray picture. That compression causes a certain amount of discomfort to women. Overall, 81 percent of women experience discomfort during mammography as a result of the manipulation and squeezing of their breasts. As many as 46 percent of women classify that discomfort as pain, and 7 percent say the pain is severe.

Pain may not be the only consequence of all that manipulation and squeezing. There is also the real possibility that compression of the breast during the test may cause the cancer cells to spread. Animal research has shown that the degree to which a cancer spreads can be increased by as much as 80 percent merely by mechanical manipulation of the tumor.

In one study, women under fifty-five who underwent mammograms experienced a 29 percent increase in the number of deaths from breast cancer during the first seven years of the research. During that period, the mammographers used "as much compression as the woman could tolerate." This may be especially important for younger women with more vascular breasts. Under compression the cells from carcinoma in situ may be spread within the interconnecting ductal system. This mechanical compression may be one reason for the high number of cancers found between mammograms in younger women.

The pain a woman experiences during mammography is a warning signal ignored by those recommending and performing the tests. By comparison, no physician would recommend compression of a bacterial abscess, for fear of spreading the disease, and pain is a warning sign, too.

Most women needlessly worry about the radiation from a mammogram. In fact, there is extremely little risk. Approximately one cancer in every 200,000 mammograms is produced by the radiation used in tests with modern equipment. Congress has passed the Mammography Quality Standards Act of 1992 in response to reports that half the facilities and technicians failed to meet minimal quality-assurance standards.

No Benefits for Elderly Women

A woman's risk of dying from breast cancer increases with age. Yet, there is no evidence to support the use of mammography in women older than sixty-nine years. Women older than sixty-nine should avoid mammograms simply because a cancer detected by mammography at that age can take ten to twenty years before it becomes lethal. Competing causes of death, such as a heart attack or stroke, would likely take her life long before breast cancer would.

Health authorities around the world have either openly or tacitly acknowledged this fact. Despite the fact that the American Cancer Society urges all women older than forty to have regular mammograms, the U.S. Preventive Services Task Force stated: "Mammography every one or two years is recommended for all women beginning at the age of 50 and concluding at approximately the age of 75 unless pathology is detected."

In 1987, the United Kingdom recommended a policy of single-view mammography performed every three years in all women between fifty to sixty-four years of age. In 1988, Canada urged that mammography be performed every two years in women between the ages of fifty and sixty-nine. Similar policies are in effect in Sweden, Finland, the Netherlands, and Australia.

The Myth of Early Detection

The whole intellectual and ethical argument for mammography rests on the singular belief that the test can discover cancer in its early stages, before it has spread to other parts of the body. If mammograms can catch the cancer early enough, the cancer can be contained within the breast and treated locally, thus saving the woman's life, or so the argument goes. This is the essential rationale behind mammography.

Unfortunately, the argument is groundless. Many laypeople, and a very few physicians, believe that breast cancer goes through a series of steps in which it remains within the breast for some time period until it migrates to the lymph nodes and then to the rest of the body. In the minds of these people, the process looks something like this:

Step 1. A cancer manifests and starts to grow slowly in the tissue (in this case, the breast).
Step 2. With time, the cancer grows into a larger tumor.
Step 3. Eventually, the cancer spreads to the lymph nodes.

Step 4. Finally, the cancer spreads from the lymph nodes to the rest of the body.

Unfortunately, this step-by-step progression from a harmless mass to a body full of disease almost never occurs. Rather, cancer spreads to other parts of the body via the blood in the very early stages of development. The spread of cancer to the lymph nodes actually occurs simultaneously with the spread of the cancer to the other parts of the body, or even after the cancer has spread beyond the breast.

So let's throw out the belief of this rather regimented step-by-step growth pattern and understand a little more clearly how breast cancer goes from being a single cell to a lethal disease.

Like other cancers, breast cancer begins with the mutation of a single healthy cell into a malignant one. Once this transformation occurs, the single cell begins to replicate, or divide without regard to the body as a whole. Normal, healthy cells multiply only when necessary, such as during growth of tissue or repair after an injury. Cancer cells not only go on multiplying, but will do so until they transform a major organ into a nonfunctioning cancerous mass and thereby kill the patient.

The time it takes one cell to divide and become two cells is called the *doubling time.* The average doubling time for breast cancer cells (as well as for most other solid tumors) is approximately one hundred days. This means that in one hundred days, a single cancer cell will have become two cancer cells. In two hundred days, that one cell will now have become four cells in a single breast that consists of about one hundred billion healthy cells.

After one year, that breast tumor now contains twelve malignant cells. At this doubling rate, it takes about six years for the single cancer cell to become one million malignant cells, which together form a tumor that is about the size of the tip of a lead pencil. A mass of this size is less than one millimeter in diameter, and is undetectable by self-examination of the breast, or by mammography.

Even though the cancer is so tiny that it cannot be seen on a mammogram, it nevertheless has already spread, or metastasized, to other parts of the body in virtually every case of true cancer (as opposed to carcinoma in situ). It is the cancer cells that have spread to the liver, lungs, bones, or brain that kill the patient, *not* the cancer cells confined to the breast.

After about ten years of growth, the average cancerous mass inside the breast is about one centimeter in diameter, or about the size of an eraser on the end of a pencil, and consists of about one billion cells. This is the earliest stage at which most tumors are discovered.

Tumors discovered by mammograms have a much slower doubling time, often over two hundred days. This means it would take on the average sixteen years for a tumor to grow from one cell to a mass of one centimeter. The very best a mammogram can do is detect a tumor mass about 2 mm in size, which means the cancer has been growing, on the average, twelve years.

After reviewing the research on mammograms and taking into account the way cancer grows, Dr. Charles Wright and Dr. C. Barber Mueller concluded in their 1995 *Lancet* review that mammography offers little hope for helping women. "About 40 doublings of breast cancer cells create a lethal tumor burden, yet mammography cannot detect a mass until 25–30 doublings have already occurred." By this time, most breast cancers have already spread to other parts of the body, which is where they will present the real threat to life.

Establishing the fact that there is a cancer present and that it has grown to a certain point may very well be helpful in some respects, but it is in no way "early detection," and should not be advertised as such. When Drs. Wright and Mueller evaluated mammography's role as an early detection device, they concluded, "We are not going to win the race by backing a loser."

To put things very simply, mammography does not find the cancer early enough.

As Dr. M. Maureen Roberts wrote in the *British Medical Journal:* "We all know that mammography is an unsuitable screening test; it is technologically difficult to perform, the pictures are difficult to interpret, it has a high false positive rate, and we don't know how often to carry it out."

The medical establishment's promotion of mammography as an early detection device puts women in an extremely difficult position. Either you go along with the cancer authorities and have a mammogram, hoping against hope that the test reveals no abnormalities, no suspicious lesions, no carcinoma in situ, and no full-blown cancer. As I have demonstrated, the chances of such a thing happening are not great, especially if you are a woman in your forties.

Or, you can choose not to have the test. But in our society, if you do not have the test and have not sufficiently educated yourself on the actual value of mammograms, you will likely face a variety of difficult emotions, especially fear and guilt. There is already a great deal of fear surrounding breast cancer. But there is also significant guilt, not only around the disease but also around the issue of whether or not to have a mammogram.

The fact is that the cancer authorities have made women feel guilty for not having mammograms, which in my view is entirely unfounded and undeserved. That guilt is especially severe for the woman who has never had a mammogram but then contracts breast cancer. Her guilt flows from the erroneous belief, fostered by our medical establishment, that regular mammograms would have saved her life.

In the absence of a true breast cancer prevention program promoted by the medical establishment, mammography has subtly and insidiously moved in to fill that void. People have come to think of mammograms as a form of cancer prevention. This is partly why women who have mammograms believe they are doing "everything possible" to prevent the disease, and therefore are acting responsibly. The truth is, they are doing nothing of the sort. A woman who gets a mammogram is not doing anything more to prevent cancer than the cigarette smoker is who gets regular chest X rays.

Mammography Is Big Business

In one way or another, everything in life has some connection with money, and medicine is no different. I get concerned when financial interests shape our presentation or perception of the truth. Mammography has a role to play in the diagnosis of cancer. I fear that this role is being inflated, and the facts surrounding the practice distorted, simply because mammography is a big moneymaker. Others share my concern.

Since 1992, 74 percent of U.S. women have had at least one mammogram and 41 percent follow the American Cancer Society's guidelines for regular mammograms. The cost of mammography varies widely, from $25 to $200.

If the average cost of a mammogram is $100 and the guidelines from major organizations are followed, the annual price tag associated with mammography would be approximately $5 billion. Add to this the cost of repeat mammograms and the related biopsies and those numbers rise to more than $15 billion annually. This much money becomes its own motivating force. As Drs. Wright and Mueller noted, "Public imagination has been captured by mammography, and all those involved in the screening industry have a major vested interest."

In the April 17, 1997, issue of *The New England Journal of Medicine,*

Suzanne Fletcher, M.D., of the Harvard Medical School, wrote: "In many cases, there are powerful financial interests involved—for example, large contingency fees for trial lawyers in the case of silicone breast implants and billions of dollars in equipment and professional incomes in the case of mammography screening. Increasingly, medical organizations themselves have engaged in lobbying to further their political and financial agendas. All these interests influence the approach to scientific reports. . . . When medical scientists disagree about the effectiveness of an intervention, it almost always means that whatever effect may be present is small."

Because mammography is a big business, it enjoys widespread media exposure: posters and brochures, articles in newspapers and magazines, and radio and television advertisements in English and Spanish that urge women to have a mammogram "once a year for the rest of your life." When updated mammography equipment was installed at my hospital, St. Helena Hospital in the Napa Valley, "educational" material was sent to all the medical doctors on staff informing them of the importance of this test for their patients. No informational material has ever been sent to me about the disappointments and potential harm that this test can bring for women.

Benefits of Mammograms

Despite its drawbacks, mammography does offer some benefit if it is used honestly and patients understand its limitations. Women must clearly be informed of all the possible harm that may result from these tests, including the technical limitations of the test, the errors in judgment and interpretation that can occur, and the needless procedures that can result from mammograms. They should also be told that there is no worthwhile survival benefit for women under fifty and older than sixty-nine, and consequently both age groups should avoid routine testing. However, for women in the middle age group, there may be a small survival benefit.

Two potential benefits result from finding tumors relatively early. The first is that even though the cancer has likely spread beyond the original site of the breast, mammograms can detect the breast tumor when it is still relatively small and subject to a more cosmetically acceptable surgery. Lumpectomy is the only scientifically supported initial treatment for most women. If the breast tumor is found early enough, the tumor size will be small enough to make that decision easier for a woman. Small tumors are more easily removed without deforming the breast.

The second benefit from having a mammogram is that once a cancer has been diagnosed, the patient has more power to assist in her own recovery than she may currently know. This is important, because it is my strong belief that a change in diet will cause women to live a longer, more healthful life.

McDougall's Recommendations

I recommend that if you're under fifty or older than sixty-nine routine screening should be avoided. If you're in the middle age group, remember that the benefits of this test remain controversial and are far fewer than advertised. In addition, there are many hazards that are not fully revealed to women who undergo this test.

I cannot enthusiastically support mammography until:

1. Studies show consistent benefits.
2. All age groups of women show benefits.
3. Women are fully informed of the related hazards of mammograms, and reasonable explanations for inconsistent benefits between studies and age groups are provided.
4. The tests can detect the majority of cancers when they are still curable.
5. Effective treatments for breast cancer are developed.
6. Efforts in early detection and treatment show a decrease in the death rate per one hundred thousand population from breast cancer; the current death rate from breast cancer is essentially the same as it was fifty years ago.

Mammography Does Not Prevent Breast Cancer

Whether or not you choose to have a mammogram, you should realize that mammograms do not prevent breast cancer—diet and lifestyle do. The relevance of these dietary benefits can even be seen on mammograms. Women consuming diets high in all kinds of fat, including monounsaturated (olive oil) and polyunsaturated vegetable fat, have shown patterns on mammograms that are more suggestive of cancer than women on low-fat diets. Not surprisingly, the benefits of a healthy, low-fat diet can be seen in a short time with the improvement of the appearance of the breast tissue on a mammogram. These changes seen on the X ray indicate there will be less chance of cancer being found in the future. A healthy diet and lifestyle are the only true forms of breast cancer prevention.

Once our society honestly acknowledges this fact, we will naturally start to divert our resources toward teaching women the benefits of a healthy diet and lifestyle, which would reduce not only their risk of breast cancer but also their risks of most other common diseases.

When our national cancer authorities put their enormous resources behind health promotion and disease prevention, the results will transform our world, and every individual life. We will see dramatic reductions in heart attacks, diabetes, obesity, rheumatoid arthritis, multiple sclerosis, and most forms of cancer, to name just a few diet-induced diseases. Unfortunately, officials who create national policy lack the foresight to recognize the kind of financial savings and economic opportunities associated with prevention.

Until they develop such a vision, the job of taking care of our health and preventing these diseases falls to each of us. The practice of pre-

---

Benefits of Mammography

- Possible improved survival for cases detected in women ages fifty to sixty-nine
- Less radical treatment for smaller tumors
- Reassurance with negative results
- Strong incentive for change in diet and lifestyle

Disadvantages of Mammography

- Increase in cancer deaths for young women
- Increased suffering with awareness of disease
- Anxiety and distress for falsely diagnosed women
- Unnecessary treatment for falsely diagnosed women
- More treatments for a longer time
- Overdiagnosis of questionable tissues
- Overtreatment for questionable tumors
- Increase in testing and treatment for all
- False reassurance for women whose cancer is not detected
- Physical discomfort
- Cost to country and individual

vention is nontoxic, cost-free, self-administered, and ecologically sound. It can save you from some of the most terrifying diseases known to humankind, including breast cancer. In the meantime, the practice of health promotion and disease prevention, as described by the McDougall Program, will dramatically improve the quality and, quite possibly, the length of your life.

CHAPTER 8

Treating Breast Cancer with Surgery, Radiation, Chemotherapy, and Drugs

No words can adequately express the shock, confusion, and feelings of loss and betrayal that accompany a diagnosis of breast cancer. Though loved ones may rally around you and express their unconditional support, some part of you may feel terribly alone and overwhelmed by fear. That fear and the desperation that comes with it may temporarily distort your judgment and give rise to the belief that everything from this moment onward will happen quickly, or must happen quickly. In your haste to find stability, you may lunge at medical treatments that you hope will miraculously return your life to normal. Read these words carefully: *Do not make any quick medical decisions.* Rather, allow yourself enough time so that your shock can heal and your clarity and stability can return. Only then can you make appropriate decisions.

The first thing you must understand is that the diagnosis is not the end. The fact is that you will go on living. Even if the diagnosis is accurate, there is time. For many women, there is a lot of time. Ten to twenty years of survival is common; some will live even longer. Right now, you may feel as if you are free-falling, but as hard as it may be to believe, life's routines, responsibilities, and mundane demands will reassert themselves. You will find stability in daily life once again.

However, you will never be quite the same, nor should you be. You will have to make crucial decisions, including the kinds of treatments you embrace and reject, how you can best take care of yourself, the ways in which you will spend your time, and how best to enhance your life.

In this chapter, I want to help you to navigate the medical maze that you face and guide you as you make your medical decisions. In the next chapter, I will show you how you can promote your own health and your body's cancer-fighting defenses. There is a great deal you can do to treat your disease; indeed, there is a great deal you *must* do if you want to embrace your chances of living a long life.

But before you can do that, there are numerous decisions you must make regarding your medical treatment, and all of them can be crucial in determining your health, the quality of your life, and longevity.

Essentially, there are two forms of treatment that you must use to adequately treat breast cancer. The first is medical treatment, of which there are several types, including surgery, radiation, chemotherapy, and drug treatment. You will have to make decisions about every form of treatment available to you.

The second involves all the ways you can promote your overall health, immune system, and cancer-fighting defenses. Within this realm, the most powerful tool you have available to you are the foods you eat each day. I will show you how specific foods can help promote your health and fight cancer. No matter whether you perceive yourself as a former junk food junkie, or think of yourself as having been on a "good" diet, the best single tool you can use to improve your health is to adopt the McDougall Program, which can have a dramatic effect on your health, no matter what your former diet was like. Once your new diet is in place, you will want to supplement it with appropriate social support. The third tool you may want to consider is the promotion of a positive relationship between your mind and body.

I'm going to deal first with the medical decisions you will have to make. Let's begin at the very beginning.

Finding a Lump

Women find more than 90 percent of breast lumps themselves. Don't panic! Fortunately, only 20 percent of these suspicious masses ever turn out to be cancer. A lump in the breast is more likely to be cancerous if it is hard, painless, has irregular borders, and is fixed (that is, attached to the skin or underlying muscle tissue). Soft, smooth, easily movable lumps are usually not cancer. Also, noncancerous masses are often painful to the touch.

The only way to determine if this mass is cancerous is to have a biopsy, a procedure by which a small sample of the tissue from the mass is removed. That sample is then examined under a microscope to determine whether or not it is malignant. The needle biopsy, the most common kind of biopsy done, leaves almost no scar.

No doubt, you and your physician will discuss whether or not a mammogram is appropriate under the circumstances. Remember, a mammogram cannot diagnose cancer; all it can do is identify dense masses of tissue in the breast that doctors must then interpret. If your doctor is encouraging a mammogram, ask him or her why such a test is necessary, especially since it will not be definitive.

If there is a high level of suspicion that the mass is cancer, you may want to forgo the needle biopsy and go directly to an excisional biopsy, an operation that will remove the entire lump, which will then be examined by a pathologist to determine if it is cancer. If you have such a surgery, ask the surgeon to be careful to get all of the tumor and to leave a margin of healthy tissue around the specimen to be sent to the pathologist. If the margins are free of cancer this may be all the treatment you need.

IF THE LUMP IS CANCEROUS

If a pathologist determines that, in fact, the lump is cancerous, do not make any rash decisions. In fact, you do not have to decide what to do today, next week, or even next month. Right now, you need to do two things: first, gather information and, second, digest that information and decide what course of action you want to take. You have time to do both. The cancerous tumor that is present in your breast has been growing on the average for ten years before it was discovered. How could taking the time to gather information and consider your options be harmful?

The first bit of information that you will want is a second opinion on the biopsied lump. The pathologist's decision, which is based on a small bit of tissue taken from your breast, will change your life forever. Don't you think that decision deserves to be reviewed by another authoritative source? Have the tissues reviewed by an independent laboratory.

If both the first and second opinions concur that the biopsy is positive for cancer, then, in most cases, no further tests on you are needed to determine the extent of the disease. Routine laboratory, bone scans, liver scans, and chest X rays are *no longer recommended*, because the detection rate of metastatic cells is extremely low, and any abnormalities found by these tests usually turn out to be "false positives," or diagnoses of cancer that later prove to be incorrect. The problem with false positives is that they trigger an array of unnecessary tests that are costly, invasive, and sometimes dangerous. Tests on the actual tumor to determine characteristics, such as whether or not it is estrogen positive, will also be done.

What you will have to do if both the first and second opinion turn out positive is to decide on a course of therapy. Let's review the options.

WHAT IS DCIS?

Because mammography has become so widespread today, the incidence of a kind of "cancer" referred to as ductal carcinoma in situ (or DCIS) has risen dramatically. The problem with DCIS is all the unknowns associated with the disease. The cells that make up the illness look like cancer, but in the vast majority of cases they remain confined to the milk ducts of the breast and do not break out into the bloodstream to form metastatic disease elsewhere in the body. It is the metastases to the liver, bone, brain, and other parts of the body that kill, not the illness confined in the breast.

Yet, how rapidly and how often DCIS progresses to invasive and life-threatening cancer is still a mystery. No one can say with certainty whether this condition will progress to that life-threatening stage or remain dormant and relatively harmless. What we can say is that the odds favor that the illness will remain DCIS and not become full-blown cancer. Unfortunately, medicine has long taken a kind of male-oriented approach to all forms of uncertainty and mystery. Faced with the unknown, modern medicine has adopted a strategy that might best be characterized as "lock and load": it directs its full armamentarium against a disease that, for all intents and purposes, it doesn't really understand. Thus, into the breach of uncertainty doctors rush with their scalpels and their radiation and their chemotherapy.

This attitude appears to be changing, however, as more and more surgeons refuse to operate on DCIS and instead take a more gentle, wait-and-see approach. In 1983, 71 percent of DCIS cases were treated with mastectomy. With the current trend toward breast-conserving surgeries, only 44 percent of all DCIS cases in the United States are treated by radical surgery today; however, thousands of women still undergo unnecessary mastectomies to remove small breast "cancers" that may not spread or threaten their lives. Recent research shows DCIS can be effectively treated with wide excision of the area, leaving clear margins, and that radiotherapy adds no benefit. The study of 694 women with DCIS showed a mortality of 1 percent with mastectomy, 3 percent with excision plus radiation, and 1 percent with excision alone.

McDougall's Recommendation: If you are diagnosed with DCIS, the only surgery you should consider is a biopsy to remove the suspect tissue. Aggressive surgery (mastectomy), radiation, or chemotherapy is not necessary. In addition, you should adopt the McDougall Program, which in turn will boost all your cancer-fighting mechanisms and support your body's efforts to overcome the disease.

If the illness is not DCIS, you will have to consider other forms of treatment, including surgery.

Treating Breast Cancer with Surgery

Breast cancer is one of the first kinds of cancers to be treated by surgical intervention. Initially, the kind of surgery used was radical mastectomy, or the surgical removal of the breast, underlying chest muscles, and lymph nodes. Over the past century, a number of new approaches have been devised to remove the tumor.

Here is a summary of the kinds of surgical procedures that have been in use.

- Biopsy: the removal of a small piece of the suspected tumor for laboratory analysis
- Lumpectomy: the removal of the entire tumor only, and not the adjoining tissues
- Partial or segmental mastectomy: the removal of a large section of the breast with tumor and surrounding tissues
- Simple mastectomy: the removal of the entire breast
- Modified radical mastectomy: the removal of the entire breast as well as the adjacent lymph nodes in the armpit (axilla)
- Radical mastectomy: the removal of the entire breast, the lymph nodes in the axilla, and the underlying chest muscles
- Extended radical mastectomy: the removal of the entire breast, the lymph nodes in the axilla, the underlying chest muscles, and the lymph nodes next to the breast bone (sternum)

RADICAL SURGERY

Radical mastectomy was introduced by Dr. William Halsted of Johns Hopkins University Medical School at the end of the nineteenth century. From that moment on, the operation rapidly became the leading form of breast cancer treatment for much of the twentieth century.

In the state of Hawaii, during the years 1960 and 1961, 78 percent of women with breast cancer were given radical mastectomies. This extreme form of surgery was altered somewhat, as surgeons began choosing the "modified radical mastectomy," which removed the breast and the lymph nodes in the armpit. With the introduction of the modified radical mastectomy, the treatment patterns changed. In 1977, when I was in the early years of my own medical practice, only 27 percent were given radical mastectomies and 65 percent underwent modified radical mastectomies. Still, greater than 90 percent of women with breast cancer were losing their breasts and their lymph nodes, and a significant number had their chest muscles removed as well.

The radical mastectomy, in fact, has been the gold standard by which all other procedures are compared. Ironically, *to date no survival advantage of one surgical approach over another has been found.* The evidence has been accumulating for decades that neither the radical nor the modified forms of mastectomy offer any better survival benefit than that of the lumpectomy. And doctors have known this to be true since 1959. (The underlying reason for this lack of survival benefit was discussed in chapter 7: by the time of diagnosis the cancer has been growing for an average of ten years. By this time, if it is truly cancer, it has already spread beyond the confines of the breast.)

To help you make a fully informed decision, and to do all I can to improve your chances of survival, I must tell you that despite improved surgical techniques, advanced methods of radiotherapy, and the widespread use of chemotherapy, the death rate from breast cancer has not changed meaningfully during the last fifty years. That raises an important question: Why add mutilation and further misery to the problems you may already face if you have been diagnosed with breast cancer? It also lays bare just how essential it is for you to do all you can to improve your chances of overcoming the illness.

McDougall's Recommendation: What is the scientifically supported decision when it comes to breast cancer surgery? In my opinion, a lumpectomy with clear margins is the only surgical treatment scientifically justifiable for most women as initial therapy.

It is important that when the lumpectomy is done that the tissue margins around the tumor are free of cancer. Achieving clear (or negative) surgical margins appears to be the single most reliable indicator as to whether or not you will have a recurrence of cancer within your breast sometime in the future. If the initial surgery left behind cancerous tissue margins, then a re-excision should be done. If this second operation successfully eliminates such cancerous tissue, then the risk of local recurrence will be almost the same as if the surgery had been successful the first time.

TIMING YOUR SURGERY TO MAXIMUM ADVANTAGE

Research has found that timing your surgery according to your hormonal cycles may extend your life. If you are a premenopausal woman, you should schedule your surgery during the second half of your menstrual cycle, known as the luteal phase (starting about fourteen days after the first day of bleeding of the menstrual period). No one fully understands why timing the operation in this way is associated with an increased length of survival, but there are theories.

According to one theory, during the first part of the menstrual cycle, when estrogen levels are rising and thus supporting the illness, many more cancer cells may spread during surgery to new tissues. At the same time, there may be a decrease in natural cancer killer cell activity, also due to higher levels of unopposed estrogen. Natural killer cells are among the immune system's most important cancer-fighting forces. Thus, the first part of the menstrual cycle, known as the follicular phase, may support the aggressiveness of the cancer, while it decreases the strength of the immune system. Having an operation during this period will stress your immune system even more, and thus weaken the body's efforts at fighting the disease.

In any case, the facts support the choice of scheduling your surgery accordingly. If you are a premenopausal woman with positive lymph nodes—in other words, you have cancer that has spread beyond your breast to your lymph nodes—the chances of your being alive and free of obvious disease five years after the surgery are 75.5 percent if you are operated on during the luteal phase, compared with 63.3 percent of women who are operated on during the follicular phase.

Hence, selecting the right time of the month for any kind of breast surgery, from a needle biopsy to a radical mastectomy, is important for premenopausal women. Waiting a few days will not make any difference in your condition, and it could extend your life.

Reducing the Risk of Recurrence

Once you are diagnosed with cancer, you must approach your treatment decisions with a clear understanding that you are dealing with two separate goals:

1. To control the disease locally, which is to say, within the breast.
2. To control the systemic disease, meaning the cells that have spread throughout the body, or metastasized. It is the systemic disease, with

its microscopic nests of cancer cells that lodge in the liver, bones, lungs, and brain, that threatens a woman's life. The local disease, while being the source of the original cancer, is not the real threat to life.

As I pointed out in chapter 7, in virtually every case, cancer cells have spread to other parts of the body by the time the disease has been diagnosed. Thus, the decisions you make to control the local disease—the cancer in your breast—will not affect the length of your survival, since the disease in your breast is not life-threatening. However, the more aggressively the breast and surrounding area are treated, the less chance there is of the disease returning to the breast area.

The fear of recurrence of cancer within the breast is often used by physicians as an argument for more aggressive treatment, especially for the use of mastectomy and radiation. It's essential for you to understand that the scientific evidence urges caution when it comes to such surgery and/or radiation, for the following reasons.

First, it's true that the use of less aggressive treatment initially raises the risk of the disease recurring in the breast. For a significant percentage of women, however, there will be no recurrence in the breast. Still, if the tumor does return to the breast, the use of additional surgery or radiation at the time of recurrence is just as effective at removing the cancer from the breast as it would have been had you had further treatment initially after diagnosis. And survival advantage is not lost by delaying treatment until the time of recurrence.

It must be remembered, however, that while many doctors and surgeons emphasize the importance of keeping the cancer from reoccurring in the breast, such a reoccurrence does not affect length of survival. Still, let's consider the methods used to prevent such a recurrence and try to put such information into perspective.

RADIATION

The research clearly shows that surgery in combination with radiation treatment significantly reduces the chance of cancer recurring in the breast. For example, treatment of DCIS with lumpectomy alone has a 16 percent chance of local recurrence in forty-three months. With the addition of radiation therapy, the risk of recurrence to the breast is reduced to 7 percent.

For invasive cancer, the risk of recurrence in the breast area after lumpectomy alone is about 25 percent within forty-three months. After nine years, the local relapse rate is about 43 percent with lumpectomy alone. With the addition of radiation after six years, the chances of a relapse occurring in the breast are reduced to 6 percent. After nine years, the chances of a relapse occurring in the breast are reduced to 12 percent with the addition of radiation.

However, clear margins were not obtained in all cases in these studies. When clear margins are obtained, shown by the experience of doctors at the Cleveland Clinic, then the risk of local recurrence is 11 percent at five years and 16 percent at ten years. These breast-cancer specialists do not consider radiation therapy necessary when the surgery is adequately performed.

Allow me to remind you that even though radiation treatment may reduce the risk of recurrence within the breast, it does not change the average length of survival according to most published studies. The chances of living with breast cancer are the same, no matter whether you receive radiation treatment or avoid it, according to a 1995 overview of 17,273 women with breast cancer in thirty-six trials. This lack of survival improvement is consistent with the commonly held belief that breast cancer is either confined to the breast or disseminated to the rest of the body at the time of diagnosis. However, two recently published studies offer some hope by showing a small survival improvement when radiation is used in the treatment of breast cancer. Long-term follow-up of these encouraging studies may eventually show previously recognized disadvantages to radiotherapy—more deaths from heart disease and other cancers. Sadly, in past studies the small reduction in death from breast cancer has been offset by an increase in radiation-induced heart disease and other cancers, and patients must endure the serious side effects of radiation.

Side Effects of Radiation

High voltage radiation to the breast area will kill the tumor left behind by the biopsy and any cells that have spread to sites within the breast. However, radiation damages the skin and surrounding tissues of the breast and results in a number of short- and long-term side effects. Early on, radiation treatment can cause radiation sickness, depression, and loss of appetite. Later, it can result in breast deformity, rib fractures, and inflammation of the lung. In most cases, the breast retains a reasonably normal appearance. However, the deeper tissues often become firmer to the touch, and the skin becomes discolored and leathery.

When the left breast is treated, the heart and coronary arteries may be damaged. This increases the risk of dying of heart disease by more than 50 percent. Radiation can also damage the immune system and thereby double your risk of dying from other forms of cancer. For example, direct damage from radiation has been found to increase the risk of cancer of the esophagus by about fivefold ten or more years after radiation.

McDougall's Recommendation: Such facts should place the use of mastectomy and radiation in a new light, especially since mastectomy is severely disfiguring and radiation has serious side effects. My question to all doctors and their patients is this: Why radiate and/or disfigure 100 percent of women, when less than 45 percent will have a local recurrence in the breast? A "watch-and-wait approach" would leave 55 percent of women with an intact breast and an undamaged heart and immune system.

In the end, you must decide what is best for you. Consider that recurrence in the breast will not affect your length of survival, nor will it prevent you from treating the disease at the time of recurrence. However, if such recurrence would be terribly upsetting to you, then aggressive treatment initially may be your best approach. On the other hand, many women would rather have as little harm done to them as possible and would prefer to deal with new issues if and when they arise.

REMOVING THE AXILLARY LYMPH NODES

The presence of cancer in the nodes that circulate lymph from the cancerous breast—the lymph nodes found in the chest and armpit—has been used by doctors to determine:

1. The aggressiveness of the disease
2. The length of time the cancer has been present
3. How long a woman is likely to live
4. Whether or not chemotherapy should be used

Having positive lymph nodes, which means that cancer has infiltrated the lymph vessels, is associated with, but does not guarantee, a shorter lifespan after diagnosis. Studies have shown that when no nodes are involved, the five-year survival rate after diagnosis is about 80 percent; ten years after diagnosis, the survival rate with no node involvement drops to 65 percent. When the axillary nodes have been infiltrated, the five-year survival rate is about 50 percent; ten years later, it's 35 percent. Thus, the presence of cancer in the lymph nodes generally indicates that the disease is aggressive and/or in its advanced stages.

Because of these associations, doctors have routinely removed the axillary nodes to see if there has been infiltration and, if cancer is present, to recommend the use of chemotherapy, or "cancer-killing" drugs. These drugs are administered after surgery. This policy has been changing of late, however, with many doctors recommending that all women with breast cancer undergo chemotherapy, regardless of whether or not they have positive lymph nodes. If all women get chemotherapy, regardless of whether or not lymph nodes are cancerous, then clearly the removal of the lymph nodes becomes unnecessary. Or, if you decide that regardless of the findings you will not accept chemotherapy because of its toxicity and very limited effectiveness, there is clearly no reason to examine the lymph nodes (unless you're simply curious).

Still, most women with breast cancer will have to decide if they want their lymph nodes removed.

There are three things you must understand when confronting the question of whether or not to have your lymph nodes removed. First, removing the axillary lymph nodes does not increase the length of survival. Women whose cancer has infiltrated their lymph nodes and who decide against removing the lymph nodes live just as long as those who have the lymph nodes removed, and maybe longer.

Second, removing the lymph nodes will not decrease the chances that the cancer will spread. By the time of diagnosis, the illness has already spread to other sites, so the removal of these lymph nodes and associated lymph vessels will not provide any protection against the spread of the disease.

The third thing you must understand is that having positive lymph nodes does not guarantee any particular outcome. In fact, even though involvement of the lymph nodes generally indicates that the disease is in an advanced stage, many women with positive nodes *live for twenty years or longer after their cancer is discovered.* In one study, 35 percent of the women who were living for more than twenty years after being diagnosed with breast cancer had lymph nodes that were positive for cancer at the time of diagnosis. That's a significant percentage of women who were defying the odds. But therein lies the problem; "the odds" are simply that: a very general guide that does not necessarily apply to you. As we will see in greater detail in chapter 9, women who do not accept the odds, but instead make their own decisions and follow their own course of action tend to live longer. They defy the odds because they do not succumb to the predictions made on the basis of the "average patient."

Does knowing that your lymph nodes are positive or negative have a real value to you? Again, you must decide for yourself. Removing the nodes will help your doctor guess how long you have had the disease, what stage it is in, and how long you may have left to live. Many women want to know such information; they feel that not knowing only contributes to their fears and diminishes the quality of their lives. Others feel that such information only detracts from the quality of their lives because it increases the burden of their fears. Along the same lines, it must be acknowledged that doctors tend to be pessimistic about a woman's chances of survival if there is positive lymph node involvement. You must decide what impact, if any, such pessimism will have on you.

If removal of the lymph nodes will not have any positive effect on the outcome of your disease and may negatively affect your own spirits and those of your doctor, what then is the benefit of taking them out? The last remaining reason for removing the lymph nodes is to help your doctor determine if, in fact, you need chemotherapy. At this stage of your treatment, you will have to decide whether or not you will benefit from such drug therapy.

CHEMOTHERAPY

By now, you realize that surgery and radiation have had a very limited impact on both cancer itself, and the longevity of people with the disease. In fact, they are largely failures when it comes to improving survival. There is no cure for breast cancer and current treatments have not appreciably extended the lives of those with cancer. The failure of cancer therapy has led to the practice of administering chemotherapeutic agents for variable periods of time after surgery. The approach, called *adjuvant chemotherapy*, is intended to enhance the effects of surgery and radiation therapy.

The purpose of the chemical agents is twofold: first, to inhibit or kill cancer cells that may have spread throughout the body; second, to affect the cancer before it seriously harms or kills the patient.

The overall benefit of chemotherapy on patients is small, I am sorry to say. Once the tumor has been removed from the breast, chemotherapy reduces the risk of recurrence of cancer by 28 percent. It reduces the risk of death by 16 percent. For patients with positive lymph nodes, overall survival may be increased by 6.8 percent over ten years. Some experts argue that as few as 6 percent of women have their lives prolonged by fourteen months.

In general, long-term chemotherapy (e.g., the use of the drugs over twelve months) appears to be no more effective than short regimens (e.g., administration over six months).

The use of several drugs as opposed to single drug therapy appears to provide better results. Also, it appears that the higher the dose, the better the results.

Side Effects of Chemotherapy

Side effects of adjuvant chemotherapy are unpleasant, to put it mildly. They include hair loss, nausea, loss of nerve function, depressed blood cell counts that result in anemia, and increased vulnerability to infections, diarrhea, cystitis, vomiting, and oral ulcers. Chemotherapy impairs concentration, memory, thinking, and language skills, and causes sexual dysfunction, poor body image, and psychological distress.

Weight gains of five to fifteen pounds are common. The added body fat that often accompanies the use of such drugs reduces the quality of life and, ironically, increases the risk of recurrence of breast cancer!

The drugs also depress the immune system, thus decreasing the body's ability to ward off infection. Viral infections are twice as common in women while they undergo adjuvant chemotherapy for breast cancer. Another irony of chemotherapy is that as it weakens the body's immune system, it also prevents the body from defending itself against the cancer.

When women who have undergone chemotherapy are asked about the effects of these drugs on their lives, 79 percent say they significantly interfered with their lifestyles, and 29 percent reported that, given the chance, they would never undergo the treatment again.

McDougall's Recommendation: Chemotherapy is an experimental agent whose benefits are so small, and its toxicity so great, that it should be restricted exclusively to further scientific study. After decades of use, chemotherapy has not proved itself sufficiently beneficial to women with breast cancer that it should warrant almost universal application. In its desire to offer women some form of therapy, medicine is administering drugs that offer little benefit, but cause great suffering. Women should be spared that suffering. Meanwhile, ongoing trials should continue until science discovers chemotherapeutic agents that are more effective against the disease, and far less toxic to the body.

CHEMOTHERAPY PLUS BONE MARROW TRANSPLANT

Another highly experimental treatment is high-dose chemotherapy followed by bone marrow transplants that have been taken from the patient prior to the use of chemotherapy. The patient is given a chemotherapy dose of two to ten times the standard levels. Such levels would ordinarily be fatal, but having bone marrow available for transplant after the chemotherapy treatment allows the patient to survive.

About four thousand women a year undergo this treatment at a cost of $80,000 to $150,000 each. Even though several studies show survival benefits for high-risk patients with a poor prognosis (those with evidence of metastatic disease or infiltration of more than ten lymph nodes), the treatment poses great risks, and its value is far from established.

HORMONE THERAPY

Quite unexpectedly, the similarity between the effects of chemotherapy and those of surgery to remove the ovaries led to an important insight by scientists. Chemotherapy often plunges premenopausal women into menopause, a transformation that has been associated with improved survival rates. Similarly, the surgical removal of the ovaries of women with breast cancer also led to improved survival. Moreover, the extent of the improvement in survival was similar in both cases. This led some investigators to believe that the improvements women experienced from chemotherapy came exclusively from the destruction of the ovaries and the resulting diminution of estrogen. The fact that breast cancer is a hormone-dependent disease supported this hypothesis. Upon further analysis, scientists realized that the survival benefits from chemotherapy are limited almost exclusively to those women who cease to have menstrual periods.

A review of 133 randomized trials involving seventy-five thousand women compared the results of chemotherapy, removal of the ovaries, and hormonal therapy and found *all* of them to have similar survival advantages. An overview of the survival benefits after the ovaries have been surgically removed reveals an improvement in survival of 6.3 percent fifteen years after diagnosis. Chemotherapy, you will recall, results in a survival benefit of between 6 and 6.8 percent over ten years.

Given that the side effects from surgery and radiation to stop the function of the ovaries are so much less severe than those of chemotherapy, the advantage of the first two treatments seems clear. Surgery or radiation are a lot more humane than subjecting a woman to the debilitating side effects of chemotherapy, especially since all three have similar results. The simplest, safest, and most economical means of removing ovary function is by laparoscopy surgery.

Antiestrogen Drugs

Using the same principle, scientists created the drug *tamoxifen* to chemically reduce the cancer-promoting effects of a woman's own estrogen on her cancer. Tamoxifen has been shown to prolong survival and to delay recurrence of disease when administered for up to five years after initial surgery. The real advantage to this hormonal approach is that the results appear to be as good as those obtained with any of the more toxic adjuvant chemotherapy programs, and the adverse side effects are far fewer. Only 2 percent of women stop taking the drug because of side effects, which are similar to those of menopause.

Tamoxifen as adjuvant therapy has reduced the risk of recurrence by 25 percent and the risk of death by 17 percent. This achievement most likely represents an extension of longevity and not a cure. Excellent results are seen in both premenopausal and postmenopausal women with either estrogen receptor positive or negative tumors. However, there are two serious drawbacks: an increase in the risk of cancer of the uterus and blood clots.

Combining chemotherapy and tamoxifen results in no further benefits, however. A seven-year study of 3,920 women who were fifty years of age and older, all of whom had positive lymph nodes, found no significant difference in the length of survival time between those women who were treated with tamoxifen alone, versus those treated with a combination of cytotoxic chemotherapy and tamoxifen.

McDougall's Recommendation: Considering the last one hundred years of scientific evidence I think the best modern medicine has to offer most women with invasive breast cancer is a lumpectomy (with clear surgical margins). More extensive surgery, such as a mastectomy, should be performed only if the tumor is so large that it cannot be removed with good cosmetic results. Radiation should not be given initially routinely but should be reserved for later if the tumor recurs in the chest area. Chemotherapy should not be given outside of experimental studies. Estrogen stimulation of the cancer must be reduced by tamoxifen and/or surgical removal of the ovaries (laparoscopy oophorectomy). Most important, as you will learn in the next chapter, the cause of breast cancer—the high-fat American diet—must be replaced by a low-fat, plant-based diet that supports a woman's healing capacities to fight off the cancer.

Supporting Prevention Is the Key to Winning the War on Cancer

In the May 29, 1997, issue of *The New England Journal of Medicine,* longtime cancer researcher J. Bailar, Ph.D., and his colleagues published a lengthy review of the data on cancer deaths from 1970 to 1994 and found that the age-adjusted mortality rate from cancer was 6 percent *higher* in 1994 than it was in 1970. Cancer deaths among both men and women fifty-five years of age and older increased 15 to 20 percent, the scientists reported.

Declines in mortality from cancers of the cervix, uterus, colon, rectum, and stomach were due to a reduced incidence (fewer of these cancers occurred for known and unknown reasons) and early detection.

Meanwhile, cancers of the brain, prostate, breast, and melanoma all increased in incidence. The researchers conclude: "The war against cancer is far from over. Observed changes in mortality due to cancer primarily reflect changing incidence or early detection. The effect of new treatments has been largely disappointing. The most promising approach to the control of cancer is a national commitment to prevention, with a concomitant rebalancing of the focus and funding of research."

My message exactly.

Like you, I've been hearing all my life that "the cure for cancer is right around the corner," and that all scientists need are "a few more dollars for research." Yet, today more people contract and die from cancer than ever before.

We have made some progress in the treatment of rarer forms of cancer, such as the leukemias and solid tumors in children. Similarly, small gains have occurred as a result of early detection of cancers of the cervix and colon. Nevertheless, we are undoubtedly losing the war on cancer, despite pouring billions of dollars into research, testing, and treatment. And there is no reason to believe that this unfortunate trend will change.

When will we learn? How many have to die before we stop believing in the public relations propaganda being fed to us via the national media?

We know that as many as 90 percent of cancers are caused by smoking, alcohol, radiation, chemicals, viruses, and unhealthy foods. We also know that most of these causes can be avoided or mitigated by changes in diet and lifestyle.

What is most distressing is that the results from medical treatment are so consistently poor. In a 1986 report published in *The New England*

Journal of Medicine, Dr. Bailar reported a similar assessment of cancer therapies, with similarly bad news. Since then, no appreciable change in the way we treat cancer, or in our government's efforts to educate people about prevention, has taken place.

Why? The answer is obvious. The resistance to new ideas, even when they are founded on solid science, arises from the fact that the current approach is so lucrative. Tests and treatments for cancer are big business, with big profits. Add to this the fact that human nature resists change and will always seek quick and easy solutions, even when they are merely cosmetic, and you get a medical leviathan trapped in its own gilded cage.

Yet, there is hope. The money is running out. Managed care (capitation) is forcing the excess cost of medical care to shift from the patient and the insurer to the hospital, clinic, and doctor. There's a new cry in hospital boardrooms across the land: "Sick patients reduce profitability!" That recognition will bring about a revolution.

All those expensive treatments that are useless or harmful or both are about to be recognized for what they are. Such routine treatments as the amputations of the breast (mastectomies), prostate (radical prostatectomy), and colon (colectomy) are about to go the way of bloodletting. Most forms of chemotherapy also will be discontinued.

With the change in profitability now on the horizon doctors will start to support prevention. Hospitals and physicians now making fortunes on mammograms, mastectomies, and chemotherapy will suddenly start to sound like your guardian angels, calling on you to improve your diet and lifestyle in order to prevent cancer and other serious illnesses. Greed, we will see, can be made to work for us, just as it does against us.

In the meantime, you must defeat cancer by preventing it. If you get cancer, refuse radical and dangerous therapies until their worth is proved to you. At the same time, do all you can to improve your health and boost your body's cancer-fighting mechanisms by adopting the McDougall Program.

In the next chapter, I'm going to show you how such a step can have a dramatic effect on your body's efforts to overcome cancer.

CHAPTER 9

Strengthening Your Cancer-Fighting Forces

One of the first hurdles a woman with breast cancer must overcome is the belief that her doctor's medical treatment is the only important method of healing available to her. This belief, which is so insidious as to go unnoticed by most patients today, turns a woman into a passive patient and prevents her from using other powerful tools for healing, the most important of which is a starch-based, high-vegetable diet. Every woman with breast cancer must realize that being a passive patient keeps her from committing all of her personal and spiritual resources to the job of extending her life. The research suggests that such passivity can be dangerous. Those patients who are engaged in their own healing process appear to live longer, perhaps because they are far more willing to make the changes that will support their body's immune and cancer-fighting defenses.

If you are a woman battling breast cancer, that, in essence, is the challenge facing you: to boost your defenses so that your body gets the maximum amount of support to fight the cancer. The struggle that rages between your body and the life of the tumor is commonly referred to as the *host versus tumor relationship*. All medical treatment, which to date includes surgery, radiation, and chemotherapy, attempts to remove or weaken the tumor. Yet, there is another side of the battle that medicine entirely neglects, which is *strengthening the host*—namely, you and your own cancer-fighting defenses that are attempting to defeat the disease.

As I showed in the previous chapter, medicine's cancer treatment has not been successful. Perhaps one reason for this failure is that medicine emphasizes the destruction of the tumor—yet fails to fully accomplish that feat—while it neglects the challenge of boosting your health and vitality. This neglect is all the more frustrating after you examine the growing body of evidence that supports the use of diet and lifestyle in the treatment of breast cancer.

If you have been diagnosed with cancer, you must be responsible for the part of your therapy that your doctor will ignore. Your efforts may well mean the difference between the unmitigated spread of the illness or a lengthy and happy survival.

One of the major misconceptions many people have about cancer, and especially about breast cancer, is that the development of the disease is steady and inexorable. On the contrary, the clinical course of the illness is highly variable, with some women dying shortly after diagnosis, and others living thirty-five years or more after the disease is recognized.

Upon hearing this, some doctors and many patients wave their hands dismissively and say, "Yes, that's true, but there are too many possible factors involved to understand why breast cancer spreads rapidly in some women and very slowly in others."

Such a statement sounds cautious and prudent, but in fact it's incorrect. The scientific evidence points directly to diet and lifestyle as possible, and even likely, reasons why the course of cancer is so quick and deadly in some women and so sluggish in others. In addition, the evidence suggests that diet and lifestyle eventually may be a proven therapy in the fight against cancer, in the same way that the two are used today in the treatment for heart disease or adult-onset diabetes.

The best way for you to boost the health and vitality of your defenses is through improved nutrition and, secondarily, with a health-promoting lifestyle. Let's examine both of these areas and the science that supports their use as part of your treatment.

Fighting Cancer with Food

The link between diet and cancer has been well known for most of the twentieth century, dating back most notably to the work of pioneer researcher Otto Warburg, who in the 1920s began showing that normal cells can become cancerous when deprived of adequate oxygen. Research has accumulated for decades showing that excess fat intake, which is one of the more powerful ways of depriving cells of oxygen, is directly associated with the onset of cancer.

The general public became aware of such evidence in 1977 when the U.S. Senate Select Committee on Nutrition and Human Needs published its landmark report, "Dietary Guidelines for the United States." The committee's findings, which at the time hit the American public like the proverbial ton of bricks, stated that six of the ten leading causes of death, including breast cancer, were directly related to the American diet, with fat intake being the primary disease-causing agent. That report was followed by a series of scientifically based government documents from such institutions as the National Cancer Institute (1979), the National Academy of Sciences (1982), the American Cancer Society (1984), and the U.S. Surgeon General (1988), all of which urged Americans to change their diets to prevent serious illness, including breast cancer, by reducing their intake of fat from meat, dairy products, and eggs, while increasing their consumption of whole grains, fresh vegetables, and fruit. The National Academy of Sciences went so far as to say that fat intake is a "causal" factor in the creation of cancer. Other aspects of the American diet that contribute to degenerative disease, including cancer, include the excess consumption of cholesterol, refined flour products, and sugar.

Clearly, these dietary constituents either cause cancer or contribute to its cause. But viewed in a slightly different way, we can also say that a diet rich in these components supports and nurtures the growth of cancer once it manifests. Such a point of view is crucial once you have been diagnosed with cancer. At that point, you're no longer interested in preventing the disease. What you are concerned about is eliminating everything from your life that encourages its growth. First and foremost among such villains are the rich foods that make up the American diet and were paramount in the cause of your cancer. The amounts and types of fats in the diet have been the focus of extensive research.

FAT AND YOUR IMMUNE SYSTEM

Fat encourages the growth of cancer in several ways. As we have already seen, fat triggers the oxidation process that deforms the DNA in cells and can cause some to become cancerous. Fat also promotes the growth of cancer by raising estrogen, prolactin, and cholesterol levels, all of which appear to act as fuels for malignant cells to multiply and spread. Other hormones, such as prostaglandins, are also adversely affected by fat intake and, scientists believe, contribute either to the cause of cancer and/or its promotion.

Fat also depresses your immune system. Immunologists have shown that fat infiltrates the cell membranes of macrophages, one of the more important soldier-cells in the immune system. Macrophages identify pathogens and cancer cells by literally bumping into them and thereby touching the disease-causing agents with their sensitive cell membranes. Once the macrophage feels the cancer cell, virus, or bacterium, it is able to identify it as "not self," or as a threat to health, and then destroy the cancer cell or pathogen in one of several ways, most notably by producing powerful chemicals capable of killing the cancer cell, virus, or bacterium. Macrophages can also "call out" other immune cells by producing chemical messengers, called cytokines, that produce changes throughout the body and signal other immune cells to help in the fight against the disease. Unfortunately, once the fat infiltrates the macrophage's cell membrane, it can prevent the cell from identifying the cancerous cell as "not self," or as a threat to health. Consequently, the macrophage does not react to the cell—it doesn't attack it, nor does it call out its friends to kill the cancer. Thus, the cancer cells are allowed to proliferate.

Perhaps the most important type of cell in the entire immune system is the lymphocyte or CD4 cell, which, like the general of an army, coordinates the entire immune system's response to any illness, including cancer. It is both CD4 cells and macrophages that are most affected by HIV, leading to the disease AIDS, which, in essence, destroys the brain of the immune system. Studies have shown that in people on high-fat diets, CD4 cells fail to proliferate as rapidly in the presence of disease, which of course prevents the CD4 cells from marshaling a full-scale attack against the cancer.

Thus, fat, which triggers the onset of cancer and then promotes its growth, also puts your immune system to sleep—obviously, a deadly combination.

Other ways in which fat intake promotes the growth of cancer are by altering the structure of cell membranes, by changing the number of hormone receptors on the cells, and by affecting the communication between cells.

Whatever the mechanisms, there is widespread agreement that fat plays a crucial role in both the onset and promotion of breast cancer.

LINKING FAT TO THE DEVELOPMENT AND SPREAD OF BREAST CANCER

The speed with which breast cancer spreads through the body and eventually kills the patient appears dependent, in part, upon the consumption of fat. Animal studies have shown an almost linear relationship between fat intake and the incidence of breast cancer. In fact, many studies have demonstrated this relationship so compellingly that the evidence suggests a "dose-relationship," meaning the higher the fat intake, the greater the incidence of breast cancer. Once the cancer manifests, animal research has shown that fats and oils promote the growth of tumors.

Animals that eat diets higher in cholesterol show a higher incidence of tumors and metastases. On the other hand, animals who have cancer and are switched to diets that are very low in fat and have no cholesterol experience a significant retardation in both the growth of tumors and their number. They also live longer than those who continue to eat a high-fat, high-cholesterol diet. Once again, scientists find a dose-relationship: the lower the fat in the animals' diets, the slower the growth of the cancer.

Such findings have been replicated in human research. Scientists from Laval University in Quebec City, Canada, found that high intakes of saturated fat correlated with much higher rates of cancerous involvement of the lymph nodes that supply the breast, a much more aggressive tumor, and a more deadly disease.

When cancerous cells are looked at under a microscope, scientists have found that the cancers in people who have maintained high-fat diets—especially diets centered around meat and few vegetables—are much more aggressive than cancers in those who ate lower-fat diets. In 1991 a study of women with breast cancer living in Hawaii found those following high-fat diets had over three times the risk of dying compared to those women with low-fat intakes. High consumers of vegetable fats had almost twice the risk of dying compared to low consumers. Hundreds of other studies have shown how vegetable fats promote cancer growth, and death in women with breast cancer.

A study of eighty-two Swedish women between the ages of fifty and sixty-five, published in a 1993 issue of the *European Journal of Cancer*, found on microscopic examination of the cancer cells that those with lower intake of total fat had tumors with more favorable DNA patterns (euploid DNA). The chances of having an unfavorable DNA tumor pattern (aneuploid DNA) increased by 16 percent for each gram of total fat and 30 percent for each gram of saturated fat. (The McDougall Program provides about 11 grams of fat all mixed up, and protected safely, in starches, vegetables, and fruits, while the American diet may easily supply a woman ten times that much fat—much of it in the form of cancer-promoting free oils.)

Eating a Low-Fat Diet Improves Your Chances of Survival

In general, patients with breast cancer who formerly ate high-fat diets tend to survive for shorter periods of time than those who ate low-fat diets.

A study of 678 women with breast cancer, who after diagnosis and treatment were given a 90 percent chance of surviving five years, found that for every 5 percent increase in their intake of saturated fat (from animal sources), their risk of dying increased by 50 percent.

Interestingly, that same study, which was published in a 1994 issue of the *Journal of the National Cancer Institute*, found that the risk of dying appeared to decrease by more than half with higher intakes of beta carotene and vitamin C (both found only in plants). The more of these vitamins in the diet, the better the prognosis, the scientists reported.

Other research has confirmed that women with breast cancer who eat low-fat diets have much higher rates of survival than those who eat high-fat diets. For example, Japanese women traditionally eat diets much lower in fat than those of American women and, not surprisingly, Japanese women in Japan with breast cancer live longer than American women with breast cancer do. Specifically, 60 percent of Japanese women with cancer who are beyond menopause but have no evidence of distant metastases are alive ten years after diagnosis of breast cancer. In Boston, the ten-year survival rate for women with the same conditions is only 31 percent.

A study of 953 women with breast cancer, published in a 1985 issue of the *Journal of the National Cancer Institute*, estimated the risk of death increased by 40 percent for each kilogram (2.2 pounds) increase in fat intake per month. The negative effects of fat were seen mostly for women whose breast cancer had already spread to other parts of the body. (On the McDougall diet you might eat ⅓ of a kilogram of fat a month, whereas the standard American diet can provide you with 3⅓ kilograms a month.)

Eating a High-Fat Diet Increases Your Risk of Recurrence

One of the reasons women on low-fat diets survive longer is because their cancers do not recur as frequently as those in women who eat high-fat diets.

A study of 240 Swedish women, published in the *Journal of the National Cancer Institute* in 1993, found that those following diets higher in total fat, including saturated fat (from animal sources) and polyunsaturated fats (from vegetable sources), had much greater rates of recurrence of cancer than those on low-fat diets. The scientists found that the risk of recurrence was increased by 8 percent for each 1 percent increase in total fat intake in their diet. The authors, who were from the Department of Cancer Prevention at Karolinska Hospital in Stockholm, concluded that "dietary intervention might serve as an adjuvant treatment to improve breast cancer prognosis." A safe statement, to be sure!

Eating a High-Fat Diet Raises Hormone Levels

Estrogen and prolactin levels are often determined by the level of fat in the diet. In chapter 5, I described how fat raises estrogen and prolactin levels, and how these hormones give rise to breast and other hormone-dependent cancers, for example, endometrial cancer.

Studies have shown that reducing estrogen and prolactin levels, either by means of drugs or surgery, can retard the growth of established breast cancer. It can also cause regression of tumors and prolong survival. A reduction in these hormones by a healthy diet and lifestyle would be expected to be at least as beneficial to women as the effects of drugs and surgery.

BEING OVERWEIGHT INCREASES YOUR RISK OF DYING

Of course, fat intake is directly related to body weight, and weight is directly related to the risk of dying from breast cancer. A study of 698 postmenopausal women with breast cancer from the Iowa Women's Health Study found that overweight women are almost *twice* as likely to die from the disease as thin women. Those women with the highest fat intake also carried twice the risk of dying.

The authors, who reported their findings in a 1995 issue of the journal *Cancer*, concluded: "Although clinical trials are required, these findings support the hypothesis that a high fat intake is associated with reduced survival of postmenopausal women with breast cancer and suggest that women with breast cancer should consider limiting their intake of fat."

Regina Ziegler, Ph.D., MPH, of the National Cancer Institute, reported a study in the May 15, 1996, *Journal of the National Cancer Institute* that showed women in their fifties who had a recent gain of ten or more pounds had three times the risk of developing breast cancer compared to those who did not gain weight. Recent weight loss was consistently associated with a reduced risk of developing breast cancer.

* * *

The fat and cholesterol content of your diet, your weight, and your hormone levels not only cause or contribute to breast cancer but also encourage its growth once it manifests. All of these factors are under your control, once you adopt a low-fat, starch-based diet. This diet will dramatically improve your chances of long-term survival, as well as enhance the quality of your life.

CONTROLLING CANCER WITH PLANT FOODS

A woman on the American diet may easily consume 50 percent of her calories from fat. The McDougall diet offers as little as 5 percent of its calories from fat. It can make an enormous difference in how long you live with breast cancer. But if I were to leave you with the impression that lowering fat is all you can do to improve your diet, I'd be doing you the kind of disservice that many of my medical colleagues are doing when they leave out the subject of diet entirely. As I mentioned earlier in chapter 6, you can lower the fat content of your diet and still consume foods that will promote breast cancer. In order to prolong your life you must do more than lower fat. You must also eat vegetables, whole grains, and moderate amounts of fruits. The reason, simply, is this: plant foods are where the cancer fighters are found.

There is an old legend told by Native Americans that describes how the plant kingdom one day realized that animal foods were harmful to humans, so the plants convened a council to decide what to do. After much discussion, the plants decided to start producing substances within themselves that would treat the animal-induced diseases and restore health to humans. This story is part of the mythology that surrounds the birth of herbal medicine among Native Americans.

The fact is that the more scientists study plants, the more they realize what powerful medicinal qualities plants possess. What they also realize is that when it comes to understanding the mysteries that lie in plant foods, science has only scratched the surface. Plants contain substances that boost immune function, fight cancer, and slow the aging process. There are literally hundreds of health-enhancing chemicals in a single plant, such as broccoli. Scientists realize that they don't understand most of them.

We have discussed how cancer is caused by free radical production, or a process called oxidation. Fat is a major source of oxidation. On the other hand, plant foods contain substances that can slow the oxidation process, and in some cases stop it entirely for short periods of time. Only plant foods contain significant quantities of the wide array of antioxidants, especially beta carotene and vitamins C and E.

In a study published in the March 20, 1996, issue of the *Journal of the National Cancer Institute*, researchers found that women who ate more than five servings of vegetables each day had half the risk of breast cancer than women who ate less that three servings per day.

"We used to think it was a particular mineral or vitamin or antioxidant," John Pierce, Ph.D., head of cancer prevention at the University of San Diego Cancer Center, said in a recent interview. "Now we know it's more complex. In effect, a variety of produce works like a soup filled with weak anticarcinogens. You need to drink the whole soup for maximum effect."

FIGHTING CANCER WITH ANTIOXIDANTS

Researchers from Queen Elizabeth II Medical Center in Australia studied a group of 103 women with breast cancer to determine what, if any, effect the level of beta carotene consumption might have on their survival. They divided the women into three groups, based on the amount of plant-derived beta carotene they consumed each day. Then they followed the women for an average of seven years, after which the scientists found that only one woman in the group with the highest beta carotene consumption had died. In the intermediate group, eight women had died, and in the group with the lowest levels of beta carotene consumption, twelve women had died within seven years.

The scientists, who published their findings in a 1994 issue of the *British Journal of Cancer*, concluded that the results may have been due to anticancer effects of beta carotene, or that perhaps the vitamin acted as a marker for some other cancer-fighting element in fruits and vegetables. Since the higher concentrations of beta carotene would have been associated with a diet relatively rich in plant foods and lower in fat, the scientists also speculated that the women's longevity may have been the result of a low-fat diet.

Still, other research has supported beta carotene as a potential cancer fighter, especially when it is derived from plant sources, as opposed to supplements. Studies have shown that beta carotene encourages macrophages to consume, or phagocytize, cancer cells. It also triggers the macrophages to produce tumor necrosis factor, a cancer-killing chemical capable of destroying both cancer cells and tumors.

A study published in the medical journal *Cancer* demonstrated that beta carotene increased the percentage of lymphocytes and natural killer (NK) cells in men with cancer. The researchers found that the beta carotene significantly improved the ability of NK cells to kill cancer cells.

A large population study of 6,500 Chinese done by Cornell University researchers found that daily consumption of foods high in beta carotene was associated with low rates of certain cancers, particularly stomach cancer.

Fighting Cancer with Phytoestrogens

In April 1993, the *Proceedings of the National Academy of Sciences* reported that a substance in soybeans and soybean products blocks blood flow to tumors, thus preventing them from getting needed oxygen and nutrition. The substance, a phytoestrogen called genistein, accomplishes this feat by preventing angiogenesis, a process by which blood vessels attach themselves to tumors. Cancer cells and tumors, like all other cells and tissues in the body, need oxygen and nutrition to survive. In this way, genistein helps to destroy cancers.

Researchers told the *New York Times* that the discovery of genistein could "have significant implications for both the prevention and treatment of many types of solid tumors, including malignancies of the breast, prostate and brain."

After studying the effects of phytoestrogens on breast tumors, researcher David Ingram reported in the October 4, 1997, issue of the *Lancet* that a "substantial reduction in breast cancer risk among women with a high intake (as measured by excretion) of phytoestrogens."

Ingram interviewed women with breast cancer and then took urine and blood samples, testing both for quantities of phytoestrogens. He then compared the women with high phytoestrogen levels to 144 women who also suffered from breast cancer and found that those women with high phytoestrogen levels had one-third to one-fourth the risk of developing breast cancer than those with low phytoestrogen levels.

To date, more than fifteen phytoestrogens have been identified in human urine. All derived from edible plants, these substances have been divided into two main groups: *isoflavonoids* and *lignans.* Isoflavonoids are found mostly in unfermented soy products, while lignans are found in the dietary fiber of many plant foods, including whole grains, berries, fruits, and vegetables. Especially rich sources are found in flaxseed.

Phytoestrogens, which have a chemical structure similar to that of estrogen and act in the body as weak forms of estrogen, occupy the cells' estrogen receptor sites. There they block the attachment of the far more powerful and disease-causing estrogens produced by a woman's ovaries and fat cells. Since these plant estrogens do not cause cancer, and in fact protect your body's cells from the cancer-causing effects of estrogens, the plant estrogens are seen as having highly protective, anticancer effects on the cells.

Asian populations, which subsist on plant-based diets, consume large quantities of phytoestrogens, especially from soybeans and soybean products. This is one reason why they are believed to have lower rates of breast cancer. Incidentally, these phytoestrogens also appear to have significant protective effects on a man's body by reducing the risk of prostate cancer.

Because phytoestrogens are proving to be important cancer fighters, they are now being extracted from plants and placed in pill form. But no one knows what effect, if any, these chemicals will have on the human body once they are removed from their plant sources and the incredible array of vitamins, minerals, and other substances that normally accompanies them. The more we discover about nature, the more we realize that everything in the natural environment, including our food, is a precisely balanced ecosystem, bringing together a staggering number of elements in perfect harmony. If you remove a single nutrient or chemical substance from a plant, you change both the plant and the substance you have stripped it of. Once a phytoestrogen is removed from its plant source, it may be useless to human health, or even harmful. No one knows. What we do know is that when people consume their vitamins, minerals, and phytoestrogens in their original plant form, their health is enhanced and their capacity to fight breast cancer is strengthened dramatically. Therefore, I advise all my readers to consume their nutrients and phytochemicals in their natural packages—as starches, vegetables, and fruits.

The Benefits of Eating Greens

Like beans and other phytoestrogen-containing foods, broccoli and other green and leafy vegetables contain substances that appear to prevent and even inhibit tumor formation, especially in the breast. Scientists have found that broccoli, cabbage, kale, Brussels sprouts, collards, and mustard greens contain a group of compounds, called indoles, that may inhibit tumor-causing estrogen from targeting the breast. In animal studies, these vegetables have been shown to switch on enzymes that prevent exposure to carcinogens. They also contain sulforanphane, another cancer fighter. Sulforanphane has been called a "major and very potent" trigger for detoxifying tissues and blood and for promoting production of cancer-preventive enzymes.

Fighting Cancer with Fiber

When you eat a wide variety of plant foods, you get lots of fiber, which is essential for any woman with breast cancer. One of the keys to prolonging your life and even overcoming your disease is to lower your estrogen levels. And one of the best ways to do that is to consume lots of fiber. A study published in the *American Journal of Clinical Nutrition* showed that daily consumption of 30 grams of fiber will lower your estrogen levels by 20 percent. Such a drop in estrogen will dramatically reduce one of the cancer's most important fuels, and thereby help to retard its growth.

The chances of having a small (2 centimeters or less) tumor in the breast compared with the chances of finding a large tumor are increased significantly when the woman consumes a high-fiber diet, according to a study reported in a 1989 issue of the *Journal of the National Cancer Institute*. Smaller tumors are more likely confined to the breast, are likely to be in the earlier stages of the illness, and are generally less aggressive.

Fighting Cancer with Exercise and Lifestyle Changes

Regular exercise independently lowers estrogen levels, while alcohol consumption raises them. Both regular exercise and the elimination of alcohol have been shown to prolong survival in women with breast cancer. Needless to say, so does quitting cigarette smoking. Cancer-causing chemicals produced by the combustion of tobacco have been found in the breast fluids.

SOCIAL SUPPORT INCREASES LONGEVITY

In 1989, Stanford psychiatrist Dr. David Spiegel and his colleague James L. Spira, Ph.D., received a great deal of press attention when they reported that women with advanced breast cancer who participated in a support group lived twice as long as those who did not participate in such a group.

Social support groups have been shown to be especially effective at improving quality of life, enhancing coping skills, and reducing anxiety and depression. Very often, they provide a sense of comfort, understanding, and information for people who share a common experience, such as cancer. They also provide a setting to discuss the emotional impact of the illness, its meaning, various family difficulties caused by the disease, such as problems of intimacy, and the common sense of isolation and stigma that frequently accompanies major illness. In general, support groups have been shown to result in fewer visits to doctors and hospitals by group participants.

Sandra Levy and her colleagues have followed a group of women with early breast cancer for seven years and found that social support predicted both higher natural killer cell activity and the rate at which the disease progressed after recurrence. Women with high natural killer cells were found to either have a later recurrence of the disease or avoid recurrence entirely.

After eating a starch-based diet, getting daily exercise, eliminating alcohol, and avoiding cigarette smoking, the next best thing you can do for yourself is to join a cancer support group.

FOLLOW-UP TESTS CONTRIBUTE TO STRESS

Most physicians favor intensive follow-up programs for women after treatment for breast cancer. Such programs include physician visits, bone scans, liver echography, chest X rays, and blood tests. However, patients who underwent such intensive follow-up did not live any longer than those who regularly saw their physicians but were tested only when an obvious need arose.

Every time a woman has to visit her doctor or undergo a test looking for a recurrence of disease she risks the possibility that something might be found, and this can cause anxiety and depression. Most recurrences are actually detected by the woman herself. One reason follow-up with doctors' visits and high-tech tests do *not* improve survival is that there are still no effective treatments for cancer once it has spread. This is true no matter whether the disease is found in its early or later stages.

Two things are certain about such attention and testing: first, patients experience significant ongoing psychological stress from the disease, especially since they are constantly being reminded of their condition by the presence of doctors and the need for further testing. Second, much more money will be spent on the disease. Both adversely affect the quality of a woman's life.

Twenty years ago, when the U.S. Senate Select Committee on Nutrition and Human Needs reported that diet was a major factor in six out of the ten leading causes of death, including cancer, most doctors and laypeople dismissed the statement. Today, of course, science has established that diet is not only a cause of such illnesses but also can be a highly effective form of treatment, as in the case of coronary heart disease and other disorders.

Although the research supporting diet as a treatment for cancer is still relatively young, there are enough clues today to provide clear guidelines and to act. I believe that better nutrition can improve the quality of life for women suffering from breast cancer. Will improving the health and vitality of your immune and cancer-fighting defenses increase your life expectancy from five years to ten or even fifteen? We don't know the definitive answer to that question yet.

A large-scale study of two thousand women with breast cancer, all of them forty-seven years of age and older, is now being conducted by the National Cancer Institute. The study will try to determine if a diet of 15 percent fat will improve the prognosis for postmenopausal women. Don't wait for the results of that study to tell you what to do. Adopt a starch-based diet today and reap all of its known and unknown benefits, including the very real likelihood that you will live a longer, healthier, and far happier life.

CHAPTER 10

Safeguarding Your Uterus

No organ in the human body, not even the humble gallbladder, faces a greater likelihood of being surgically removed than a woman's uterus. The womb that made physical existence possible for each one of us is under siege. Consider the following statistics:

- One-third of American women lose their uteruses by the age of sixty. Barely half of the women in California will carry their uterus to the grave.
- About 500,000 hysterectomies are performed annually.
- Hysterectomy is second on the list of the most common operations performed in the United States (cesarean section is in first place).
- A woman's chances of having a hysterectomy double if her doctor is a gynecologist instead of an internist or general practitioner.
- Less than 10 percent of hysterectomies are considered medically necessary.
- The cost of hysterectomies performed each year is $3 billion.
- Your chances of having heart disease increase threefold after you have had a hysterectomy.

The vast majority of hysterectomies are performed to *improve the quality of a woman's life*, rather than as treatment for a life-threatening disease such as cancer. Has medicine failed women so completely that there is nothing else that can be done, short of surgically removing the uterus, to improve the quality of a woman's life?

For more than fifteen years, Barbara Williams, of Arizona, suffered from severe pain in her genital area, incontinence, "burning" urine, and painful intercourse. The cause of her disorder, called vulvodynia, is unknown and there is no cure, according to medical science. Unlike cystitis, it is not caused by bacterial infection. Because of the extremely painful symptoms and disruption to her marriage, Barbara actually considered having a hysterectomy when one of her doctors recommended the surgery.

In 1996, Barbara read my book *The McDougall Program for a Healthy Heart*, part of which covers women's heath issues, and decided to adopt my diet program. Within two weeks of eating a diet composed exclusively of fresh vegetables, whole grains, and fruits, all of her symptoms of vulvodynia disappeared.

Barbara wrote to me after her remarkable recovery. "My experience indicates that perhaps a diet too high in protein [causing a depletion of calcium and other minerals], combined with the ingestion of too much fat [upsetting hormonal balances], may cause the symptoms of vulvodynia in susceptible individuals, and that the pain disappears rapidly when healthy balances are restored. I originally went on your diet because of extremely heavy menstrual bleeding. My last period was the easiest I've ever had; no cramps, no clots."

Barbara also experienced a variety of other improvements in her health. "Not only has the vulvodynia disappeared, but my cholesterol is down, my energy is up, I'm losing weight and my menstrual periods are lighter and no longer painful . . . every good thing that you say will happen is happening to me, and more."

Because of the improvements in her condition, Barbara's husband also adopted the McDougall Program and experienced similarly dramatic benefits. "My husband went on your diet with me for his weight, blood pressure, cholesterol, and arthritis," Barbara wrote. "They're all responding as you say they will, and he's feeling like a spring lamb. He's looking great, too," she added.

Seven Reasons to Safeguard Your Uterus

For me, there are no disposable organs. The human body was designed to maintain its health and integrity from birth until death; no part of us was designed to be removed at a certain age. Unfortunately, many of us today, including most doctors, think of the body as having some less than important parts. Thus, we have come to believe that we can lose the spleen or gallbladder or uterus, and that such losses have little, if any, effect on the quality of our lives. Such attitudes are part of the reason why there are so many unnecessary hysterectomies performed each year.

This attitude is ingrained in medical students while they are young and still forming their values and attitudes toward the human body and their patients. Like most doctors, I was taught a number of phrases during my medical school training that were intended to help me sell women on a hysterectomy:

"Since you aren't going to have any more children, there is no reason for you to keep your uterus."

"This is a simple, safe way to be free from monthly periods."

"A hysterectomy will free you from the risk of cancer."

"You have had enough children—a hysterectomy is a good method of birth control."

"Your sex life will improve now that you don't have to worry about pregnancy."

"If your fibroids grow any bigger, the operation will be more dangerous."

"Your fibroids are so big they will press on other organs, possibly causing your kidneys to fail."

"Hormone pills will replace everything after your ovaries are removed."

"You have early cancer (precancerous lesions). Surgery is the only way to save your life."

During my twenty-five years of medical practice, I have learned that all of these statements are factually incorrect. No one loses an organ without suffering a variety of physical and psychological side effects. Sometimes this operation is essential for a woman's health and longevity, but in a great many cases, it is not. In this chapter, I want to describe the appropriate and inappropriate reasons for having a hysterectomy.

Let me begin by saying that if you are a woman who is considering an "elective" hysterectomy—one that is not essential for the treatment of a life-threatening disease—and believe that the loss of your uterus will have little or no consequence on your life, consider the following seven reasons for keeping your womb.

1. PROTECTION FROM HEART DISEASE

At least five recent studies suggest that retaining the uterus protects premenopausal women from heart disease. Research indicates that the uterus produces hormones (prostacyclins) that may reduce the risk of a heart attack. Such beneficial hormones act to preserve cardiovascular health in ways that are quite independent from the effects of estrogen, which is produced by the ovaries.

Premenopausal women who have undergone a hysterectomy experience a threefold increase in heart disease, even when they have retained their ovaries, according to research from the Framingham Heart Study. The risk of hypertension is also increased after a hysterectomy.

2. PRESERVING SEXUAL RESPONSE

Women report a general loss of sexual desire and response following a hysterectomy.

3. AVOIDING A SENSE OF LOSS

Quite naturally, many women feel a disturbing sense of loss after removal of their uterus. Something uniquely female is gone forever. In hindsight, many woman realize that they associated youthfulness, good health, sexual vitality, and fertility with their uterus. Only after the surgery did they realize how much the uterus contributed to their sex lives, their self-image, and their feelings of attractiveness. Once the irrevocable surgery has been performed, some women experience depression, anxiety, and difficult sexual relations.

4. IRREVERSIBLE CONTRACEPTION

Once the uterus is removed, a woman has no chance of conceiving and giving birth to children. When you consider that many women have elective hysterectomies at the age of thirty-five, such a loss can prove especially significant later in life.

5. RISKS OF SURGERY

Although the risk of death from the operation is only 1 percent, approximately five hundred women die each year while undergoing the operation, most often from anesthesia and postoperative infections. Complications after surgery occur in 25 to 50 percent of cases, though most of these are minor. Typical postoperative problems include fevers and urinary tract infections, but major problems, such as serious infections, bleeding, and bowel perforation, can occur that have a long-lasting, adverse impact on your health.

6. ANATOMIC CHANGES

Removal of the uterus may result in some form of altered anatomy, including the prolapse (sagging or falling) of the vagina, the bladder, or the rectum. An increase in the need to strain for bowel movements (constipation) is reported by about one-third of women after a hysterectomy.

7. HORMONE CHANGES

For reasons that are not fully understood, the ovaries sometimes fail in women who have had hysterectomies, causing premature menopausal symptoms and bone loss. This deficiency may be due to loss of important hormones contributed by the uterus. Another reason may be that blood supply to the ovaries has been reduced as a result of the surgery, which requires that certain arteries be cut and tied off during the operation.

Interestingly, a survey of 6,622 women ranging from thirty-nine to sixty years of age found, in all age groups, that women who had had a hysterectomy, with one or both ovaries preserved, had experienced more severe flushing, sweating, and vaginal dryness than women who had not had the operation. Forty-year-old women report severe flushing and sweating after surgery similar to that of fifty-year-olds who have not had surgery. The forty-year-old women also report even more vaginal dryness than sixty-year-old women who have not had a hysterectomy.

Unfortunately, many doctors do not understand that such changes can occur and dismiss women who make these complaints after the surgery has been performed. After undergoing hysterectomies, women have reported being told by their doctors to "see a psychiatrist. You still have your ovaries."

Appropriate Reasons for Hysterectomy

There are various kinds of surgeries performed to remove a woman's uterus and other sex organs. The first, of course, is a partial hysterectomy, which is the removal of only the uterus. The second is a total hysterectomy, which involves the removal of the uterus and cervix. This operation can also involve the removal of one or both ovaries, as well, though the removal of just the uterus and cervix still qualifies as a total hysterectomy. An oophorectomy is the removal of one or both ovaries, also called an ovariectomy, and a salpingo-oophorectomy is the removal of one or both fallopian tubes and ovaries.

Among the most important and appropriate reasons surgeons perform hysterectomies is to treat cancer of the uterus, referred to medically as adenocarcinoma of the endometrium. Cancer of the uterus is rare in women younger than thirty-four and, in fact, most surgeries for cancer are performed in women older than fifty-five. Cancers of the cervix, ovaries, or fallopian tubes usually require a hysterectomy as part of their treatment.

Cervical cancer is believed to be caused by a virus (human papillomavirus) that is transmitted during intercourse. Therefore, a woman's first line of defense against infection, and resulting cancer, is to practice safe sex.

Interestingly, new research suggests that differences in diet may explain why some women who are infected with the virus contract cervical cancer, while others don't, even after viral exposure and infection. A plant-based diet may confer some protection against cervical cancer.

Still, given the threat of infection, every woman should have regular Pap smears to determine the presence of cervical cancer. I recommend two consecutive years of negative Pap smears, by which I mean two annual tests in which the Pap smear shows no sign of cancer. After these two tests are performed, she should have the test every three years until she is fifty. Regular Pap smears will be able to detect changes in the cervix sufficiently in advance to allow simpler, milder forms of treatment, and help a woman to avoid potentially deadly cancer and a hysterectomy.

Hysterectomies are also used appropriately to stop hemorrhaging during childbirth, when the uterus ruptures, or when laceration of major blood vessels causes bleeding that cannot be stopped; the surgery is often necessary to save a mother's life. Life-threatening infection after an abortion is sometimes an absolute indication. Infections too severe to be eradicated by more conservative treatments (antibiotics and drainage) may require removal of the uterus. Early treatment of pelvic infections may therefore make the difference between a simple problem and one that requires the most drastic solution. There are a few other legitimate but comparatively rare reasons for performing a hysterectomy.

Hysterectomy to *prevent* cancer cannot be justified, however. Estimates are that an elective hysterectomy at age thirty-five would result in an overall gain in life expectancy of 2.4 months by saving 1.3 percent of women who would have otherwise died of cervical or endometrial cancer. Appropriate use of hysterectomy accounts for less than 10 percent of all the hysterectomies performed.

Factors Other Than Health
That Influence Hysterectomy

You might think that postmenopausal women would be most at risk for hysterectomies, since these women are beyond their childbearing years, but in fact hysterectomies are most commonly performed on premenopausal women between the ages of forty and forty-five. It's true that these years are not the primary childbearing years, but they are nonetheless the prime years of a woman's life. Women in this age group are still far too young to be manifesting such significant symptoms that require surgery.

The relative youth of women who undergo this operation is only one of its bizarre aspects. Twice as many hysterectomies are performed in the United States as in England and Sweden. Within the United States, the surgery is more common in the South than in the Northeast. In fact, the location of your home is only one of the variables that increase the likelihood that a hysterectomy is in your future.

YOUR DOCTOR

Having a male doctor substantially increases your risk of having the surgery. In an ongoing Swedish study, female gynecologists recommend *half* as many hysterectomies as male gynecologists do. The same pattern holds true in communities in the United States. Research has shown that male gynecologists in North Carolina routinely order more hysterectomies than do female gynecologists.

Although we could speculate forever about the psychological and chauvinistic reasons for this disparity, you are probably better off choosing a female gynecologist, especially if you want to protect your uterus.

The older your doctor is, the greater your chances of having the operation. Perhaps old habits or old attitudes die hard. Doctors graduating from medical school during the eighties and nineties are more reluctant to recommend hysterectomies than those trained during the sixties and seventies. Not surprisingly, the number of hysterectomies peaked in 1975, when 725,000 were performed. Since then, that number has fallen and leveled off at its present annual level of 500,000.

Having a gynecologist as your primary care physician also increases the likelihood of having a hysterectomy. Women who make frequent visits to a gynecologist stand a greater chance of being targeted for hysterectomy than those who rarely or never see a gynecologist, simply because gynecologists are trained to recommend hysterectomies.

HEALTH INSURANCE

One study showed that a woman with health insurance has a 40 percent chance of having a hysterectomy during her lifetime. If you have the money, there are doctors who will perform the surgery, whether you need it or not. Such a state of affairs prompted one physician to write in a recent issue of the *Lancet*, "More often, the indications [for a hysterectomy] are a cooperative patient and a uterus and good health insurance."

AGE

The older you get, the greater your chances of undergoing a hysterectomy. In fact, age as a risk factor cuts both ways. The older you get, the greater your chances of developing a condition that truly warrants the operation. On the other hand, many doctors see older women as no longer needing their uteruses; consequently, the organ becomes expendable as a woman ages. Many women view their uteruses in much the same way.

EDUCATION

The less you know about the pros and cons of a hysterectomy, the more likely it is that you will have one. A media campaign to increase the knowledge of residents in Canton Ticino, Switzerland, about hysterectomies decreased the rates of the operations by nearly 26 percent. We live in a culture in which hysterectomy has become accepted. How many women realize that nine out of ten hysterectomies are medically unnecessary? If you ask women who have had the surgery if they needed it, nine out of ten will tell you that it was essential. That's called good salesmanship.

In too many instances, a kind of blind acceptance sets in when a doctor "recommends" a specific medication or operation. This is especially true of hysterectomies. However, studies have shown that when women seek a second opinion regarding whether or not they should have a hysterectomy, the number of operations is reduced by as much as 28 percent.

Remember, all doctors do not think alike. When a doctor recommends that you have a hysterectomy, get a second opinion.

One of the primary reasons why there is such an excess of unnecessary hysterectomies is that many doctors do not really know when this operation is truly necessary and what the alternatives may be to surgery. As a patient, you must educate yourself on both of these points.

Conditions for Which Hysterectomy Is Recommended but Not Always Necessary

Barbara Williams's vulvodynia and heavy menstrual bleeding responded so quickly and so positively to the McDougall Program because the typical Western diet, rich in fat and low-fiber foods, is the primary cause of female problems that lead to a hysterectomy. High-fat, low-fiber foods combine to raise estrogen levels. The standard American diet commonly raises estrogen levels by as much as 150 percent above normal.

Each month, during a woman's menstrual cycle, estrogen levels increase and stimulate the lining of the uterus, called the endometrium, to grow. That blood vessel–rich tissue will provide nourishment in the event that a fertilized egg implants in the uterine walls. If a woman does not become pregnant, the endometrium is shed during the woman's monthly menstrual period, releasing the accumulated blood, tissue, and unfertilized egg. When estrogen levels rise and fall within healthy ranges, this process is efficient and largely free of discomfort.

However, when estrogen levels are excessive, they overstimulate the endometrium, causing it to become excessively thick. The resulting period is therefore associated with excessive amounts of blood loss, clots, and pain. When estrogen levels persist at high levels, bleeding can become very heavy and sometimes it occurs in midcycle. This common condition of heavy bleeding is known as dysfunctional uterine bleeding or abnormal uterine bleeding (AUB).

Estrogen also has the capacity to stimulate cells to multiply. Excessively high estrogen levels can overstimulate the endometrium, causing the overgrowth of cells within the lining of the uterus, a condition called endometrial hyperplasia. Eventually, this can lead to uterine cancer.

Far more common than uterine cancer, however, is the development of fibroid tumors. In this case, excess estrogen overstimulates the cells of the muscle tissue that makes up the body (walls) of the uterus. Such stimulation causes smooth muscle cells to proliferate and form nonmalignant tumors that are the size of a golf ball to the size of a basketball. These growths are commonly known as fibroids.

Fibroid Tumors

One in four women have fibroid tumors, or uterine leiomyomas. Seventy-five percent of these women do not experience any symptoms. Research has shown repeatedly that fibroid tumors are related to diet. The incidence of fibroid tumors is highest among African-American women; however, they are uncommon in African women who remain in Africa and continue to eat their traditional plant-based diet.

A low-fat, high-fiber, high-carbohydrate diet will lower hormone levels rapidly and dramatically, thus relieving most of the symptoms affecting female sex organs. Periods become lighter, shorter in duration, and further apart. In my experience, many of the symptoms associated with fibroids simply disappear, even though the fibroid tumors do not shrink with a change in diet. Still, fibroids will shrink once menopause starts and estrogen levels fall. The best approach most often is simply to wait for menopause to cause fibroids to disappear naturally rather than have a hysterectomy. Unfortunately, a great many women and doctors do not wait, which is why the removal of fibroids is the reason behind about 30 percent of all hysterectomies.

Appropriate Reasons for Hysterectomy to Remove Fibroids

There are several appropriate reasons that support a hysterectomy to remove fibroid tumors. Doctors are often forced to remove the uterus to control excessive bleeding caused by the fibroids; such bleeding can cause significant and even life-threatening anemia. Other reasons include pelvic pain brought about by the tumors, and symptoms arising from pressure on the surrounding tissues, causing back pain and disorders of the urinary tract.

Inappropriate Reasons for Hysterectomy to Remove Fibroids

On the other hand, the presence of one or more fibroids is often used inappropriately to perform hysterectomies. Indeed, most gynecologists automatically recommend a hysterectomy when fibroids cause the uterus to enlarge to the size of a twelve-week pregnancy (about the size of a softball), very often with little discussion. If there is a discussion, the doctor will usually offer one or more of the following reasons, even though each one is refuted by the scientific evidence.

1. *The fibroid is too large to allow the doctor to examine the ovaries.* Very often, doctors want to perform a hysterectomy when fibroids reach the size of a twelve-week pregnancy because they can no longer directly examine the ovaries, which, some physicians argue, prevents them from detecting the possible presence of ovarian cancer.

Ultrasound can safely and effectively examine the ovaries to determine their health. Furthermore, there is no evidence that removal of the enlarged uterus improves your chances of surviving ovarian cancer. In fact, ovarian cancer rarely occurs in women before the age of fifty, and most hysterectomies for fibroids are done in women between the ages of thirty-five and forty-four. Thus, hysterectomy as a prevention for ovarian cancer is unsupported by the scientific research.

2. *The doctor is unable to rule out cancer of the uterus because of the presence of the large fibroid.* This is not true for women who have not yet entered menopause. First, endometrial cancer appears mostly in postmenopausal women, usually in women older than fifty. Moreover, for most women with endometrial cancer, the uterus is of normal size. Therefore, the presence of a large fibroid, especially in a younger (or premenopausal) woman, makes uterine cancer highly unlikely.

However, there is one valid concern: the presence of a new or enlarging mass in a woman who has passed through menopause, especially one who is not taking hormones, must certainly be viewed with concern.

3. *The large fibroid may harm other organs.* Blockage of the urethras, which are the tubes that run from the kidney to the bladder, is very rare, and the likelihood of damage to the kidneys is extremely low. Urinary frequency and constipation can occur, but generally do not lead to illness worthy of a hysterectomy.

4. *The size of the fibroid and the enlarged uterus may increase the risk of surgery; therefore, it is better to remove the uterus entirely before the fibroid becomes too large and too dangerous to operate on later.* At this point, the research has not shown that the size of the uterus is associated with an increased risk of death, blood loss, or complications at the time of surgery. Sometimes the location of the fibroids, such as in the cervix,

can make removal more difficult, but even this has not been associated with any negative side effects.

5. *Removal of the fibroid, while leaving the uterus intact, increases the chances of becoming pregnant.* The scientific evidence on this point is conflicting. There is no strong evidence, however, that operating on the fibroids will increase a woman's chances of becoming pregnant. Meanwhile, women with fibroids become pregnant every day.

6. *If you do not remove the fibroids and uterus, you will not be able to take synthetic hormones.* There are other better ways to prevent heart disease and osteoporosis, such as through diet and exercise (see chapters 11 and 12).

Alternative Treatments for Fibroids

The first and most reasonable alternative is to do nothing, especially if there are no symptoms, or if the symptoms can be relieved by simpler means. If you can put off surgery until menopause, fibroids will likely regress as the function of the ovaries decreases and estrogen levels fall. If symptoms prevent you from waiting, there are surgical procedures and drug therapies that are far less severe than the irrevocable hysterectomy.

Surgical Alternatives: The fibroids themselves can be removed with the use of a hysteroscope, an instrument inserted into the uterus that is able to remove the tumor only. The excessive menstrual bleeding that often occurs with fibroids can be controlled in 75 to 90 percent of cases. Complications occur in fewer than 5 percent of cases, and the need for repeat procedures or for actual hysterectomy is less than 20 percent.

If a hysteroscopy cannot be performed, a procedure called myomectomy may be done. Physicians remove only the fibroids through the abdomen; the operation has shown good results. In many cases, the fibroids can be removed through a small incision by using a laparoscope, a narrow tubelike instrument often used to examine the inside of the abdomen.

Drug Therapy: A drug called gonadotropin-releasing-hormone agonist (GnRH agonist), which causes the ovaries to decrease production of estrogen, can shrink fibroids between 20 and 60 percent. This prescription medication is available as nasal spray, injection, or implant under the skin. Unfortunately, when the GnRH agonist is stopped, the fibroids typically grow back because of the presence of high levels of estrogen. However, this temporary help may be all that is needed if menopause is close.

The drug may be used effectively in combination with a low-fat, high-fiber diet. Once the fibroids have been reduced significantly, a healthful diet may be enough to keep estrogen levels sufficiently low to prevent them from regrowing.

Other Tests: If these methods are unsuccessful and excessive bleeding continues, the condition of the uterus should be evaluated with the use of D & C (dilation and curettage or a scraping-out procedure) and biopsy. The patient should also be examined for the possibility that the blood may not be coagulating, resulting in excessive bleeding. These procedures and tests should be done before a hysterectomy is performed.

DYSFUNCTIONAL UTERINE BLEEDING

Approximately 20 percent of all hysterectomies are performed to treat dysfunctional uterine bleeding, also known as abnormal uterine bleeding (AUB). The diagnosis is made indirectly, by excluding other possible causes of excessive bleeding, such as fibroids, cancer, pregnancy, or a blood disorder that prevents coagulation.

Alternative Treatments for AUB

If AUB is sufficiently severe to cause anemia and, as a result, disrupt a woman's life or even threaten it, the first step is to treat the condition medically. Nonsteroidal anti-inflammatory drugs such as Advil and Motrin can be the first line of treatment. After these are used, progestin with or without estrogen, danazol (a male hormone), and/or a GnRH agonist should be used for at least a month to try to control the bleeding. A hormone-releasing IUD (levonorgestrel-releasing intrauterine device) has been shown to decrease menstrual loss by more than 90 percent in women with confirmed heavy bleeding.

If these methods are unsuccessful, ablation of the endometrium with the use of laser technology or electrocauterization can be effective ways to stop blood loss. This approach is faster, cheaper, and safer than a hysterectomy, and has been shown to work in up to 90 percent of reported cases. However, as with hysterectomy, the woman is left sterile.

A low-fat diet will reduce hormone levels and help control bleeding in many women. In fact, a change to a healthy diet seems obvious and necessary.

PRECANCER OF THE CERVIX

Before cervical cancer invades the tissues and blood vessels, there is a stage when it is confined to the outer surfaces of the cervix. This precancerous condition is called carcinoma in situ, and is often detected by a Pap smear, which must then be confirmed by a follow-up biopsy. Once the cancer invades the deeper tissues, a hysterectomy is the recommended form of treatment.

Alternative Treatments for Carcinoma in Situ

Early cancers can be effectively treated with laser or cryosurgery (freezing the cells with liquid nitrogen) to destroy the precancerous tissue. These treatments result in cure rates that are similar to those associated with hysterectomy. Less costly and less risky, they are performed exclusively on the cervix.

PRECANCER OF THE UTERUS

Approximately 6 percent of hysterectomies are done for endometrial hyperplasia, a condition in which cells inside the lining of the uterus proliferate. Hyperplasia is believed to be a precancerous condition.

If the proliferating cells are the type that are typical of a normal uterus, the condition is *not* the basis for a hysterectomy. The presence of atypical cells in increasing numbers is considered an indication for hysterectomy by some doctors, particularly when the patient desires the surgery or is postmenopausal.

Alternative Treatments for Hyperplasia

When cancer is ruled out by D & C, hormone therapy can be used to treat the hyperplasia. Progestin, a synthetic version of progesterone, and natural progesterone both oppose estrogen activity and either can be given to reverse the hyperplasia. Careful monitoring is required.

GENITAL PROLAPSE

Prolapse is a condition in which the tissues of the birth canal move downward, or sag, toward the outside of the body. When this happens, the ligaments and muscles that keep the uterus suspended within the body are stretched beyond their normal shape and integrity. Various kinds of prolapse are described by physicians: uterine prolapse, cystourethrocele (prolapse of the bladder and urethra), and rectocele (prolapse of the rectum). Uterine prolapse accounts for about 15 percent of hysterectomies.

Symptoms include pelvic pressure, urinary incontinence, rectal discomfort, and difficulty with intercourse. A woman can also experience significant pain when the internal tissues have moved outside the body, thus exposing the cervix through the vaginal opening.

Prolapse is believed to be caused by the intense pressure placed on the uterus and its muscles and tendons during the birth process. Lifting heavy objects or coughing places additional strain on these muscles, which can stretch them beyond their normal limits and eventually weaken them.

What most physicians and laypeople fail to understand is that the most destructive pressure brought to bear on the uterine muscles and surrounding tissues is from chronic constipation and the routine straining that normally is required to move dry, rock-hard stools. This condition, of course, is caused by the standard American diet, loaded with low-fiber foods and animal tissue remnants that cannot be easily eliminated. Decades of such straining bring enormous pressures to bear on pelvic organs, stretching ligaments and muscles, and moving them from their normal positions. This repeated, mechanical distortion of the tissues cannot be reversed by changing to a high-fiber diet, but further progression may be halted.

Alternative Treatments for Genital Prolapse

Whether or not you need treatment for genital prolapse depends on the degree and severity of the symptoms. If there are no symptoms, or if the existing symptoms can be controlled by simple measures, then a hysterectomy can be avoided. One time-honored treatment, called a pessary, involves the insertion of a specially designed ring into the vagina to support the uterus and correct any displacement. Such rings are made of rubber, plastic, or metal and are sometimes inflatable.

In addition, estrogen vaginal creams can sometimes be used to strengthen vaginal tissues. Kegel exercises—in which a woman repeatedly contracts and relaxes the perineal (pelvic) muscles, such as when she is through urinating—can also be effective. Surgeries designed to pull back the uterus into the pelvis and support the bladder and rectum can also be effective at replacing the uterus in its proper place. Such procedures are preferred to hysterectomy.

ENDOMETRIOSIS

Approximately 20 percent of hysterectomies are performed to treat endometriosis, a condition in which the endometrial tissue inside the lining of the uterus grows unchecked beyond the uterus, spreading to the intestines and other organs within the abdomen. It occurs almost exclusively in women in their reproductive years. Common associated problems include pelvic pain, especially during periods and intercourse; ultimately, the condition can lead to infertility.

Alternative Treatments for Endometriosis

Progression of endometriosis depends on the presence of high levels of estrogen. Medical treatment, therefore, is directed at reducing estrogen levels to stop the excessive stimulation of uterine tissues. Hormone suppression can be accomplished with GnRH agonist and danazol. Remember, a healthy low-fat, high-fiber diet will cut estrogen levels by one-third to one-half in a few weeks. I have seen many women who are suffering with endometriosis get dramatic benefits with the McDougall Program. A change in diet should be a fundamental part of treatment.

Surgical treatments using a laparoscope destroy or remove large areas of endometriosis. Open abdominal surgery has also been used to clean up these lesions.

CHRONIC PELVIC PAIN

About 10 percent of hysterectomies are done to alleviate pain in the pelvic area that has no apparent correctable cause. Sadly, a history of childhood sexual abuse is found in many of these cases.

Alternative Treatments for Chronic Pelvic Pain

If you suffer from chronic pelvic pain, you should ask yourself if the pain is sufficiently severe to warrant major surgery, especially if there is no guarantee that the pain will be alleviated with removal of the uterus. If the answer is no, then avoid the surgery. Nonsteroidal anti-inflammatory medications such as Advil and Motrin are often helpful.

When the pain is associated with menstrual periods, it may be effectively treated with birth control pills. A multidisciplinary approach using physical, psychological, and dietary care has been shown to be effective.

Strategies to Consider if You Must Have a Hysterectomy

Even if you must have a hysterectomy, you still have important decisions to make. There is the choice of abdominal, vaginal, and laparoscopy-assisted hysterectomy. There are strong arguments for each of these approaches, but you will have to discuss these options with your doctor in order to decide which approach is best for you. Vaginal hysterectomy is associated with fewer complications than an abdominal operation.

In addition, try to adopt the following strategies:

1. Keep your cervix if possible. The cervix, which produces natural lubricants that are especially important during intercourse, may play an important role in a woman's sexual response. One study found that women who had their cervixes removed during hysterectomy had a greater reduction in orgasms than those whose cervixes remained after surgery.

Removal of the cervix increases the length of the operation, thereby boosting the chances of encountering complications during surgery. There is also an increased risk of infection when the cervix is removed. In Sweden, 21 percent of hysterectomies leave the cervix, while only 1 percent of hysterectomies in the United States leave the cervix.

2. Keep your ovaries. Many doctors recommend removal of the ovaries during a hysterectomy to prevent ovarian cancer. However, the actual risk of ovarian cancer in such cases is extremely small. One estimate is that seven hundred women would have to have their healthy ovaries removed to prevent one case of cancer.

Your ovaries are important. Because they produce and release important hormones, including estrogen and male hormones, they reduce your risk of heart attacks, osteoporosis, and menopause-associated discomforts. The hormones produced by the ovaries improve your feelings of well-being and your sexual desire.

3. Educate yourself. Most hysterectomies are considered to be "elective" surgeries. *They don't have to be done.* You have a choice. By

being informed and working with your doctor, you have a very good chance of saving your uterus, cervix, and ovaries in most cases.

After giving birth, many women believe that the uterus is a vestigial organ, a part of their bodies they no longer need. I have tried to show you that this is not the case. Every part of your body plays an important role in your health and well-being from the moment of your birth to the moment of your death.

CHAPTER 11

Building Strong Bones

"**I** am a fifty-year-old woman who started menopause about five years ago," Karen Melbourne wrote to me in 1996. "When I had my annual physical, I persuaded my doctor to send me for a bone density test which confirmed my fears—I was in the beginning stages of osteoporosis with significantly weakened bones for my age group.

"My doctor had put me on Premarin for menopause symptoms, but I had stopped taking it when I found out about the cruelty issues related to the horses they gather it from." [Premarin is a form of estrogen made from the urine of pregnant mares.]

However, Karen's ceasing to take Premarin only increased the likelihood that she would develop even more severe osteoporosis. The female hormone estrogen is essential for maintaining bone density. For the first five years after menopause, women commonly lose anywhere from 4 to 8 percent of their bone mass each year. After that five-year period, women typically lose about 1 percent of their bone mass annually. Unfortunately, osteoporosis was not the only problem that Karen needed to worry about. Because estrogen reduces a woman's risk of heart attack and stroke, she also faced an even greater risk of suffering from heart disease when she stopped taking Premarin. When estrogen levels fall as a result of menopause, the incidence of heart disease among women jumps immediately to equal that of men. Estrogen also reduces the common symptoms of menopause, including hot flashes, sweats, fatigue, and mood swings. Of course, hormone replacement therapy (HRT) has a price: it significantly increases a woman's risk of uterine and breast cancer. (I discuss the issues related to menopause and HRT in chapter 13.)

Right around the time of her bone density test, Karen, a resident of California, attended one of my lectures in the San Francisco area, a presentation that, quite by coincidence, was on the subject of osteoporosis. In the course of my talk, I said that the primary cause of osteoporosis is a high-protein diet, which is abetted by several other factors, most of which are related to lifestyle. Those words piqued Karen's concern, because, as she later wrote, "Since I was a teenager, I followed a very high-protein diet (lots of red meat, chicken, fish, cottage cheese, and eggs), thinking that this was the way to keep my weight down. Of course, it never worked. I also did very little in the way of exercise."

Immediately, Karen bought several of my books, including a cookbook by my wife, Mary, and began following the McDougall diet.

Meanwhile, Karen was being pressured to resume her HRT. "My doctor insisted that my only hope of avoiding disabling bone loss was to get right back on the estrogen with calcium supplements." Because Karen had already lost significant amounts of bone, the continuation of the disorder would likely result in devastating fractures within the next decade of her life, her doctor told her.

Karen was afraid, but her fear did not prevent her from studying the reasons why she had lost so much bone at a relatively young age, and why she continued to lose it so rapidly. In order to thoroughly educate herself, Karen bought several more of my books and attended three more of my workshops. "I also heard a discussion on your radio show encouraging women in my situation to follow a low-protein diet, exercise, and use a natural progesterone cream to treat menopausal symptoms and osteoporosis," Karen later wrote to me.

Karen told her doctor all of the information she had gathered, but her physician still insisted that she should resume taking Premarin. Karen now had a decision to make. Based on all she had read and heard, the McDougall Program seemed like the most prudent approach. As she later wrote, "I continued to eat the diet you recommend. I took no calcium supplements, and, of course, used no dairy products. My doctor gave me a prescription for natural progesterone cream . . . I also began an exercise program—daily half-hour walks and twice a week moderate weight training.

"After eighteen months, I went back for another bone density test. Not only had I not lost more bone, I had actually started to reverse the process. I certainly bet on the right doctor! Now I tell every woman who will listen: to prevent or reverse osteoporosis, eat a low-protein

diet, exercise, use natural progesterone cream during and after menopause. It works!"

What Causes Osteoporosis?

The primary cause of osteoporosis is the high-protein diet most
Americans consume today. As one leading researcher in this area said,
"Eating a high-protein diet is like pouring acid rain on your bones."
The effects of that acid rain diet are made even worse by a handful of
other bone-depleting factors, including a sedentary lifestyle, cigarette
smoking, excess consumption of salt and caffeine, and the reduction in
estrogen at the time of menopause. Following the popular beliefs that
chicken, fish, and low-fat dairy products are "health foods," the diet becomes even higher in protein. Because the vast majority of women follow the high-protein American diet and a "bone-weakening" lifestyle,
millions of them suffer from osteoporosis. That enormous population
of women is viewed by many physicians and scientists today as a consumer group, one that very easily can be guided into undergoing tests
that establish the presence of the disorder. Once a woman finds out
that her bones have been weakened or, indeed, that she has osteoporosis, she can be placed on drug therapy for the rest of her life. Testing is
expensive and profitable. Drug therapy is even more so. Osteoporosis is
big business, involving billions of dollars and employing many thousands of health care professionals, businesspeople, and administrators.
Consider the following statistics:

- More than 25 million Americans suffer from osteoporosis; ap-
  proximately 22 million are women.
- Osteoporosis causes 1.5 million fractures each year.
- The annual cost for treatment of the disorder in the United States
  alone exceeds $10 billion.
- Average length of hospitalizations for a hip fracture is twenty to
  thirty days.
- As many as 21 percent of nursing home patients are admitted for
  hip fractures.
- Half of all patients with hip fractures do not recover the ability to
  walk independently.
- The odds of dying from a hip fracture are about the same as those
  for dying from breast cancer.

The diagnosis and treatment of osteoporosis is so profitable because millions of people unwittingly weaken their bones, making them dependent for life on diagnostic tests and drug therapy that slows the disorder or, at best, restores some bone tissue, but never cures it. For many people, the drugs are ineffective and cause harmful side effects.

The best advice is to do all you can to avoid the traps of the system by maintaining the strength, durability, and density of your bones through appropriate diet and exercise. If you already have the disorder, you must prevent further bone loss while doing all you can to promote the strength of your skeleton. In the end, only you can prevent yourself from suffering from this life-threatening disorder.

Building and Losing Bone

Contrary to what many of us believe, bones are not sticks of concretized calcium, but dynamic tissue that is constantly breaking down and rebuilding itself. Each year, about 10 percent of your entire skeleton is broken down in a process called *resorption* and then rebuilt. Bones are composed of several layers, starting with a thin outer membrane that contains blood vessels and nerves. Beneath that is a thick, hardened shell composed primarily of protein, calcium, and phosphorous. The protein at this layer, which is called collagen, forms a lattice-like structure that holds both calcium and phosphorous; the two minerals act as a mortarlike material to make bones hard and resilient. At the center of bones is a spongy marrow containing tissues that produce red and white blood cells, called the bone marrow.

The skeleton starts to develop as cartilage while each of us is still in the womb and grows to its maximum thickness by about age thirty-five, at which point we all start to gradually lose bone—about 1 percent a year, on average, for both men and women.

Bone loss is accelerated for the first four to eight years after menopause, when a woman's body dramatically reduces its production of estrogen. Estrogen is essential for maintaining healthy bones in women. (In men, testosterone serves the same function.) During this time, a woman can lose as much as 10 to 15 percent of her bone mass in the arms and legs, and up to 15 to 20 percent in her spine. Once that four-to-eight-year period is over, bone loss slows once again to about 1 percent each year, on average. While all people experience the thinning of bones, not everyone suffers from osteoporosis and osteoporosis-related fractures. Many factors influence the development of the disorder, especially the overall strength and density of bones at their peak and one's diet and lifestyle.

Apart from hormone levels, there are two other primary ways of developing and strengthening your skeleton. The first is by eating a plant-based, low-protein diet; the second is by getting regular exercise. Bones grow thicker and denser with all forms of weight-bearing exercise, including walking and weight training. As one researcher said, "You only have the bones you need. The more demands you make of your body in the form of exercise, the more bone you produce." Whenever bones are stressed through exercise, the rate at which they break down and rebuild is increased; however, the exercise causes bones to rebuild even stronger to meet the demands placed on them by regular exercises. Scientists at the U.S. Department of Agriculture's Human Nutrition Research Center at Tufts University recommend walking at least four days per week, and preferably more, along with three sessions of weight training. The weights can be small handheld weights that can be carried and lifted regularly while walking.

Obviously, the stronger your skeleton is at the time you reach peak bone mass, the greater your chances will be that you will avoid the thinning of your bones, or osteoporosis, later in life.

Osteoporosis is formally defined as the thinning of bones, resulting in the loss of bone density and strength, which in turn leads to fractures from even minimal trauma. The disorder occurs from the loss of all bone material, not merely from the loss of calcium. The myth that osteoporosis is caused by a calcium deficiency was created to sell dairy products and calcium supplements. There's no truth to it. American women are among the biggest consumers of calcium in the world, and they still have one of the highest levels of osteoporosis worldwide. And eating even more dairy products and calcium supplements is not going to change that fact.

During the fifteen to twenty years after she experiences menopause, a woman can lose as much as 50 to 75 percent of her skeleton, at which point fractures start to develop. The most common fracture sites are the hip (at the head of the femur bone), spine (in the vertebrae), and wrist (in the radius bone).

A fifty-year-old woman faces a 17.5 percent chance that she will fracture her hip sometime during the remainder of her life. What that means is about seventeen women out of one hundred suffer an osteoporosis-related hip fracture sometime between the age of fifty and the time of death. When you think about it, you realize that that's quite a lot of women, especially when you consider that about half of all hip fractures are crippling and about 20 percent are fatal. That same fifty-year-old woman has an 11 percent chance of suffering a fracture in her spine, and a 13 percent chance of fracturing her wrist.

Destroying Your Bones

Osteoporosis has many causes, but a flaw in the female design is not one of them. What's the sense in designing a body intended to last eighty-five or more years and then equipping that body with a set of bones that holds up for only sixty years? In fact, the primary cause of osteoporosis, like that of most degenerative diseases, stems directly from the way we take care of our bodies.

Worldwide analysis reveals that hip fracture rates increase as a population's animal protein intake increases. The data are straightforward and unequivocal: in rural Africa and China, where people live mostly on vegetables, hip fractures are rare to nonexistent. In countries where meat, poultry, fish, and dairy products dominate meals, hip fractures are common. Why would the excess consumption of these foods destroy bones?

Meat, poultry, fish, eggs, and dairy products are all rich sources of protein. The building blocks of proteins are substances called amino *acids*. Animal foods are rich sources of these amino acids. Most plant foods, on the other hand, are composed of alkaline substances.

The acid-alkaline, or pH, balance of the human body is slightly alkaline. The body protects this acid-base balance carefully so that biochemical reactions can occur properly. A diet rich in animal foods provides an abundance of acids that must be neutralized, or *buffered*, in order for the body to function properly and health to be maintained. The body's primary buffering system is its bones, or, more specifically, the phosphorus in its bones. When excess acids pour into the body, the pituitary gland signals the bones to release calcium and phosphorus into the blood. These minerals combine to form alkaline phosphates, which are used by the body to neutralize the amino acids. Unfortunately, the freed calcium and other bone materials that were washed out from the bone are then excreted by the kidneys and lost to the body. The net effect is a loss of bone and the first link in a chain of events that leads to osteoporosis.

The next link involves changes in the way the kidneys function. In health, the kidneys normally retain the minerals the body needs, including calcium. Unfortunately, the excess consumption of animal proteins causes the kidneys to get rid of calcium from the body. It works like this. When animal proteins are broken down, they give rise to by-products called urea. Urea causes the filtration rate of the kidneys to increase, which causes more calcium from the blood to be lost into the urine. The acids from animal proteins can cause the kidneys to excrete large amounts of calcium into the urine. And then there's the element sulfur, a constituent in three of the twenty amino acids. These three sulfa-containing amino acids inhibit the reabsorption of the calcium back into the bloodstream from the microscopic urine-collecting tubules in the kidneys. Animal foods are rich in proteins that contain these amino acids. Methionine, a sulfur-containing amino acid, is twice as prevalent in meats as it is in grains. There is five times more methionine in beef as there is in beans.

Thus, the more animal foods you eat, the more you trigger your kidneys to pump out calcium from your body. It's a well-researched mechanism: excess animal protein in, calcium out. The result is a net loss of calcium, or what doctors refer to as a negative mineral balance. That's the way it works. Researchers estimate that when you double the amount of protein you consume, you lose about 50 percent more calcium in your urine.

Not surprisingly, osteoporosis has reached epidemic proportions in countries where meat, poultry, eggs, fish, and dairy foods are consumed abundantly.

Many other investigations have found that people with higher intakes of animal protein have greater loss of calcium into their urine and/or thinner bones [lower bone mineral density (BMD) or fractures].

- In a study of thirty-eight white women between the ages of twenty-four and twenty-eight years, protein intake was found to be negatively associated with radial (wrist) bone mineral content and bone density.
- In five districts of China where residents had markedly different diets and lifestyles, 764 middle-aged and elderly women were studied. Calcium loss in the urine was found to be associated with animal protein consumption, but not plant protein.
- A study of 886 men and women found the more protein consumed, the more calcium lost in the urine.
- The Nurse's Health Study recently found that women who consumed 95 grams of protein a day compared with those who consumed less than 68 grams a day had a 22 percent greater risk of forearm fractures.

DIETARY CALCIUM

One of the most telling ironies in all of health care is that osteoporosis is most prevalent in countries that have the highest consumption of milk and calcium. I realize that that statement flies in the face of a hundred television commercials, but it's true. What is also true is that the people in these countries also consume diets rich in animal food. The bottom line is that even if you are chasing your steaks and Big Macs with milk and calcium supplements, you're still going to lose your bones.

Worldwide, osteoporosis is most common in developed countries where dairy products and calcium supplements are consumed in the largest quantities: the United States, Sweden, Finland, England, Canada, Australia, and New Zealand. Likewise, the occurrence of osteoporosis appears rarely in Asian and African countries, where milk is not consumed because it is not available, not a customary drink, and/or because of a very high incidence of lactose intolerance. On the basis of this evidence I must conclude that calcium intake per se does little or nothing to protect the bones from the true causes of this disease. And high calcium intakes are totally unnecessary to form strong healthy bones that will last a woman her lifetime.

In fact, most of the world's population consumes only 300 to 500 milligrams of calcium each day, yet manages to grow and maintain normal adult skeletons. These people get their calcium from diets composed primarily of plant foods. They do not suffer from any "calcium deficiency disease." In fact, no such disease exists, even among people who do not eat any dairy products.

Drinking Milk Does Not Build Strong Bones

Milk has long been universally recommended for strong bones. However, only one properly designed study has ever tested the effects of milk supplementation on the bone health of women at an age when they are most likely to suffer from osteoporosis. That study, which ironically was funded by the National Dairy Council, fed a group of postmenopausal women three eight-ounce glasses of skim milk per day for one year. The researchers then compared these women with a control group that did not receive the three glasses of milk each day. The results were disappointing, at least for the dairy interests.

The women fed the extra milk consumed more than 1,400 milligrams of calcium a day and still remained in negative calcium balance. They also lost bone at twice the rate of those who did not receive the extra calcium. According to these investigators, "this may have been due to the average 30 percent increase in protein intake during milk supplementation." Needless to say, this finding did not reach the six o'clock news.

OTHER CAUSES OF OSTEOPOROSIS

As I said at the outset of this chapter, diet is the primary cause of osteoporosis, but there are also numerous other contributing factors that promote the disorder. Among the most important of these are cigarette smoking, salt intake, and caffeine consumption. In a large study of 84,484 nurses, researchers found that nurses who drank the most coffee had three times the risk of hip fracture when compared with those who drank the least. Excess use of salt has also been shown to promote calcium loss and thus contribute to bone loss. Finally, women who smoke one package of cigarettes each day throughout adulthood will lose an average of 5 to 10 percent more bone mass than nonsmokers by the time both groups reach menopause.

The role of dietary calcium remains controversial, but at this point it appears that taking a supplement won't do much harm. Taking a 300 mg calcium pill each day will decrease your iron absorption by 60 percent; this, of course, will increase your risk of suffering iron deficiency anemia. That same 300 mg calcium supplement will also increase your risk of kidney stones by about 20 percent. Supplements labeled "bonemeal," "dolomite," "oyster shell," or "natural" are contaminated with

PROTEIN CONTENT OF FOODS*			
Food	*% of Calories from Protein*	*Food*	*% of Calories from Protein*
Bananas	5	Egg (whole)	32
Beans (navy)	25	Egg whites	82
Beef (ground)	32	Fish (tuna)	65
Chicken (light, without skin)	71	Potatoes	9
Corn	13	Rice (brown)	9
Cottage cheese (nonfat)	75	Turkey (light, without skin)	76
Cow's milk (skim)	39	Yogurt (nonfat, plain)	41
Cow's milk (whole)	21		

*Lower-fat animal products are higher in animal protein. See appendix C for more information on the hazards of some low-fat foods.

significant amounts of lead and/or aluminum. Calcium citrate is advertised as the best form of calcium to prevent osteoporosis. Unfortunately, this form of calcium increases the absorption of aluminum from
dietary sources. Aluminum is believed to play an important role in the
cause of Alzheimer's disease, and is the most important substance for
you to avoid in order to prevent this severe form of dementia. Higher
consumption of animal fat may also play a role in the loss of mental
function from this disease.

Still, on balance, such consequences are small when compared with
the risks of trying to get calcium from dairy products: heart disease,
cancer, obesity, diabetes, infectious diseases, and autoimmune diseases,
just to name a few.

Osteoporosis is not an inevitable consequence of aging. No matter
how strong or weak your bones are today, you can do much to avoid further deterioration and bone loss by adopting the McDougall Program.
Many people who follow my recommendations develop stronger and
denser bones, even after they have been diagnosed with osteoporosis.

CHAPTER 12

Monitoring Bone Health and Choosing Treatment

This chapter focuses on the diagnosis and treatment of osteoporosis. The difficult task facing any woman with osteoporosis is discerning which tests and treatments are essential and therapeutic, and which ones are not.

Diagnosing Osteoporosis

When osteoporosis is suspected, your doctor will begin her or his investigation by taking your medical history. Your doctor will then do a thorough physical examination and follow with a basic array of laboratory tests to rule out the possibility of other diseases, such as hyperthyroidism, hyperparathyroidism, adrenal cortisol excesses, gastrointestinal diseases, or possible bone cancers.

Your physician very likely will recommend that X rays be taken of certain bones to see if there are any existing fractures. Half of all spinal fractures are asymptomatic, meaning that there is no pain associated with the break, or any other outward indication of their presence. Therefore, X rays are needed to determine if any bones have been broken. Fractures are regarded as a "flag," or risk factor, for future breaks, simply because one or more fractures suggest the possibility of weakened, fragile, or osteoporotic bones. They also indicate a possible tendency to injure oneself. Women with a single spinal fracture have about three times the risk of incurring a future fracture compared with women with no spinal fractures. Women with two or more spinal fractures have six to nine times the risk of future fractures.

X rays help your doctor determine the possible presence of osteoporosis, but the degree of the illness, the density of your bones, must be established by other tests.

BONE MINERAL DENSITY (BMD) DIAGNOSIS

The density of your bones, or their mass, can be measured by a variety of techniques. The results of these tests are expressed as *bone mineral density* (BMD). American women and men lose significant amounts of bone density during their lifetimes. For example, scientists have discovered that the average American woman loses about 50 percent of the bone mineral density in her hip over the course of her lifetime, while the average American man loses about 35 percent of the BMD in his hip.

Scientists can determine the mineral density of any bone by shooting a beam of photons through the bone and determining how much that beam is reduced when it exits through the other side. Strong, healthy bones will be dense, and therefore will block much of the photon beam from passing, while porous bones will allow more of the beam to penetrate and exit. The greater the strength of the beam exiting through to the other side, the weaker or more porous the bones.

This test has been standardized, so that scientists know how much the beam is reduced by healthy bones and by bones that suffer from various degrees of osteoporosis. BMD is then expressed in relation to reference data known as "standard deviation scores." These scores represent the density of the bone being testing compared with reference values—usually the bones of young adult women. Standard deviation (SD) scores range from strong, healthy bones, which get a 1, to low bone mass—a condition known as *osteopenia*—with scores that range from −1 to −2.5. Bones that receive a score of −2.5 indicate osteoporosis. A person is said to have severe osteoporosis when they score a −2.5 and have a history of fractures from nonviolent trauma. Women in the lowest BMD group (those with scores of −2.5) have 8.5 times the risk of fracture compared with those in the highest density group (women with BMD scores of 1). A woman with a low BMD and a history of just one fracture is extremely likely to have another fracture. In fact, her risk is about twenty-five times higher than that of the woman with a higher BMD who has not had any fractures.

For most women, the best age for the BMD test is anytime between sixty and sixty-five. At this point, there are still ten to fifteen years before a woman is likely to suffer a serious fracture and still plenty of time to allow treatment, if necessary, to restore lost bone.

Many women, concerned about osteoporosis, wonder if they shouldn't start hormone replacement therapy immediately after menopause to protect themselves against the disorder, as opposed to starting later in life, say around the age of sixty. Research has shown that it doesn't make any difference on bone strength. A study in the February 1997 issue of the *Journal of the American Medical Association* found no significant difference in bone mineral density at any site between women who started estrogen therapy at menopause and those who started after sixty years of age.

Jean Parker, age thirty-two, came to my clinic at St. Helena Hospital in 1992 with elevated cholesterol, frequent headaches, and mild arthritis; all problems easily solved by a change in her diet. She had one other concern that was not so readily fixed. Several months back she had her bone density tested at her local shopping mall and the results suggested severe bone loss. Further testing by her personal physician confirmed results of −2.5 SD that put her in the "fracture zone." The diagnosis of osteoporosis was particularly disturbing to her because she had been exercising for years and trying to eat healthy (mostly chicken and fish—no red meat).

Since she was still menstruating and had a family history of breast cancer her doctor decided to forgo a recommendation of hormone replacement therapy and instead prescribed Fosamax. After reading the side effects and refusing to believe someone as young and healthy as she was could possibly have a serious disease, she decided to postpone treatment.

I told her that the BMD test was just one of the many bits of information used to help determine the need for treatment, and was only a comparison of her results with those of many younger women. The results could not tell her individual risk of fracture or if she was actually losing bone. Her BMD test may have always been less than the "golden standard," and at her age she almost certainly had perfectly healthy, strong bones. My recommendation was for her to continue her exercise, eat a lower-protein diet (no chicken and fish), and not take any medication. Because she needed reassurance I also suggested she repeat the BMD test. The next year's results were the same, and so were those of the following year. Fortunately, in Jean's case the common tendency in medicine is to treat test results rather than the patient.

BONE-MEASURING MACHINES

When it comes to measuring bone mineral density, any skeletal site—heel, wrist, hip, vertebrae—is equally useful for making the diagnosis of osteoporosis or osteopenia. Still, it's a good idea to measure the actual site of a potential risk, especially if it involves the hip or spine. Such measurements will provide the clearest and most accurate indicators for the potential risk of suffering a fracture in one of these important sites.

There are a variety of methods for assessing bone density, and all of them produce reliable results. BMD testing can be obtained at your local hospital with a doctor's prescription. Very often, the test can also be obtained without a prescription at many local shopping centers or malls. Here are the most commonly used tests.

Dual Energy X-ray Absorptiometry

The most popular method for measuring bone mineral density, dual energy X-ray absorptiometry, not only is very precise but also allows doctors to determine very small changes in bone density. The test uses two photon beams of different energies; the comparison between how these beams are affected by bone and soft tissue allows doctors to make more accurate estimates of BMD. For this reason, dual energy X-ray absorptiometry is the most common tool used to assess both the spine and the limbs. The test uses a low dose of radiation—about 20 percent of the dose used for a chest X ray—and the results taken over time, and for many different patients, are highly consistent. The test requires about ten to fifteen minutes to take and costs between $100 and $200.

Single Energy X-ray Absorptiometry

Single energy X-ray absorptiometry is used to measure only the limbs, and most often the forearm. The machines are portable and less expensive, the results are highly consistent, and the radiation dose used is very low.

Quantitative Computer Tomography

This test uses a CAT scan machine to more clearly identify individual bones. The equipment is expensive and the radiation dose is relatively high. Results are also less consistent and reproducible. Also, the machine can measure only the wrist and spine; it does not test the hip.

Broadband Ultrasound

Broadband ultrasound transmits sound waves through bones to determine their relative density. It is accurate and radiation free; the machines are cheap and portable. Unlike the other tests, ultrasound provides additional information about the quality of the bone and strength.

MEASURING THE RATE OF BONE RESORPTION

Besides knowing the mineral density of your bones, you and your doctor may also want to know the rate at which resorption is taking place in your bones—or how rapidly you are losing bone mass. Such bone turnover speeds up at menopause and peaks between one and three years after cessation of ovarian function. Once resorption peaks, it gradually slows over the next eight to ten years, which means that your loss of bone is also slowing.

The rate at which resorption is taking place can be detected directly if you undergo a bone biopsy, which removes a small amount of bone tissue that is then examined under a microscope by a pathologist. Such a test is painful and invasive, which, of course, makes it unattractive.

However, the rate of bone resorption can be measured indirectly by determining the quantities of particular substances released from the bones during resorption. One substance commonly measured is a by-product of bone collagen called deoxypyridinoline crosslinks (also called Pyrilinks-D, or simply crosslinks). After release from the bones it makes its way into your blood and eventually into your urine. These crosslinks increase significantly after menopause, indicating increased resorption, and return to premenopausal levels within a few months of hormone replacement therapy, indicating stabilization of bone turnover.

The test, which is highly accurate, is the single most effective method of monitoring short-term changes in bone metabolism. It is noninvasive and easy to take. You can order the deoxypyridinoline crosslinks (Pyrilinks-D) test for about $80 without a doctor's prescription by calling Aeron LifeCycles at (800) 631-7900.

Combining BMD and Crosslinks

Even though this crosslinks test yields important additional information, most doctors do not use the test because they believe that BMD provides all the information they need to determine if treatment is necessary. I believe the combination of both tests can be helpful in determining whether or not you need treatment. Anyone concerned about osteoporosis wants to know how strong her bones are, and what is the likelihood that she will suffer a fracture in the future. BMD testing alone can tell you a lot about the present condition of your bones.

Urinary deoxypyridinoline crosslinks can tell you about the present rate of bone turnover, which can be used to extrapolate how rapidly you are losing bone. Combined, these tests can help predict the future. A recent twelve-year study found that women classified as "fast losers" of bone, based on urinary crosslinks testing, lost 50 percent more bone than slow losers. In that instance, a combination of a low bone mineral density and high levels of crosslinks provides strong evidence of need for treatment.

Another study looking at the use of crosslinks testing predicted which women would respond to the hormone calcitonin. Those with high bone turnover, based on crosslinks testing, showed a significant increase of bone in the spine after one year of therapy, whereas no increase was seen with the same therapy in the low bone turnover group.

Concerns About BMD Testing

Medical tests offer your doctor vital information about your health that he or she needs to provide you with the right form of therapy. In the best of all possible worlds, tests should be performed only on people with symptoms of illness, and only those tests that are essential should be done.

However, to put things bluntly, BMD testing has become big business. The more people you test, the more you can treat, which means profits all around. Manufacturers of BMD testing equipment are in business to make money. Medical doctors, clinics, and hospitals that own BMD testing equipment have made an investment for which they want a return. Thus, more and more women are being tested for bone mineral density, even those who are healthy and have no other risk factors for osteoporosis.

As more women are tested, more women are treated with drug therapy. That means profit potential for the pharmaceutical companies that make the drugs to treat osteoporosis. In fact, the biggest promoters of BMD testing are the drug companies. As with so many other forms of medical technology, BMD testing—an inherently useful and valuable tool—has been overused because it can generate profits.

The truth is, BMD is only one of many risk factors that can predict an osteoporosis-related fracture in women; others with similar predictive value include a history of maternal hip fracture, weight loss since age twenty-five, and the habit of standing for less than four hours a day—data easy to obtain without expensive testing. Interestingly, many doctors are beginning to question not only the testing but also the use of drugs to treat osteoporosis.

Dr. Deborah Marshall of the Swedish Council of Technological Assessment in Health Care wrote in the August 31, 1996, issue of the *Lancet:* "There are no data from controlled clinical trials about the consequences of screening by measuring BMD in terms of fractures averted, although trials are in progress in Britain and Sweden. Furthermore, it is not enough to identify individuals correctly as being at high risk: one must be able to treat those identified with effective treatments. There are currently too many unanswered questions about available treatments—including their effectiveness in terms of preventing fractures, compliance rates, and the loss of benefit after treatment is stopped—to justify endorsing a screening programme."

Like most physicians, I believe that estrogen therapy is effective at strengthening bones and preventing fractures, but too few of us recognize that there is very little hard scientific evidence proving the effectiveness of the therapy. The many unanswered questions that remain should encourage every doctor to be cautious when it comes to prescribing hormone replacement therapy. Patients need to be examined and screened carefully; they must also be educated about the side effects related to the drugs. Finally, they should be given the tools for strengthening their own health and preventing disease, including further deterioration of their bones.

As one writer put it in a 1997 issue of the *British Medical Journal,* "Until results of the first randomized study primarily investigating the protective ability and the detrimental effects of hormone replacement therapy, one should be cautious about suggesting the use of hormone replacement therapy for women without symptoms of estrogen deficiency."

The case for screening large numbers of healthy women at menopause is not strong, and the consensus view is that population-based screening cannot be justified at present. A related grave concern for our health-cost-conscious country is that it would cost $6 billion to "screen" every woman in the United States near menopause for BMD. Health care providers interested in cost effectiveness are thus locked in combat against those purely interested in the potential profits of such "preventive" medicine.

Guidelines for Appropriate BMD Testing

When should BMD testing be done? I believe that assessment of bone mass is most justified in those cases in which results obtained will influence decisions about the treatment, and for monitoring bone loss caused by disease. Here are my guidelines for the use of BMD testing.

When to Use BMD Testing

- To determine whether hormone replacement therapy (HRT) or other therapy may be indicated for a woman who has lost her ovaries at a young age.
- To determine the amount of bone damage that has occurred and whether treatment, such as surgery, needs to be done for a person with long-standing hyperthyroidism or hyperparathyroidism.
- To determine whether the steroid dose should be reduced for a person on corticosteroid therapy because of bone loss.
- To determine whether a fracture was likely due to bone loss (low BMD).
- To determine whether spine deformity is due to bone loss (low BMD).
- To motivate patients (or to help them decide) to accept, or to continue with, a therapy.

When Not to Use BMD Testing

- To determine whether someone who is already known to have osteoporosis is in need of treatment. For example, a seventy-five-year-old woman with a history of spinal fractures or loss of height would be adequately diagnosed from her history alone and would warrant aggressive treatment. BMD would add no useful information for management of her disease.
- To diagnose someone at a very low risk of fracture, such as a thirty-five-year-old woman who is concerned about osteoporosis, but has no history of unusual fractures and is otherwise healthy. In such a case, BMD would be a waste of money; it would only add to her worry; and it would not be the basis for any treatment, regardless of the findings, because nonviolent fracture is so unusual in someone this young. In the worst case, the test might encourage her doctor to place her on a lifetime of expensive and potentially toxic drug therapy.
- To determine the outcome of treatment that is known to work. Frequent monitoring is routinely recommended to determine the effect of bone-building drugs like estrogen (HRT), bisphosphonates (Fosamax), and calcitonin (Miacalcin). This doesn't make sense, since these drugs have almost always been demonstrated to work: 97 percent of the time Fosamax increases BMD and 95 percent of the time HRT increases BMD. Any variance seen would more likely reflect machine error than actual changes in bone.

Consideration must be given to the potential risks and harms of screening, including anxiety and distress, job discrimination, inability to obtain health and life insurance, and dependency on medications with serious side effects.

Treatments for Bone Loss

All drugs have adverse side effects, though some have more than others. Do not make a hasty decision to begin drug therapy, because these treatments will likely continue for the rest of your life.

I highly recommend that women who decide to begin drug therapy also adopt the McDougall Program, because it will reduce their risk of cancers of the breast and uterus and gallbladder disease—all of which are side effects of estrogen therapy.

HORMONE REPLACEMENT THERAPY

Hormone replacement therapy (HRT) does prevent further deterioration of bones and very often replaces lost bone in women with osteoporosis. The November 6, 1996, issue of the *Journal of the American Medical Association* published the results of the Postmenopausal Estrogen/Progestin Interventions Trial, in which two groups of women were compared—one was given HRT and another was given a placebo. Both groups were followed for three years. At the conclusion of that period, the women who were given the placebo lost 1.8 percent of their spine's bone mineral density, and 1.7 percent of their hip BMD. Those on estrogen alone, or on a combination of estrogen and progestin (Provera), gained about 3 to 5 percent BMD in the spine and 1.7 percent in the hip. Other studies have shown that estrogen replacement therapy for six years or more leads to BMD values 10 percent higher than those of untreated women, and reduces the risk of hip and other fractures by about 50 percent. But there *are* potential side effects, including cancer (see chapter 13).

DESIGNER ESTROGENS

An optimal hormone replacement therapy would retain the benefits of estrogen while being free of the adverse side effects. Drugs have been designed to specifically effect different tissues in different ways. The first such successful "designer drug" was the antiestrogen tamoxifen used for the treatment of breast cancer for the past two decades.

This drug suppresses breast cancer, but increases hot flashes. In addition to its antiestrogen effects, it also has estrogen stimulating effects on the uterus, bones, and LDL (bad) cholesterol, resulting in more endometrial cancer, but stronger bones and lower cholesterol.

Recently a new designer drug, raloxifene (Evista), was introduced to the market, which does not stimulate the uterus and may not stimulate the breasts. Breast tenderness is not a side effect, and an increase in breast and uterine cancer, as seen with estrogen, is not expected. The positive effects on bone density are about half those of estrogen. LDL cholesterol is lowered as much by raloxifene as by estrogen, but other heart disease preventing factors are improved much less by raloxifene. Only one of three trials has shown a reduction in heart disease with raloxifene. Like estrogen and tamoxifen, raloxifene increases the risk of blood clots. Leg pain and hot flashes are also increased over placebo. Raloxifene does not decrease the ovary's production of estrogen, and premenopausal women who take raloxifene will continue to ovulate and therefore may become pregnant. The drug can harm the unborn fetus.

Overall, raloxifene's major benefit of not stimulating the uterus may help a few women; however, this is offset by the fact that it probably does not reduce the risk of heart disease. Side effects are fewer, which will improve compliance. Many women use estrogen for strengthening and moisturizing their vaginal tissues. Raloxifene does not appear to offer these benefits. The long-term safety and effectiveness of the drug has not be established, and direct comparisons with other drugs are still lacking. The dosage of raloxifene is 60 mg a day and a thirty-tablet bottle costs about sixty dollars.

BISPHOSPHONATES

Bisphosphonates, such as Fosamax, prevent bone mineral loss and even replace lost bone. In one study, 994 postmenopausal women with osteoporosis were treated with Fosamax or a placebo. Those receiving the drug showed progressive increases in BMD at all skeletal sites, whereas those receiving the placebo lost bone. The difference between the two groups was 8.8 percent in the spine and 5.9 percent in the hip. The findings also measured a 48 percent reduction in spinal fractures and a reduced loss of height in the women taking the drug. However, no significant difference was found in the number of other (nonvertebral) fractures between the treated and placebo groups.

Among the most commonly reported side effects of bisphosphonate treatment are abdominal pain, muscle pain, nausea, esophagus and stomach irritation, constipation, and diarrhea.

CALCITONIN

Calcitonin is a hormone produced by the thyroid glands of mammals, but similar substances have been found in birds, fish, fungi, and bacteria. Calcitonin inhibits the activity of cells involved in bone resorption. Because it is digested in the intestines, the medication must be given by injection or by nasal spray. Patients with fast bone turnover rates seem to benefit most from taking this drug. Long-term calcitonin treatment results in measurable increases in BMD of the spine and hip; it has also been shown to reduce the number of fractures at both sides.

Calcitonin also appears to decrease bone pain, reduce the amount of time patients are confined to their beds, and reduce the use of pain medication by patients with fractures. So far, it appears to be safe and is seen as having no long-term side effects.

Calcium supplements have been shown to be of value in some studies; however, their actual benefits are much less than advertised. Because taking calcium has so few side effects, you may want to add this mineral to your treatment program as a supplement. (There are some problems with taking calcium supplements—see chapter 11. Remember not to get your calcium from dairy products because of the serious health hazards—see chapter 2.) Other highly promoted treatments, like vitamin D and fluoride, are of questionable benefit, and fluoride has severe side effects. Therefore, these two treatments should be avoided.

DIET AND EXERCISE

You should adopt a very low animal protein diet, because meat, poultry, fish, and eggs are the biggest causes of bone loss. The benefits of following the McDougall Program range far beyond the health of your skeleton—it will also dramatically lower your risk of heart disease and cancer—but that benefit alone should be enough to get many people to change what they eat.

Start an exercise regimen. In adults, physical activity has been shown to increase or maintain BMD at the site of greatest physical force and to reduce fracture risk. Most studies also indicate that magnitude of force is actually more important than frequency of exercise. Therefore, walk daily and do some other mild, weight-bearing aerobic exercise, such as aerobic dancing. Training with light weights is an ideal supplement to a bone-strengthening program.

The benefits of a healthy diet and exercise program extend well beyond the issues related to a specific illness or disorder. They enhance your entire life.

CHAPTER 13

Balancing the Positives and Negatives of Hormone Replacement Therapy

Susan Cole of Denver, Colorado, had been expecting some mild night sweats and occasional hot flashes when she entered menopause at the age of fifty, but she never expected both symptoms to be so intense. "My hot flashes were like someone plugged me into an electrical outlet," she said. "Suddenly, I got this surge of intense heat. These episodes appeared randomly, too, which really bothered me. Out of nowhere, boom, I'd get a hot flash." Not only were the hot flashes intense, but they were frequent: Susan got between ten and fifteen hot flashes per day. She also would sweat profusely at night. "For a while I was soaking my nightgown." Finally, her doctor recommended hormone replacement therapy (HRT). The hormones have been shown to significantly increase the risk of breast cancer. Susan worried that the drugs would act as a catalyst for the onset of cancer, especially since she had a history of fibrocystic breast disease.

Because she had always believed that diet played a major role in her health, Susan decided to change her way of eating. At that point, she had been avoiding red meat, but was still eating eggs and lots of dairy products, especially cheese. Thus, even though she had given up red meat, her diet was still rich in animal protein and fat. Perhaps a change in diet might reduce the severity of her menopausal symptoms, she thought. In 1995, she found my book *The McDougall Program—Twelve Days to Dynamic Health* and adopted the diet.

"I began to feel better within the first week of adopting Dr. McDougall's diet," she said. "My hot flashes and night sweats were reduced by about

90 percent. They were also less frequent. My symptoms were so mild that I decided that this was manageable."

They were manageable as long as she remained on the diet, Susan said. "I realized that my symptoms became more intense when I went off the diet. Every time I ate a high-fat or high–animal protein food, I'd have far more intense symptoms the next day. But as long as I stay on the diet, I feel great."

Women approach menopause today as if it were a dangerous road hazard, a place where life goes out of control and painful experiences are not only unavoidable but anticipated. Menopause arrives on its own timetable and forces each woman to provide answers to serious, even life-altering, questions: Will I need hormone replacement therapy (HRT)? Will the drugs' benefits outweigh their potential side effects? If I avoid HRT, will I suffer a premature heart attack or osteoporosis? Will I have to endure nerve-racking night sweats or debilitating depression? How will I cope with these changes?

The good news is that menopause is a normal, natural stage of life, through which women have been passing without the aid of doctors and pharmaceutical companies for several million years. Women today can experience a relatively mild menopause simply by adopting a diet and lifestyle that lead to a more balanced hormonal condition. If HRT is needed, a healthy diet and lifestyle will mitigate the illness-producing side effects of the drugs.

This chapter offers you a balanced perspective and shows you how you can use diet, exercise, HRT when necessary, and herbal remedies to navigate the challenges and overcome the symptoms of menopause with the fewest possible side effects.

What Is Menopause?

In the largest sense, menopause means the end of childbearing, but it specifically refers to the final period, or the end of menstrual bleeding. Menopause occurs when the ovaries stop producing eggs and dramatically reduce their production of the female hormones estrogen and progesterone. Many women experience a gradual reduction of these hormones, which is why menopause is often experienced as a transition period rather than an abrupt change in a woman's life. That transition, which for some women can last as long as ten years, is usually referred to as perimenopause.

The change in a woman's hormone levels at menopause is dramatic and involves estrogen, progesterone, and many types of male hormones, called androgens. These hormones are created not only by the ovaries but also by other tissues in a woman's body, including fat cells. This is why estrogen continues to be produced by the body even after the ovaries reduce their production of the hormone after menopause.

The primary function of estrogen is to promote the development of a young girl into a woman. The hormone stimulates the growth of her uterus, vagina, and breasts and maintains these tissues throughout her life.

There are three types of estrogen: *estradiol,* which is the most potent form of estrogen; *estrone,* the principal hormone present in women after menopause; and *estriol,* the weakest of the three, and the one most active during pregnancy.

Progesterone is called the pregnancy hormone because it prepares the uterus for the implantation of the fertilized egg. Progesterone is produced after ovulation by the developed egg follicle, known as the corpus luteum. Although small amounts are made by the adrenal glands, the production of progesterone essentially ends at the time of menopause.

While estrogen levels fall off dramatically at menopause, and the production of progesterone all but stops, the male hormone, testosterone, continues to be produced at premenopausal levels for at least ten years after menopause. That means that testosterone now makes up a greater percentage of a woman's hormonal balance. As you may know, testosterone is responsible for stimulating sexual desire, which is why many women actually enjoy sex more after menopause. This fact also puts an end to the age-old myth that women somehow are less sexually alive after menopause. Although testosterone levels may increase, those other male hormones, which are at their highest levels during a woman's reproductive years, are reduced after menopause.

Once a woman passes through menopause, these powerful estrogen hormones do not stimulate the hormone-sensitive organs—the breast, the uterus, and the ovaries—as much. That's good, since the overstimulation of these organs can lead to disorders including uterine fibroids, fibrocystic breast disease, and cancer. This also explains why uterine fibroids and fibrocystic breast disease naturally regress and usually disappear after menopause (unless you use estrogen).

Your estrogen levels and the amounts of fat and fiber in your diet will determine when you experience menopause. Women who eat a high-fat, low-fiber diet or are overweight typically experience menopause much later in life, on the average between the ages of fifty and fifty-one, while those who are lean and on low-fat, high-fiber diets usually experience menopause about two years earlier. About 10 percent of women enter menopause before the age of thirty-eight; another 30 percent before forty-four. By the age of sixty, virtually all women have passed through menopause. Alcohol consumption raises estrogen levels and delays menopause, while exercise and cigarette smoking reduce estrogen levels and bring about an earlier menopause.

SIGNS AND SYMPTOMS OF MENOPAUSE

I have found that virtually all of the common symptoms associated with menopause are either reduced or exacerbated by diet and lifestyle. Therefore, menopausal symptoms vary tremendously among women, depending on the kinds of foods they eat and how they live each day.

The most common menopausal symptoms include hot flashes, thinning of the genital tissues, vaginal dryness, pain with intercourse, loss of muscle mass and tone, fatigue, insomnia, and night sweats. Hot flashes occur in about 75 percent of menopausal women who eat a Western diet. For more than half of these women, the hot flashes will last less than two years, and most will only experience them once or twice a day. Between 15 and 20 percent will be forced to endure them for more than five years. A study reported in the June 1987 issue of the *Journal of Behavioral Medicine* showed that stress was also a factor in the frequency and endurance of hot flashes. Many women find that the use of alcohol, which dilates blood vessels, makes hot flashes more intense.

Other menopausal symptoms include an increase in anxiety or nervousness, irritability, forgetfulness, and bouts of depression. Actually, depression as a symptom of menopause is not as common as many women believe. Research has shown that premenopausal women are far more likely to suffer from severe bouts of depression that require hospitalization than women who are in the throes of menopause.

Many women gain weight during and after menopause. The increase in weight appears to be the result of a decrease in physical activity, as well as a decrease in the amount of energy, or calories, burned during rest. Some may notice a decrease in scalp, pubic, and auxiliary hair. After menopause, thinner skin, a decrease in the size of the breasts and uterus, and various degrees of osteoporosis are commonly noted.

Natural Treatments for Menopause

Overall health affects every aspect of life. Therefore, it shouldn't be surprising that it also can determine the kind of menopause you experience. Women who are lean, exercise regularly, and eat a nutritious, starch-based diet experience significantly milder menopausal symptoms. The exercise can be as simple as a daily walk of two miles, or at least twenty to thirty minutes. Many women experience more intense hot flashes when they exercise vigorously, but when they walk to burn calories and maintain a low body weight, their menopausal symptoms are reduced.

There may be no better natural treatment for menopause than a healthy diet, however. Japanese women who live in Japan and eat the traditional Japanese diet composed chiefly of rice, vegetables, and soybean products rarely complain of unpleasant menopausal symptoms. As one author noted in the *Journal of the American Medical Association:* "There appears to be no 'midlife crisis' for the majority of Japanese women, who regard the end of menstruation as one small part of a normal mid-life transition associated simply with aging, which few women approach with dread." In fact, hot flashes are so rare among Japanese women who live in Japan that there is no word in their language to

---

SIGNS AND SYMPTOMS OF MENOPAUSE

Vagina
- Painful intercourse
- Bloodstained discharge
- Itching
- Smaller size

Bladder
- Increase in frequency and/or urgency of urination
- Stress incontinence
- Bacteriuria

Uterus
- Uterine prolapse

Skeleton
- Fractures

Breasts
- Reduced size
- Drooping

Skin
- Dryness and/or itching
- Easily injured
- Hair loss
- Facial hair
- Dry mouth

Heart
- Coronary disease
- Elevated cholesterol

Psychological disturbances
- Hot flashes
- Anxiety
- Depression
- Insomnia
- Altered libido

describe them. Unfortunately, such immunity does not exist for women who eat a diet higher in fat and lower in fiber, even if they are Japanese.

There are reasons why a healthy diet and lifestyle are associated with mild menopausal symptoms. A plant-based diet is low in fat, which means that it will promote ideal body weight and a balanced hormonal environment. It is also rich in plant foods, which contain an abundance of phytoestrogens, a much milder form of estrogen, one that promotes cellular health. Every cell in the body has within it estrogen receptor sites where the estrogen molecules bind and produce their activity. Phytoestrogens also bind to the cell's estrogen receptor sites, thereby blocking the activity of the more powerful, disease-causing estrogens produced by your own body.

Phytoestrogens have other beneficial activities, including boosting immune function and fighting cancer. Laboratory tests have shown that phytoestrogens directly inhibit the growth of human breast cancer cells. Other research has demonstrated that when women are given daily doses of 60 grams of soy protein, which is a rich source of phytoestrogens, their hormonal balance changes to one that is less favorable to the development of breast cancer.

Because most plant foods contain phytoestrogens, vegetarians have been shown to have much higher levels of these substances than meat eaters. When researchers compared the phytoestrogen levels of three groups of women—those who followed a macrobiotic diet (very similar to the McDougall diet), lacto-ovo-vegetarians, and meat eaters—they found that those who ate a macrobiotic diet had by far the highest levels of phytoestrogens; not surprisingly, meat eaters had the lowest.

Other research supports these findings. Scientists compared the respective quantities of three phytoestrogens—genistein, daidzein, and equol—excreted in the urine by Japanese and Finnish women. The Japanese women were found to have sixty to one hundred times higher levels of these powerful health-promoting chemicals in their urine than the Finnish women.

Among the foods with the highest concentrations of phytoestrogens are soy products, such as tofu, tempeh, and miso. Boiled beans of any kind are also abundant sources of these protective chemicals. They are also plentiful in most other unrefined plant foods, including whole grains, seeds, berries, and nuts. In addition, plant foods contain an abundance of other compounds that support a woman's hormonal balance, her hormone-sensitive organs, and her overall health. And as you would expect, studies show that vegetarians have much higher levels of these protective chemicals than do meat eaters.

The McDougall Program emphasizes a broad approach to menopause, starting with a nutritious, starch-based diet, which is the foundation of good health. Women should be active and walk twenty to thirty minutes at least four to five times per week. If you decide to take hormone replacement therapy to alleviate your menopausal symptoms, I encourage you to adopt the McDougall Program as well. Many women take HRT to reduce the severity of their symptoms and don't make any changes in their diets and lifestyle; however, HRT carries significant risks. A woman who eats a nutritious, starch-based diet and gets regular exercise reduces those risks and, at the same time, improves the quality of her life.

Hormone Replacement Therapy

Hormone replacement therapy can benefit many menopausal women, especially if they are experiencing unpleasant symptoms that detract from the quality of their lives. HRT can relieve hot flashes and prevent thinning and drying of the vaginal tissues. It measurably reduces the risk of osteoporosis and its resulting bone fractures. Certain forms of HRT may lower cholesterol and protect against heart attack and stroke. However, a significant amount of the reduction seen in heart disease is due to the fact that women who use HRT have healthier lifestyles rather than the hormone itself.

Taking these drugs involves significant risks. HRT increases your risks of gallbladder disease and breast and uterine cancer. A less threatening but nonetheless distressing side effect for many women is the resumption of monthly menstrual periods. To date, only 20 to 30 percent of all menopausal women actually begin HRT, and of those who do, about half stop the drugs shortly after starting. The most common reasons for ceasing the therapy include the fear of cancer and a lack of any perceived benefits from the drugs.

There are many forms of HRT and not all of them are appropriate for every woman. If you decide to begin HRT, you must choose the form that best suits your needs and particular condition. You should also monitor yourself consistently to determine if HRT is having the desired effects, and whether or not you continue to need the drugs. Menopausal symptoms, such as hot flashes, have a limited duration—they will pass naturally. Many physicians, in their enthusiasm for these drugs, simply prescribe the most popular forms of HRT and expect the woman to remain on them indefinitely. If you are taking HRT to relieve menopausal symptoms, you may eventually give up the hormones, but *you* must be the one to determine when to stop HRT. Hormones should be used to improve the quality of your life. If you are feeling good already, leave well enough alone.

PRETREATMENT EVALUATION

Before beginning HRT you should have a complete history and physical examination. Your breasts should be checked for possible tumors by physical examination and a mammogram. These tests are necessary to rule out the possibility that hormone therapy may stimulate the growth of breast cancer.

A vaginal exam should be performed to determine whether or not you suffer from fibroid tumors, which may be encouraged to grow even larger with the use of HRT. A Pap smear and a biopsy of the endometrium should be performed to check for existing cancer. You should tell your doctor immediately if you experience any severe or unusual bleeding while taking HRT. If such bleeding occurs, you should probably have your doctor perform a biopsy of the inside lining of the uterus.

Though there are numerous forms of HRT, there are no agreed-upon clinical or laboratory tests to determine which form will be most effective for you. Many doctors will measure the estradiol levels in your blood or saliva in order to guide them in their recommendations.

The amount and type of estrogen needed varies greatly among patients. Reduction of hot flashes and improvement in vaginal symptoms are the most reliable indications that the treatment is correct.

WHEN HRT IS NOT RECOMMENDED

You should not consider HRT if you have (or have a history of) the following:

    Known or suspected pregnancy
    Cancer of the breast or uterus
    Known or suspected estrogen-dependent cancers
    Acute liver disease
    Active thrombophlebitis or thromboembolic disorders
    Undiagnosed genital bleeding
    Hypersensitivity to hormones

HORMONE PILLS

The pill form of HRT, taken orally, is the most popular way of administering the drugs. Oral estrogen appears to slow the body's rate of fat burning and consequently tends to increase body fat, so many women experience weight gain when they take estrogen therapy. Estrogen therapy also increases the risk of gallbladder disease by 2.5 times. Dosages depend on the kind of medication prescribed. When the prescribed dose is too high, you will likely experience headaches, nausea, vaginal bleeding, and breast swelling and tenderness.

Taking estrogen alone significantly increases the risk of uterine cancer. Women who have had a hysterectomy usually receive estrogen therapy alone—for all or part of each month. Women who still have a uterus take estrogen plus progestin, which mitigates the cancer-causing effects of estrogen on the uterus. (Progestin is a term used to describe natural or synthetic chemicals that cause some or all of the same biological changes produced by the hormone progesterone.)

The belief that progestin will completely reverse the cancer-causing effects of estrogen on the uterus is a myth that is promoted by most doctors; it is not supported by the scientific literature. Women who use estrogen with synthetic progestin for more than five years have an increased risk of contracting endometrial or uterine cancer compared with those who do not undergo HRT, according to a study published in the February 15, 1997, issue of the *Lancet*. The degree of that risk varies depending on how often progestin is used each month. For women who use the synthetic progestin less than ten days per month, the risk of contracting uterine cancer was 3.1 times greater than that for women who do not take either hormone. For those who take progestin between ten and twenty-one days per month, the risk was 2.5 times greater than for those who do not take the hormones.

Still, if estrogen is given, the best approach is to take progestin, too. The study found that women who took estrogen alone, without the progestin, were four times more likely to have uterine cancer. The risk of endometrial cancer is reduced by progestins, but there is still a substantial risk of contracting cancer.

CHOOSING CYCLIC OR SUSTAINED THERAPY

Sequential Therapy

Estrogen and progestin are given in two ways. The first is called *sequential* therapy, which has the woman taking estrogen each day for the entire month and then adding progestin for the last ten days or two weeks. The second is called *continuous* therapy, which has the woman taking both hormones each day of the entire month.

For women with a uterus, sequential therapy is the most common way to prescribe estrogen and progestins. However, these women often experience menstrual periods while on this form of therapy. Although some women prefer to continue having periods, most do not. Therefore, most women will choose continuous therapy.

Although progestin reduces the risk of endometrial cancer, it does not reduce your chances of contracting breast cancer. In fact, studies suggest that synthetic progestin, known as medroxyprogesterone (Provera), may actually increase the risk of breast cancer. This form also has an adverse effect on blood cholesterol and triglyceride levels.

Continuous Therapy

Continuous therapy is becoming more popular because it eliminates the common side effect of a monthly period that occurs with sequential therapy. However, the long-term effects of continuous therapy are still largely unknown. Normally, a woman's hormone levels rise and fall each month according to the natural rhythms of her body and her environment. With continuous therapy, which sustains the same hormone levels throughout the month, doctors have dramatically changed this cycling or rhythmic activity. No one knows what effect that will have on the body, but I am concerned that the unnatural hormone environment created by continuous hormones, especially when it is maintained for years, will have a significant and adverse effect on health.

TRANSDERMAL ESTROGEN PATCHES

When hormones are taken by mouth, they are absorbed by the intestines and taken by the bloodstream directly to the liver where they are metabolized. Most of the hormone is removed and the remaining amount may be chemically changed. Therefore, it is hard to tell what the effects of a given dose of hormone will be when given by mouth.

Transdermal estrogen patches allow the hormone to enter the body through the skin, which avoids initial removal of the hormone by the liver. Without the liver's involvement, one of the major benefits of HRT is lost—namely, the improvement in blood cholesterol levels. When HRT is taken orally, the drugs trigger the liver to raise HDL, the "good" cholesterol, and lower the "bad" LDL. This does not occur when the drugs do not pass through the liver. This fact is relatively unimportant for those of us who know that diet and exercise are the real keys to a healthy heart.

On the positive side, the skin patch does not raise the levels of blood fats, or triglycerides, which, when elevated, can increase the risk of cardiovascular disease. Women using the patch also avoid the weight gain associated with taking oral estrogen.

TRANSDERMAL GELS AND CREAMS

Transdermal gels and creams are made up by a pharmacist for the specific needs of the woman and provide the same advantages as the patches. Estradiol is added to a cream or gel base. The usual dose is 0.05 to 0.1 mg in 1 gm of cream base (measured in a syringe or spoon and applied to the skin). The gel base breaks down slowly on the skin and therefore is more gradually absorbed into the system throughout the day than the cream.

VAGINAL ESTROGEN CREAMS

Application of estrogen directly to the vaginal tissues is particularly effective at preventing the atrophy, or thinning, of the vagina; it also helps to rebuild these tissues, which relieves stress incontinence in about 50 percent of women and prevents inflammation of the urethra, the tube that carries urine from the bladder to the opening near the vagina, thereby aiding in preventing recurrent bladder infections.

If you are using the drugs specifically to improve the strength of your vaginal tissues, low doses will do just fine. As little as 0.3 mg of conjugated estrogen will strengthen the vaginal tissues. There are conjugated estrogens (Premarin, 0.625 mg/gram) and synthetic estradiol vaginal creams (Estrace, 0.1 mg per gram). Half a gram daily used two to four times a week will usually be enough to improve the strength of the vagina and surrounding tissues.

ULTRALOW-DOSE ESTROGEN THERAPY

Very low doses of estrogen applied to the skin or vaginal tissues can have a very positive benefit on bone health. One recent study found as little as 7.5 micrograms (mcg) of estradiol administered through the vaginal tissues resulted in a 2.1 percent increase in forearm bone density compared to a 2.7 percent loss in nonusers. Furthermore, no proliferation of the endometrium, as measured by ultrasound, was found after six months, suggesting no increase in risk of uterine cancer from this small dose. The dose I currently recommend to use as a cream applied to the vagina or skin is 50 mcg (.05 mg). This is very small compared to the dose of 300, 625, or 1,250 mcg (0.3, 0.625 and 1.25 mg) often given by mouth. As we've discussed, estrogen given through the skin and vaginal tissues is much more effective and reliable than estrogen taken by mouth. Even though these ultralow doses appear to be effective for increasing bone strength and treating vaginal atrophy, larger doses may be necessary for treating hot flashes and other symptoms that detract from a woman's feeling of well-being. However, increasing the dose increases the risk of side effects and the risk of cancer. Further reduction in your exposure to estrogen can be accomplished by starting estrogens later in life. As I discussed in the last chapter, bone density is just as great for women who start estrogens at age sixty as those who start at menopause. I will probably reduce my recommended dose of estrogen in the future if the research continues to suggest lower doses are effective in relieving signs and symptoms of menopause.

PROGESTIN

Provera, a synthetic progestin, is available as pills to be taken orally, creams, and vaginal suppositories. Provera is not the same as progesterone, the natural hormone, and causes more adverse side effects than progesterone. Synthetic progestin raises triglycerides and lowers HDL cholesterol, while natural progesterone does not. Scientists believe that progestin acts synergistically with estradiol to increase the risk of breast cancer, while natural progesterone may lower the risk of breast cancer.

Progesterone reverses the precancerous changes in the uterus caused by estrogen. Doctors have been encouraged by a recent study showing that progesterone cream can reverse the precancerous changes in breast tissue caused by transdermal estrogen patches. If additional research supports these findings, then virtually all women (with or without a uterus) who are on estrogen replacement should also take natural progesterone.

In the future, physicians may argue that all women eating a rich Western diet should be using progesterone to help counteract some of the effects caused by the overabundance of estrogen produced by the diet and excess body fat. If that day should come, then doctors will certainly be recommending a change to a low-fat diet as well.

PROGESTERONE PILLS

Progesterone is prescribed to help offset the cancer-promoting side effects of estrogen on the endometrial tissues of the uterus. Doctors assess the cancer protection conveyed by progesterone by ultrasound tests or endometrial biopsy.

Natural progesterone, which is made from soybeans, is the same as the chemical made by a woman's ovary and conveys many of the health-promoting effects that a woman's own progesterone does. Taken as a pill in doses of 200 mg daily, natural progesterone can relieve many menopausal symptoms.

In fact, since the principal hormone lost at menopause is progesterone—there's usually sufficient estrogen still circulating in the body—restoring adequate progesterone levels is often the key to alleviating menopausal symptoms. For many women, this step alone relieves hot flashes and restores feelings of well-being. Studies indicate that progesterone reverses some of the adverse side effects of estrogen therapy, relieving breast tenderness and lumps associated with fibrocystic breast disease. Vaginal progesterone creams were found to relieve breast pain in 65 percent of menstruating women. Progesterone may also be beneficial for fibroids and endometriosis. Progesterone has bone-building benefits as well, but it does not prevent atrophy of the vaginal tissues.

When progesterone is taken orally, much of it is metabolized by the liver, which reduces the amount that reaches your tissues and other organs. Therefore, the effects of oral hormones vary. Breakthrough bleeding may be one sign that you're not taking enough progesterone.

PROGESTERONE CREAM

A recent study found that applying progesterone to the skin (a dose of 25 mg for ten to thirteen days) prevented estrogen-induced precancerous changes in the breast tissue of women. This form of progesterone is readily absorbed through the skin and passes to the hormone-sensitive organs via the blood. It is not initially metabolized by the liver. Your doctor can write a prescription for progesterone creams and gels. Normal doses range from 20 mg to 100 mg daily.

Many effective preparations can be bought without a prescription. For example, Pro-Gest cream can be purchased in natural foods stores or by telephoning (800) 888-6814 or (800) 888-6814. Using one ounce of this cream over a twenty-four-day period (20 mg/day) should prove effective at relieving menopausal symptoms and for helping to prevent many of the side effects of estrogen therapy. Premenopausal women who need more progesterone can use the cream from day twelve to day twenty-six of their menstrual cycle. This dose is approximately one-quarter teaspoon (2 cc) daily—a large dab on the tip of your finger—which you rub into a soft area of your skin (such as the abdomen or thigh). Preliminary research suggests that progesterone cream can also help rebuild bone lost to osteoporosis.

McDougall's HRT Recommendations

PROGESTERONE ONLY

For troublesome hot flashes, try an effective over-the-counter progesterone cream first. Many are ineffective because the progesterone content is too low, but the ones recommended in the list below should provide enough progesterone to have a positive effect. If these prove too weak, have your doctor write a prescription for a stronger cream or gel that offers 20 mg to 100 mg per dose, per day. Surprisingly, prescription creams are often less expensive than the over-the-counter varieties.

PROGESTERONE CREAMS

(Effective creams with more than 450 mg progesterone per ounce)

Product	Manufacturer
Angel Care	Angel Care USA
DermaGest	Broadmoore Labs
EssPro 7	Young Living
Fair Lady	Specialty Items
Femarone-17	Wise Essentials
Fem Creme	Pure Essence
Fem-Gest	Bio-Nutritional Formulas
Marpe	Green Pastures
NatraGest	Broadmoore Labs
ProDerma	Phillips Nutritionals
Progesta-Care	Life-Flo Health Care
Today's Man	Specialty Items
Wild Yam Cream with Progesterone	Wise Woman Essentials
Woman Wise Progesterone Max	Jason Natural Products
Yamcon (Pro) Extra	Phillips Nutritionals

Prepared by Aeron LifeCycles March 15, 1998

If you do not like to apply creams and gels, take progesterone orally each day, in pill form, in doses of 200 mg of micronized progesterone. This dose can be increased to 400 mg daily. However, because oral doses are metabolized by the liver before they reach your tissues, taking progesterone by mouth tends to be less effective than using a skin cream. Sustained-release formulations in pills can deliver a consistent dose of progesterone that is absorbed throughout the day.

ANDROGEN PILLS, CREAMS, AND GELS

Administering male hormones, or androgens, to women is not widely recommended by doctors. Possible adverse side effects include elevation of blood cholesterol levels and the development of male cosmetic features, such as the growth of facial hair (a condition referred to as virilizing). The notion of ingesting male hormones strikes many women as odd, at best, and downright repulsive, at worst, but in fact women make plenty of male hormones on their own.

A combination of estrogen and androgen has been helpful for relief of hot flashes. Androgens also seem to relieve estrogen-induced breast pain and seem to prevent bone loss. The best known and frequently the most desired effect of androgen therapy is an improved sexual appetite, though this should not be expected.

A dose of synthetic methyltestosterone of 2.5 mg per day is commonly prescribed by doctors. However, this synthetic form has many more serious side effects than natural testosterone. Methyltestosterone is toxic to the liver (it has been shown to cause cholestatic hepatitis) and can create liver tumors. The natural form of the hormone does not have these effects.

Natural testosterone can be prescribed by doctors in the form of pills taken daily in doses of 2 mg to 10 mg. Testosterone cream in doses that range from 0.25 mg/2 cc to 2.5 mg/2 cc can be applied to the skin or vaginal tissues to help with libido and thickening of vaginal walls.

Younger women who have lost their ovaries, which are a major source of the hormone, should seriously consider taking testosterone.

Also, women who are more than ten years past menopause (approximately sixty years of age) may benefit from testosterone since their ovaries have likely reduced production of the hormone. It may be added right to the estrogen-progesterone cream or gel, making for simple application. Once again, the criterion to use to determine the right dose and even whether or not you should continue taking the hormones is how you feel.

ESTROGEN THERAPY

If you're troubled with symptoms of genital atrophy (vaginal dryness and tenderness), then you may need estrogen. (Progesterone may do nothing to help your vaginal problems.) Pharmaceutical vaginal estrogen cream (Premarin or Estrace) used in small quantities (half a gram) two to four times a week will thicken and moisturize the vaginal tissues. Pharmacies can also make up a vaginal cream for you. Use only the amount necessary to accomplish the desired effects. Because vaginal creams may not provide sufficient quantities of estrogen to relieve hot flashes, you may have to use the transdermal skin patch or the oral therapy.

As discussed earlier, the transdermal method is generally preferred over pills for estrogen delivery since it avoids liver metabolism of the hormone. As a result, a much smaller dose can be used, and the effects of the medication will be more predictable. However, you must be careful to use the right amount when applying the treatment. Some women fail to realize how powerful transdermal delivery of estrogen really is. If you use this drug recklessly, you may suffer very serious and life-altering consequences, including the possibility of developing breast cancer. If the transdermal method is not effective or acceptable, then pills may be the last choice for estrogen treatment.

ESTRADIOL

Which form of HRT is "best" is anyone's guess. I believe that the more you mimic nature, the better your health will be. Estradiol is preferable over conjugated estrogens, which are estrogens taken from the urine of pregnant horses. (The word *Premarin* is derived from the words: *pre*gnant *mare*s' ur*ine*). Of the seven estrogens contained in the urine and in the pills, five are unique to horses; only two are shared with women. However, this preparation has been used safely for many years. But some ethical issues have been raised concerning the welfare of the horses.

Estradiol is the form of estrogen women make naturally. Transdermal application is the preferable route. Dosages should be tailored to your response. The goal is always to improve a woman's feelings of well-being by relieving hot flashes and the symptoms of vaginal atrophy.

For women without a uterus, or those who do not object to monthly menstrual periods, the most natural way to administer HRT is estradiol cream or gel (0.05 to 0.1 mg) applied to the skin every day. Progesterone must be added for those women with a uterus. It may also be of value for women without a uterus, for the breast benefits. Starting on the first day of the calendar month (day 1), use 20 mg of progesterone cream or gel once or twice a day. Continue until day 14. A menstrual period should follow in about five days if you have a uterus. This cycle is repeated monthly. Any bleeding before day 11 or after day 21 is considered abnormal, and should be investigated by your doctor.

Continuous therapy with a fixed combination of estradiol and progesterone may be preferred by women who do not want periods. Apply the combination estradiol-progesterone cream daily for the entire month.

POSSIBLE HRT PRESCRIPTIONS

Vaginal Creams

Estriol suppositories, 1 to 2 mg (up to 5 mg); use daily or as needed
Estriol cream, 1 mg per gram; use daily or as needed
Estradiol cream, 0.1 mg per gram; use daily or as needed

Transdermal

Progesterone Alone: a gel or cream of 20 to 100 mg of progesterone in 1 gram of cream (¼ tsp.) daily. A one month's supply is 1 ounce; however, 1⅓ ounces (40 grams) is usually dispensed because of wastage. A spoon measuring ¼ teaspoon is included with the jar of cream.

Sequential Therapy: a gel or cream of 0.05 to 0.1 mg of estradiol used once a day the entire month. Calendar days 1 through 14 apply 20 mg of progesterone once or twice a day in a cream. To the estradiol cream can be added 0.25 mg of testosterone. The daily dose is mixed in 1 gram (¼ tsp.) of cream and a one-month supply of the estradiol is 1 ounce. However, 1⅓ ounces (40 grams) is usually dispensed because of wastage, and the progesterone is ½ to 1 ounce (with extra dispensed because of wastage).

Continuous Therapy: a gel or cream containing a mixture of 0.05 to 0.1 mg of estradiol with 20 mg of progesterone in 1 gram (¼ tsp.), sometimes adding 0.25 mg of testosterone, daily. A one month supply is 1 ounce; however, 1⅓ ounces (40 grams) is usually dispensed because of wastage.

Pills

Estradiol 0.5 to 1 mg with 200 mg of progesterone (sometimes 1 to 2 mg of testosterone is added)

For most women, hot flashes only last for a year or two after a woman enters menopause. You should periodically consider stopping the medications to see if the discomfort is gone. Likewise, vaginal symptoms may need only intermittent treatment. Your goal is to use the least amount of the medication to control your symptoms, and to discontinue its use as soon as possible.

There is no agreed-upon clinical or laboratory way to assess the most effective dose of estrogen to be given; however, many doctors find measurement of estradiol blood or saliva levels helpful. (You can order saliva hormone tests for about $80 without a doctor's prescription by calling Aeron LifeCycles at [800] 631-7900.) The amount and type of estrogen needed varies among patients. Reduction of hot flashes and improvement in vaginal symptoms are the most reliable indications that the treatment is right. The progesterone dose must be sufficient to prevent bleeding between periods, called breakthrough bleeding, and suppress precancerous endometrial changes.

Although many pharmacies are unfamiliar with the "natural" gels, creams, and pills for women, there are a few that specialize in these natural products. You can fill your doctor's prescriptions at the Woman's International Pharmacy, (800) 279-5708; the Madison Pharmacy Association, (800) 558-7046; and The College Pharmacy, (800) 888-9358.

COMBINING THE McDOUGALL PROGRAM AND HRT

Andrea Pine of Tampa, Florida, began having hormonal problems at the age of thirteen, when her menstrual periods became "unusually heavy" and were accompanied by intense cramps and nausea. Her symptoms were so severe that she was forced to spend a week out of every month in bed and out of school. In an attempt to treat her symptoms, her doctor placed her on birth control pills to regulate her menstrual periods and her distressing symptoms. The birth control pills caused her breasts to become swollen and tender and her moods to fluctuate, but her menstrual symptoms did alleviate.

Andrea married in her twenties and had two children. She experienced her first premenopausal symptoms at the age of forty-seven, which included hot flashes, sweats several times per day, and mood fluctuations. She also suffered from chronic depression that ranged in intensity from mild to severe. She tried every herbal remedy and vitamin supplement she could purchase, including melatonin, yet none provided relief.

Andrea's doctor prescribed HRT in the form of Premarin and Provera (Prempro), taken together each day in pill form. These drugs only intensified her existing symptoms and added two new ones: nervousness and spotting between periods. Thus, even though she was taking HRT, her suffering only increased.

And then for reasons she didn't even understand, Andrea began to question the high-fat diet she was on. She began to talk about her diet with her doctor, who recommended the McDougall Program. Andrea adopted the diet and saw an immediate reduction in the severity of her symptoms. They did not disappear completely, however. Andrea was getting my *McDougall Newsletter* at the time and read one of my articles on hormone replacement therapy. In the article, I recommended that women who have severe symptoms that are not relieved by diet alone should consider a combination treatment of estradiol, progesterone, and testosterone that was applied to the skin.

Andrea wrote to me later that the combination treatment "has literally been a miracle in my life. . . . My hormone-related symptoms are now gone. I feel better than I have in my entire life. I decided to cut out all oil (in addition to not eating meat or dairy). I had always been told I needed some oil and fat . . . to be healthy. I now realize that this is nonsense. The 'hormone-related' acne (actually more related to fats and oils) I had all my life is now also gone. I have more energy than I ever thought possible. I had never exercised in my life. I now work out daily."

For Andrea, menopause has become "just another stage of my life," and she calls it "one of the happiest and most productive periods of my life."

Herbal Treatments for Menopause

What can be done for women who fear taking HRT but still suffer? Herbal preparations are commonly recommended as a "natural treatment" of menopause. Unfortunately, there are currently no government standards on the quality of herbal products in the United States, and little is known about them scientifically. While most have few adverse effects, some can be unsafe.

How do you tell if the herbal medication is worthwhile? You are the best judge, based upon how it makes you feel. This is no different than how you determine the value of HRT. Guidance for the proper dosage is obtained with the package instructions. These preparations should not be taken by women who are pregnant or nursing or by anyone known to have adverse reactions to any of these herbal preparations.

Some herbs are said to affect female hormones and some relieve mental and emotional distresses associated with menopause. The following are some of the commonly self-administered herbs used by women for menopause symptoms:

HORMONALLY ACTIVE HERBS

The estrogen and progestin bioactivity of foods, herbs, and spices was recently reported on over 150 herbs traditionally used by herbalists for treating a variety of health problems. They were tested for their relative capacity to compete with estradiol and progesterone binding to intracellular receptors for progesterone (PR) and estradiol (ER) in intact human breast cancer cells (this does not mean these herbs cause or promote cancer). The six highest ER-binding herbs commonly consumed were soy, licorice, red clover, thyme, turmeric, hops, and verbena. The six highest PR-binding herbs and spices commonly consumed were oregano, verbena, turmeric, thyme, red clover, and damiana. However, modifying estrogen and progesterone activity is probably only one role herbs play in helping women with menopausal symptoms.

Black Cohosh (*Cimicifuga racemosa*)

Other names: baneberry, squawroot (from treating women's disorders), bugbane, black snake root (treating snake bites by Native Americans), rattle weed

General Description: Black cohosh is a flowering plant that grows to eight feet tall in the Northern Hemisphere. The best-studied herb for relieving menopausal symptoms, it is obtained from the rhizome (a creeping stem with scales, leaves, and roots lying horizontally at or under the surface of the soil).

Medical Background: Traditionally, it has been recommended for female problems, indigestion, and arthritis. Benefits for women during menopause are supposed to come from its estrogen-simulating effects. Black cohosh has been studied mostly in Germany, where it is used to treat hot flashes. Experiments have shown that the herb has substances that bind to estrogen receptors in animal models and lower pituitary hormones in both animals and humans. However, a recent study from Denmark found no sign of estrogen activity on the uterus and vagina of rats. The authors conclude that this herb's benefits for menopausal symptoms cannot be explained as a traditional estrogen effect as measured in biological experiments. Therefore, the herb may work by other means, such as influencing pituitary hormones.

Elevated levels of a pituitary hormone, known as luteinizing hormone, is thought to contribute to hot flashes, insomnia, and depression in menopause. When 110 women took black cohosh or a placebo for two months, luteinizing hormone was decreased by 20 percent for those taking the herb. Two studies compared black cohosh to conjugated estrogens and diazepam (Valium). Women in the black cohosh group had greater relief of menopausal symptoms and greater reduction in anxiety and depression than those taking the prescription drugs. Vaginal atrophy also improved. Other research has found significant relief of menopausal symptoms such as hot flashes, profuse perspiration, headache, dizziness, heart palpitations, ringing in the ears, nervousness, depression, and sleep disturbances.

Side Effects: Few side effects are reported with recommended doses. Ingestion of large doses of leaves may result in nausea and vomiting, and may induce miscarriage. This herb may have additive blood pressure–lowering effects, so people taking blood-pressure pills should be cautious.

Chaste Berry (*Agnus castus*)

Other names: Vitex, Chaste Tree

General Description: As its name suggests, chaste berries, the fruit of a small Eurasian tree, were once believed to suppress the libido. The berries and leaves are used in the herb preparation. The chaste berry was well known to many of the ancients. Hippocrates (460–377 B.C.) stated, "If blood flows from the womb, let the woman drink wine in which the leaves of the Vitex have been steeped."

Medical Background: Chaste berry extracts inhibit prolactin secretion of rat pituitary cells. A randomized placebo-controlled, double-blind study of 52 women with elevated prolactin production (hyperprolactinemia) using a daily dose of one capsule (20 mg) of a chaste berry preparation found after three months of therapy that prolactin release was reduced and estrogen (17 beta-estradiol) production increased. Side effects were not reported. Therefore, this herb has effects on female pituitary and ovarian hormones and has some scientific support for use in menopause. In addition, it is an alternative treatment for elevated prolactin production in women in their reproductive years.

Side Effects: It may cause itching, rash, or nausea, and is not recommended for use in pregnancy.

Licorice (*Glycyrrhiza glabra*)

General Description: Say "licorice" and most people think of a candy, but it is also a powerful herb. Licorice is derived from a perennial plant native to southern Europe, Asia, and the Mediterranean; it is distinguished by tiny violet flowers. One of the most popular and widely consumed herbs in the world, it is said to be fifty times sweeter than sugar.

Medical Background: The main constituent found in the root is glycyrrhizin, which stimulates the secretion of the adrenal cortex hormone aldosterone. The root extract produces mild estrogenic effects, and it has proved useful in treating symptoms of menopause. Licorice is found to bind to estrogen receptors in the cells of the uterus of experimental animals.

Side Effects: Headaches, diarrhea, lethargy, fluid retention, weakness, or shortness of breath. Heavy use of licorice can affect the production of adrenal hormones (aldosterone) causing electrolyte imbalance with sodium retention and loss of potassium. This in turn can lead to high blood pressure and edema.

Ginseng (*Panax ginseng*)

Other names: Ren Shen, Chinese Ginseng, Korean Ginseng

General Description: Ginseng is native to China, Russia, North Korea, Japan, and some areas of North America. Ginseng is the most famous Chinese herb, and its use dates back seven thousand years. The name *panax* is derived from the Greek word *panacea*, meaning "all healing." It was first cultivated in the United States in the late 1800s and it takes four to six years to become mature enough to harvest. The root provides the herb.

Medical Background: Ginseng is known to have estrogenic activity. Ginseng face cream has been reported to cause vaginal bleeding in a postmenopausal woman, demonstrating its potential for powerful estrogenic activity.

Side Effects: Very rare

Hops (*Humulus lupus*)

General Description: The female flowers of this climbing shrub are used to make the herb. Historically hops has been used as a sleeping aid and to flavor beer.

Medical Background: Hops appears to have an estrogen effect and bind to estrogen receptors of human cells.

Side Effects: Nontoxic

Dong Quai (*Angelica sinensis*)

Other names: Chinese Angelica, Dong Guai, tang-kuei, Dang-gui, Umbelliferae, toki, Japanese angelica, tanggwi

General Description: The Chinese have been using this herb for more than two thousand years to treat gynecological problems. The rhizome is the source of the herb.

Medical Background: Stimulation of uterine tissue has been observed. Dong quai does not act like an estrogen, but may have some direct action on the reproductive organs (uterus) and possibly on other hormones. A recent double-blind, placebo-controlled study examined the effects of dong quai on the vaginal cells and endometrial thickness in 71 postmenopausal women, and found no statistically significant differences between the endometrial thickness, vaginal cells, or the number of hot flashes between the herb and a placebo.

Side Effects: Components of this herb may interact with sunlight to cause rashes. There is also concern that some of the chemical components may cause cancer. The *Lawrence Review of Natural Products* reports, "The potential toxicity posed by the coumarins and safrole in the essential oil outweigh the benefits of ingesting this plant, and its use cannot be recommended."

MOOD-ALTERING DRUGS

St. John's Wort (*Hypericum perforatum*)

Other names: Goat weed

General Description: St. John's wort is a bushy perennial plant with numerous yellow flowers. It is native to many parts of the world, including Europe and the United States, growing wild in northern California, southern Oregon, and Colorado. The herb comes from the flowering plant.

Medical Background: St. John's wort is licensed in Germany for treatment of anxiety, depression, and insomnia. There are at least ten compounds that may provide effects, but hypericum appears to be the most active ingredient. This compound changes the neurotransmitters in the brain, resulting in emotional benefits. There have been 23 randomized trials done on a total of 1,757 outpatients with mild to moderate depression. Hypericum extracts after two to four weeks were found to be more effective than a placebo, and about as effective as standard antidepressants. Two to four weeks are required to develop mood-elevating effects.

Side Effects: Some patients report dry mouth, dizziness, constipation, gastrointestinal upset, and confusion. In trials, fewer than 2 percent stopped taking the herb because of side effects. One patient reported photosensitivity (reaction with sunlight). Depression is a serious illness and should be treated by a doctor. Do not combine this herb with other antidepressant medication.

Ginkgo biloba

Other names: Maidenhair Tree, Bai Guo

General Description: Ginkgo biloba is extracted from the leaves of cultivated maidenhair trees.

Medical Background: A traditional Chinese medicine used to treat asthma and bronchitis, gingko is licensed in Germany to treat cerebral dysfunction with, for example, memory loss, dizziness, ringing in the ears, hearing loss, headaches, emotional instability with anxiety, and for intermittent claudication (leg pain with walking due to arteries narrowed by atherosclerosis). Benefits have been reported for poor circulation to the brain, hands, legs (intermittent claudication), and feet. Ginkgo has been shown to improve memory and to slow the progress of dementia. Four to twelve weeks of treatment are usually required to see results.

Side Effects: There are no serious side effects. In rare cases mild stomach upset, headache, and allergic skin reactions have been reported.

Kava (*Piper methysticum*)

Other names: Kava kava, Kawa

General Description: More than twenty varieties have been identified. Prepared from the rhizome of a sprawling evergreen shrub found in Polynesia, Melanesia, and Micronesia, Kava has traditionally been used as a beverage to induce relaxation. It produces mild euphoric changes characterized by feelings of happiness, more fluent and lively speech, and increased sensitivity to sounds. Chewed, it can cause numbness of the mouth. The most effective way to use kava is as a ground rhizome powder mixed with cool water.

Medical Background: A study of women with menopausal complaints found reduced symptoms after only one week, with improvements in feelings of well-being and less depression. A multicentered, randomized, placebo-controlled, 25-week outpatient trial of the active ingredient of kava compared to commonly prescribed antidepressants and tranquilizers found kava to have superior benefits over the drugs, with rare adverse effects. The authors suggested kava as a treatment alternative with proven long-term benefits and none of the tolerance problems associated with antidepressants (tricyclics) and tranquilizers (benzodiazepines). Other research has shown similar benefits. Use for treating alcohol abuse and some forms of psychosis also have been suggested.

Side Effects: Even when administered within its prescribed dosages, this herb may adversely affect motor reflexes and judgment for driving. It may also elevate effects of alcohol. Chronic ingestion causes dry, flaky, discolored skin and reddened eyes. Heavy kava users are more likely to complain of poor health and a "puffy" face, and about 20 percent are underweight.

OTHER HERBS FOR MENOPAUSE

Other herbs commonly recommended to treat some of the symptoms of menopause include: bilberry, black currant, bitter melon, chamomile, damiana, echinacea, feverfew, flaxseed, goldenseal, hawthorn, horsetail, motherwort, oat straw, pasque flower, passion flower, sage, saw palmetto, uva ursi, valerian root, and wild yam. Their benefits and risks have not been sufficiently tested.

What to Do?

To have a happy and healthy life around the time of menopause, focus on a healthy starch-based diet, exercise, stress reduction, and quitting bad habits, like daily use of coffee, tobacco, and alcohol. Next you may want to try herbal treatments. The herb most likely to give relief from menopausal symptoms like hot flashes is black cohosh. Chaste berry would be the second choice. Ginseng is relatively safe and has many positive effects on a person's state of well-being. The additional estrogen effects may be particularly helpful for postmenopausal women. Licorice has definite hormonal effects, but sometimes undesirable and serious side effects, so this herb should be used with caution. Hops hasn't been studied enough, so its effects are still to be determined. Because of lack of effectiveness and potential toxicity you should not use dong quai.

There are four alternatives to doctor-prescribed drugs to relieve depression. Exercise relieves mild depression and anxiety by producing endorphins in the nervous system. A healthy, low-animal-protein diet allows the production of neurochemicals, like serotonin, that elevate mood. Avoiding too much sleep is one of the most powerful antidepressants, because for many people too much sleep produces depressogenic substances.

Herbs can also provide effective mood-altering therapy. Three such herbs have proven effective and relatively safe: St. John's wort for depression, ginkgo biloba to help with memory and confusion, and kava for a relaxant. Use all of these herbal preparations for their desired effects, but look for side effects and discontinue use if they occur.

Make Your Postmenopause the Best Time of Your Life

A woman's life can be thought of as having three distinct physical stages: from birth to first menstruation, the period that marks her development into early womanhood and her ability to conceive children; from menarchy to menopause, a time when, among other things, she is able to give birth and raise her children; and from menopause onward, when she is free of monthly periods, the prospect of unexpected pregnancies, and the responsibilities of raising young children. Since women are now living, on average, to nearly eighty years of age, and since a great percentage of women still possess good health and vitality well into old age, this third period of life offers women the opportunity to use their accumulated experience and wisdom in altogether new, inspiring, and creative ways.

In order to make maximum use of all your resources, you should begin by adopting the McDougall Program. This will give you a foundation for good health, abundant energy, optimal weight, improved appearance, and hormonal health. If necessary, take herbal supplements and/or small doses of HRT, and only for a limited amount of time.

This formula alone can make your postmenopausal years among your best and most rewarding of your life.

CHAPTER 14

Breaking the Cycle of Cardiovascular Disease

In July 1992, Anita Fink, fifty-seven years old, of Greensberg, Pennsylvania, was told that if she did not have bypass surgery immediately she would very likely be dead within six months. The main branch of her coronary artery was 95 percent blocked, her doctors told her, and she had no collateral circulation going to that part of her heart. Her cholesterol level was 300 mg/dl, a level so high that it almost guaranteed coronary artery disease and an eventual heart attack. She was also about twenty-five pounds overweight.

Anita didn't have to be told the specifics to know that she was in grave danger. The exertion of brushing her teeth and then getting into the shower brought on severe angina, or chest pain.

"I was getting chest pain even at rest," she said recently. "I was taking nitroglycerin constantly. I couldn't shop or do any of the normal things of life anymore. I also had zero energy; any little bit of activity left me feeling exhausted and struggling with chest pain. I lived in constant fear of a heart attack."

One of Anita's two daughters told her about the McDougall Program at St. Helena Hospital in northern California. When Anita talked to her doctors about my program, they were vehemently opposed to Anita's going. For one thing, she could not walk the distance from her car to the airport without putting her life in danger. Her doctors believed that the stress of the trip alone might kill her. They also believed that using a dietary program to treat her disease was foolhardy. Anything short of immediate surgery was irresponsible, they said.

Still, there were complications. Anita had contracted Hodgkin's disease, a form of cancer, eleven years before. Her treatment had included high doses of radiation to her chest and abdomen that had depleted her sternum and ribs of calcium and left her bones porous and brittle. Doctors weren't sure if they could open her chest without causing irreversible damage to her rib cage. As Anita recalled, "They were going to do the surgery and deal with things as they went along."

Severe coronary illness and Hodgkin's disease were not Anita's only problems, however. In May of 1992, she had suffered a stroke, which left her temporarily paralyzed on the left side of her body. "I lost all control of my left arm and leg," Anita recalled. "I had to learn to walk again." She was being treated with the drug Coumadin to thin her blood, which would further complicate the proposed surgery.

"I had a gut feeling," said Anita, "that I should try Dr. McDougall's Program. If it didn't help me, then I would have the surgery done, but I thought it was worth a try." Thus, in September 1992, Anita arrived at St. Helena Hospital with her husband, David, pushing her in her wheelchair.

Even our doctors at St. Helena were skeptical that Anita would make it through our twelve-day program. After examining Anita, one of our cardiologists at St. Helena, Dr. Pieter VandenHoven, told her that she should consider having the operation at St. Helena immediately. "I told him that I wanted to try the McDougall Program first," Anita said. "Then I would decide on the surgery."

For the next twelve days, Anita ate the McDougall foods with great enthusiasm, but did only the smallest amount of exercise she could tolerate before her angina started up again. "I rode the stationary bicycle for about two minutes," Anita said. "After that, the pain came back and I became afraid, so I would stop. But after about a week on the diet, something inside of me made me realize that it could help me." While at St. Helena, Anita made a commitment to the program and never looked back. "I decided to stick strictly to the diet, which I have done religiously, and then very slowly increase the exercise that I could do," she said.

True to her word, Anita went home and ate nothing outside the McDougall regimen. She also began to walk a little bit each day. "I walked to the corner of my street. There's a little incline there and I would stop at the bottom of the incline and then turn around and come home. I did that every day for a while until I started to feel a little stronger. Then, little by little, I started to go up the incline, a little more each week, until I was able to make it all the way up and then back down."

By Christmas, Anita was off her medication and feeling as if she had been reborn. "I no longer had to take any nitroglycerin or Coumadin," she said. "Gradually, I had realized that I could do more and more without any pain. One day, I said to myself, 'Gosh, I've got a lot more energy. I'm walking up and down the stairs; I'm going to the store and running errands. I'm doing all the things I couldn't do before and I'm not experiencing chest pain."

Meanwhile, she was making regular visits to her cardiologist, who found that her heart was getting stronger and stronger. "My doctors looked at me and just marveled. They couldn't believe this."

Today Anita likes to refer to herself as a poster girl for the McDougall Program. She travels widely, especially to visit her daughter in California, and she is healthier than she's been since she was a young woman.

Her doctors are astounded. Her cholesterol level is 181 mg/dl. She walks and rides her stationary bicycle daily; she also swims regularly. "I have a tremendous amount of energy," Anita says. "My daughter has trouble keeping up with me when we're together." She has also undergone a radical physical transformation. Anita is now a well-toned 114 pounds, dresses in a petite size 6, and doesn't look anywhere near her sixty-three years of age. "My doctors just look at what has happened to me with awe," Anita said. "They cannot understand how a diet and exercise program could possibly have these kinds of results. This program saved my life."

Nature has blessed women with a certain biological protection against heart disease—at least until the time of menopause, after which estrogen levels fall, cholesterol levels rise, and heart disease rates start to climb. By the time a woman reaches the age of sixty-five, she is as likely to suffer a fatal heart attack as a man. Each year, 500,000 women die of cardiovascular disease and 250,000 die of heart attacks. Indeed, heart disease is the number one killer of women.

Somehow, women and a great many doctors forget these facts. It's almost as if a woman's temporary built-in protection against heart disease casts a spell over women and their physicians. Both have been lulled into believing that women are unlikely candidates for heart attacks, or heart disease in general. Thus, when women with clear symptom of heart disease arrive at their doctors' offices, or at their local hospitals, they are often dismissed as having indigestion or gallbladder disease or anxiety. This may partly explain why women do not get the same kinds of treatment for heart disease that men do; in some cases, this treatment could save their lives. For example:

- Women are less likely than men to be sent to the hospital when complaining of chest pain or other cardiovascular symptoms.
- Fewer women than men are sent to the coronary care unit; therefore, they are less likely to receive potentially life-saving treatments, such as blood clot–dissolving drugs (thrombolysis) given soon after the onset of a heart attack.
- Some studies show that women are four times less likely to be given bypass surgery than men, even though the incidence of chest pain is the same in both sexes and their respective needs for the surgery are comparable.
- Women have twice the risk of dying during bypass surgery, possibly because they are sicker and weaker by the time they go to surgery.
- The prognosis for recovery from heart disease is worse for women than for men.

You must protect yourself against heart disease. If you have the disorder, you must educate yourself to demand high-quality treatment.

The Genesis of Cardiovascular Disease

Most illnesses of the heart and arteries, collectively known as cardiovascular disease, arise from an underlying disorder called atherosclerosis, in which cholesterol plaques clog arteries throughout the body, including those that bring blood to the heart or brain. Atherosclerosis is the cause of most heart attacks and a great many strokes. What most people do not realize is that it affects many other arteries throughout the body: it can cause loss of hearing or sight; reduce kidney function and lead to kidney failure; result in claudication and gangrene in the legs; lead to ruptured discs in the spine and to back pain; and cause impotence.

Atherosclerosis begins when tiny globules of cholesterol in your blood become oxidized, or decayed. These rancid cholesterol balls are gobbled up by macrophages, a type of immune cell. Once these macrophages are engorged with cholesterol, they sink into the walls of your arteries, where they form a fatty streak, the first stage of atherosclerosis. The process continues and the fatty streaks grow into full-blown plaques as more cholesterol is consumed. Eventually, the plaques themselves become engorged with cholesterol, making them bigger and highly unstable.

A heart attack or a stroke can occur when a plaque becomes overstuffed with cholesterol and then ruptures, spewing vicious cholesterol, fat, and hardened debris, which acts as a catalyst to form a blood clot, medically known as a *thrombus*. That thrombus can become so large that it blocks blood flow in the artery. If that artery brings blood and oxygen to the heart, a part of the heart will suffocate and die, resulting in a heart attack, or what is often referred to as *coronary artery thrombosis*. If such a rupture occurs, and a blood-blocking clot forms in an artery that leads to the brain, it is called a stroke.

Considering their actual makeup, these plaques that sometimes rupture should be pictured as festering sores, or boils. They are not unlike the boils that would form after having a splinter of wood stuck in your hand. The affected area becomes swollen and red. Soon, pus accumulates within the sore. If left untreated, the infection grows larger until it may burst open, or spread. In many cases scar tissue becomes incorporated into the sore. One of the big differences between having such a boil on your hand and one in your arteries is that your hand contains pain nerves, which alert you to the fact that there is a problem. Your arteries contain no such nerves, which is why heart disease is often referred to as the "silent killer." You don't know the disease process is developing until it is very serious, and an artery becomes completely blocked and tissue dies—a potentially fatal situation.

Controlling Cholesterol Is Crucial

The whole process of atherosclerosis and the slow destruction of the human body begins with the consumption of foods rich in fat and cholesterol, ordinary foods that people eat every day, such as steaks, hamburger, hot dogs, french fries, milk shakes, eggs, cheese, milk, chicken, and fish. Cholesterol is a waxy substance used to make bile acids, reproductive hormones, vitamin D, and cellular parts. It is produced only by animals. Plants do not make or contain cholesterol.

Human beings make approximately 1,000 milligrams of cholesterol each day. We make all the cholesterol our bodies require, which means there's no need for us to eat cholesterol. (This is the reason cholesterol is not referred to as a nutrient, since only substances that are essential, but that we cannot make ourselves, are called nutrients.)

Your blood cholesterol level can serve as the crystal ball into your future, predicting your chances of having a heart attack and an untimely death. The average cholesterol level for people living in the United States is about 210 mg/dl. Such a cholesterol level means your chances of having a premature heart attack or stroke are about fifty-fifty, which is lousy odds when your life is on the line. A cholesterol level 260 mg/dl or above is, to me, suicide. At this level, atherosclerosis is likely to be so advanced that it can kill you in any number of ways, including a heart attack, stroke, or kidney failure.

An ideal cholesterol level is below 150 mg/dl. Studies have shown that people with cholesterol levels of 150 mg/dl or lower have a very low risk of heart disease, and are considered by some experts to be almost "immune" from the ravages of atherosclerosis.

Interestingly, it isn't just your current cholesterol level that determines your health, but also whether it is rising or falling. People who bring down their cholesterol levels from, say, 260 or 300 mg, to 200 or 180 mg experience a significant reduction in their risk of heart disease, even though they have not hit the magic number of 150 mg. The reason for this improvement is that as your blood cholesterol level falls, the plaques inside your arteries are being drained of cholesterol and fat, and they begin to heal, making them much more stable and less likely to rupture. Ruptured plaque, you will recall, is the cause of almost all heart attacks, or coronary thromboses. This is why I tell people that they will experience a significant benefit within the first few days to weeks of adopting the McDougall Program, because when your cholesterol starts dropping, your plaques are stabilizing and your risk of heart attack is rapidly decreasing. More and more, scientists are emphasizing the stabilization of plaque, as opposed to reversal of atherosclerosis, because stabilization takes you out of danger within a short period of time.

Nevertheless, measurable reversal has been shown among people who accomplish such a dramatic lowering of cholesterol levels. In fact, studies have shown that people who were able to lower their cholesterol by more than 60 mg/dl were the ones most likely to show healing in their arteries and reversal of disease.

Unfortunately, the opposite is also true: A rapid increase in cholesterol level dramatically increases your risk of heart disease. When cholesterol rises 60 mg/dl, say from 200 to 260 mg/dl, your risk of dying from heart disease increases fivefold. Therefore, the direction of any change in cholesterol—whether it goes up or down—can be very important in determining your health.

For most Americans, there's no question of where their cholesterol levels are going. The standard American diet derives more than 35 percent of its total calories from fat (most of that being saturated fat). It also provides an additional 300 to 1,000 mg of cholesterol each day from animal foods. Under such conditions, there's nowhere for cholesterol levels to go but up.

About 40 percent of the cholesterol you consume makes its way into your bloodstream. The liver attempts to remove as much of that cholesterol as it can, but the liver's capacity to do that is limited. Consequently, cholesterol builds within the system and is deposited in our body fat, tendons, skin, and artery walls.

HDL CHOLESTEROL

There is a lot of confusion today about HDL cholesterol, or high-density lipoproteins, commonly referred to as "good" cholesterol. It is just one of several fractions of cholesterol that include VLDL, or very-low-density lipoprotein; LDL, low-density lipoprotein; and MDL, or medium-density lipoprotein. HDL cholesterol has been referred to in the press as the "good" cholesterol because it is the form in which cholesterol is eliminated from the body. Thus, HDL has been associated with a lower risk of heart disease.

It's important to realize, however, that as your total cholesterol goes up, so too do all the fractions of cholesterol, including HDL. One reliable but unhealthy way to raise HDL cholesterol is to have people eat a high-fat, high-cholesterol diet.

Many people today rationalize their high cholesterol levels by saying that they also have high HDL levels. This rationalization occurs not just among laypeople, but also among physicians. I have met people with total cholesterol levels of 285 mg/dl who were told by their doctors not to worry because their "good" HDL cholesterol is also high—75 mg/dl or higher. Unfortunately, tens of thousands of people have heart attacks and eventually go to their graves each year with this false assurance ringing in their ears.

Just as HDL goes up as total cholesterol rises, so too do HDL levels fall as total cholesterol drops. This is the case for anyone who adopts a low-fat, low-cholesterol regimen. In our study of patients at St. Helena Hospital, we have found that, on average, people reduce their overall HDL levels by 19 percent in eleven days. This same effect takes place worldwide. Those populations with low blood cholesterol levels also have correspondingly low HDL levels. Yet, these same people have the lowest incidences of heart disease, because they have a low total cholesterol and a low LDL "bad" cholesterol from eating near-vegetarian diets.

Unfortunately, many physicians do not understand this. People on healthy vegetarian diets are sometimes told to eat meat because their HDL is only 25 mg/dl. Yet, their total cholesterol is only 125 mg/dl, a cholesterol level that makes them virtually immune from heart disease.

Total cholesterol is the number that matters most to me. Don't be misled by uninformed people. When you adopt the McDougall Program, you will watch your total cholesterol fall dramatically. As it does, both LDL and HDL levels will also drop. And as they do, so too will your risk of heart disease.

Reducing Triglycerides

Triglycerides are fats that are found in your blood. For many people, triglycerides are so high that these tiny globules of fat turn their blood milky white. As they fill your blood in sufficient quantities, triglycerides reduce the flow of blood and oxygen to tissues and contribute to a number of diseases, including heart disease.

As you might expect, triglycerides rise and fall, depending on what you eat. Fats of any kind raise triglycerides. Surprising to many people is the fact that simple sugars, including the sugars in fruit and fruit juice and alcohol, elevate triglycerides, as well as blood cholesterol levels, in sensitive people. On the other hand, unrefined whole grains, such as corn, brown rice, and beans, lower triglycerides. They also lower cholesterol and body weight. Exercise lowers triglycerides.

A certain segment of the scientific community has criticized diets low in fat and high in carbohydrates, saying such diets cause cholesterol and triglyceride levels to rise to unhealthy levels. Such scientists fail to discern the difference between simple carbohydrates—meaning simple sugars—and complex carbohydrates found in whole grains and fresh vegetables. In order to get triglyceride and cholesterol levels to rise, investigators add simple sugars and refined flours to their study diet—and then, to make matters worse, they overfeed their subjects. As a result both triglyceride levels and weight increase.

On the other hand, when people are allowed to eat a low-fat, high–complex carbohydrate diet to satiety, their cholesterol levels and weight fall. Their triglycerides either fall or remain stable, depending on how high those triglycerides were when they adopted the diet.

Our data from the McDougall Program at St. Helena Hospital clearly show that when people are allowed to eat as many unrefined carbohydrates as they want, cholesterol goes down and triglycerides stay the same or fall. People on the McDougall Program also lose weight without ever needing to go hungry. The McDougall Program causes profound improvements in triglycerides, especially for those most in need of it. The average drop for the entire group is 10 mg/dl in eleven days. However, for those who start with a significant elevation in triglycerides, say over 600 mg/dl, the reduction is, on the average, 311 mg/dl.

Still, it's important to keep in mind that when you adopt a low-fat, high-carbohydrate diet, you also want to get regular exercise. Walking at a brisk pace for a minimum of thirty minutes at least four to five days a week is sufficient to reduce triglycerides.

Lowering Homocysteine Levels to Keep Your Arteries Healthy

Another clear indicator of cardiovascular health is the level of the amino acid homocysteine in your blood. Elevated homocysteine levels are associated with a significantly increased risk of heart disease, atherosclerosis of the carotid artery, and deep vein thrombosis.

For a variety of reasons, homocysteine has long been suspected to be an important risk factor in the etiology of heart disease. Human and animal studies have shown that when this sulfur-containing amino acid is elevated, the incidence of artery damage increases substantially. Scientists believe that homocysteine has a toxic effect on the inside linings of the arteries, which is where atherosclerosis begins. In addition, the amino acid also stimulates the growth of muscle cells within the artery walls—a key step in the development of atherosclerosis. High levels also raise the tendency of the blood to clot, thus increasing the risk of thrombosis formation within the arteries. Apparently, even small elevations in homocysteine levels are dangerous. A 12 percent rise above normal increases the risk of artery disease by more than threefold.

By now, you can probably predict which kinds of foods raise homocysteine and which lower it: red meat and other animal foods elevate the levels of this dangerous amino acid in your blood, while vegetables, especially green, leafy vegetables, and fruit lower them.

Homocysteine levels depend on the amounts of folate and vitamin B_6 in your bloodstream. When folate and B_6 are high, homocysteine is low, which means your risk of artery disease is also low. When folate and B_6 are low, homocysteine is high, which means your risk of disease is also high.

Actually, homocysteine only collects in significant quantities when another amino acid, called methionine, is inadequately metabolized to cysteine. The process of turning methionine into cysteine requires vitamins B_{12}, B_6, and folic acid. If the transformation of methionine into cysteine is incomplete, then homocysteine, an intermediate by-product, collects. Thus, homocysteine levels become elevated only when there are inadequate quantities of these B vitamins. Research has shown that when people increase their levels of B_{12}, B_6, and folic acid, homocysteine levels fall.

Of the three B vitamins, folic acid intake seems to be the most important in determining the extent of the artery damage caused by homocysteine. Approximately 40 percent of our population does not consume enough folic acid to keep their homocysteine levels at a safe, low level. The principal source of folic acid is plant foods, especially green leafy vegetables and fruits. Processing, refining, overcooking, and packaging, especially canning, all destroy folic acid in plant foods. Thus, the rich Western diet is deficient in folic acid, which promotes higher homocysteine levels.

The rich American diet raises homocysteine in another way—by raising methionine. The higher the methionine, the more homocysteine by-product will be produced. Red meat, poultry, and fish are all high in methionine. Conversely, starches, fruits, and vegetables are low in methionine.

Thus, the same foods that raise your blood cholesterol levels also raise artery-damaging homocysteine, which is why eating the typical American diet results in such a high incidence of coronary artery disease.

How to Lower Cholesterol

REDUCING CHOLESTEROL BY CHANGING YOUR DIET

The first and best way to lower your cholesterol level is with the McDougall diet, which contains no cholesterol and is exceedingly low in fat. It is rich in folate and B_6, and low in methionine. Low-fat, no-cholesterol, high-fiber diets lower cholesterol levels, while high-fat, high-cholesterol, low-fiber diets raise cholesterol levels.

The McDougall Program, which is free of all animal foods, and therefore completely free of animal fats and cholesterol, derives approximately 7 percent of all its calories from fat. When people adopt the McDougall Program, their cholesterol levels drop radically, which is why so many experience such a dramatic transformation in their health. People experience that transformation during the first week they follow the program. From there, the benefits just snowball.

When patients at my program at St. Helena Hospital are placed on a low-fat, no-cholesterol diet, their blood cholesterol levels plummet. In the first five days of my program, cholesterol levels fall 15 mg/dl. That's 3 mg lower each day. By the eleventh day, my patients, on average, reduce their cholesterol by 29 mg/dl. However, patients with very high blood cholesterol—that is, greater than 300 mg/dl—experience an average drop of 65 mg/dl. And they accomplish this dramatic turnaround in their health in less time than most people spend on their summer vacations.

Sarah Hendricks, thirty-five, of San Francisco, began the McDougall Program in 1995 when her cholesterol level was 240 mg/dl. At five feet six inches, Sarah weighed 208 pounds. Her doctor already had warned her that if she didn't bring down her cholesterol level and her weight, she was in jeopardy of suffering significant heart disease, and possibly a premature heart attack.

Sarah wrote to me in 1997, after being on the program for nearly two years. "I just wanted you to know that I have lost seventy-five pounds and my cholesterol level is 170 mg. This past spring, my husband and I rode our bicycles from Santa Monica to San Francisco [a distance of more than four hundred miles]. I never would have attempted it when I weighed 208 pounds."

As Sarah and so many others have discovered, the McDougall Program does more than just lower blood cholesterol levels. It transforms every aspect of your health.

In addition to changing your diet, you will want to do some regular aerobic exercise, such as walking, bicycling, or swimming, or take up a health-promoting sport, such as tennis or golf. Daily exercise is ideal for lowering triglycerides, raising HDL cholesterol, and improving circulation, especially to the heart. If you have a heart condition, avoid competitive sports. Competition can cause us to stress the heart beyond its limits and therefore can be dangerous.

"NATURAL" MEDICATIONS

If your cholesterol is still too high after you adopt the McDougall Program, or you want to lower your cholesterol level even more rapidly, you may want to use any of a variety of "natural" cholesterol-lowering medications that are highly effective, relatively nontoxic, inexpensive, and easy to administer. Here is a sampling of foods and substances that will lower your cholesterol level.

- *Garlic:* one-half to one clove of garlic lowers cholesterol by 9 percent. Even odorless aged garlic, Kyolic, will lower cholesterol by 7 percent.

- *Vitamin C:* 2 grams daily will lower cholesterol by 12 percent.
- *Vitamin E:* 200 IU daily lowers total cholesterol by 15 percent. For patients starting with values exceeding 300 mg/dl, vitamin E can cause a decline in cholesterol by as much as 31 percent.
- *Oatmeal:* daily consumption of a three-ounce bowl of oatmeal can cause total cholesterol levels to decline between 3 and 10 percent; LDL cholesterol falls by 10 to 15 percent. Daily consumption of two ounces of oat bran will achieve the same results.
- *Activated charcoal:* 1½ to 2 heaping teaspoons (8 grams), taken three times a day, lowers cholesterol about 23 percent. These results are comparable to doctor-prescribed cholesterol-binding resins, colestipol and cholestyramine. Caution! Charcoal must be taken alone, because it absorbs and deactivates other medications.
- *Gugulipid:* this plant extract lowers cholesterol by 21 percent and triglycerides by 25 percent in three to eight weeks. It works by inhibiting the biosynthesis of cholesterol by the liver.
- *Niacin:* lowers cholesterol and triglycerides, but has many side effects, including flushing and raising blood sugar. Long-acting, sustained-release forms of niacin can cause chemical hepatitis in about half of its users. *Take niacin only under a doctor's supervision.*

DRUG THERAPY

I sometimes prescribe pharmaceutical drugs to lower cholesterol, especially if the person is in immediate danger and needs additional support while changing diet and lifestyle. Like it or not, drugs cause far more dramatic effects—both positive and negative—than natural approaches. Therefore, you should monitor both the benefits and the side effects carefully while taking prescription medication and inform your doctor of any changes you experience while taking the drug.

I like to start with the cholesterol-binding resins, such as Questran (cholestyramine) or Colestid (colestipol). These powders are dissolved in liquid (you can use juice or water) and taken two to four times a day. These resins attach themselves to cholesterol and bile acids in the intestine and cause them to be removed from the body. Since these medications do not escape the intestine, and therefore do not enter the bloodstream, they have few systemic side effects. Constipation, indigestion, and bloating have been the most common complaints from people who use these drugs.

The next class of drugs I use to help lower cholesterol is called HMG CoA enzyme inhibitors, like Mevacor (lovastatin,), Zocor (simvastatin),

Lescol (fluvastatin), Pravachol (pravastatin), and Lipitor (atorva-statin). These powerful drugs slow the synthesis of cholesterol by the body. They are much more effective when combined with a very-low-fat diet. In my practice I have not yet found a need to employ any of the other commonly prescribed medications, such as Lopid (gemfibrozil).

I have been using the McDougall Program to treat cholesterol levels and heart disease for more than two decades and I have seen the following three-pronged approach work wonders:

1. A very-low-fat, no cholesterol diet
2. "Natural" cholesterol-lowering medications
3. Prescription medications

With this approach, virtually anyone can bring down his or her cholesterol to the ideal levels of 150 mg/dl, or even lower.

HORMONE REPLACEMENT THERAPY

Hormone replacement therapy increases HDL cholesterol and lowers LDL somewhat, thus providing some protection against heart disease; however, these benefits are small. Women who take HRT tend to take better care of themselves anyway, so it is difficult to know for sure whether HRT actually confers any real protection against heart disease.

Even more important, the potential benefits of HRT to the cardiovascular system must be weighed against the increased risk for the development of breast and uterine cancers caused by the drugs. No informed scientist would argue that heart disease is due to "estrogen pill deficiency," which means that HRT is not the fundamental answer to cardiovascular disease. The most important and effective approach to heart disease is to eliminate high-fat foods from the diet, stop smoking, and exercise.

The Dangers of Hypertension

High blood pressure, also known as hypertension, is not a disease in itself, but an indicator of an underlying disorder in the circulatory system. Just as a fever is a sign of pneumonia, or swelling a sign of a broken bone, high blood pressure is a sign of an underlying sickness in your blood vessels.

A normal blood pressure for a person not taking medication is

110/70 or below. This value is associated with the lowest risk of cardio-vascular disease. As your blood pressure rises, your likelihood of suffering a heart attack or stroke increases dramatically. People with hypertension are seven times more likely to suffer a stroke, four times more likely to have a heart attack, and five times more likely to die of congestive heart failure.

In third world and traditional societies that subsist on plant-based diets, which are low in sodium, blood pressure remains stable throughout life. In wealthy nations that subsist on diets high in fat, processed foods, and salt, blood pressure increases as we age. In the United States, at least one in three adults has elevated blood pressure. Half of Americans sixty-five and older are hypertensive.

Doctors typically recommend that people lose weight, restrict salt in their diets, quit coffee and alcohol, and increase exercise as ways of decreasing blood pressure. A diet rich in fruits and vegetables and low in fat can substantially lower blood pressure. In addition, doctors very often place patients on blood pressure–lowering medication. Most people who start taking blood pressure medication remain on the drugs for life. These drugs are renowned for their side effects, however.

One of the most troubling classes of blood pressure medications is called calcium channel blockers. The short-acting forms of this drug have been shown to increase the risk of dying of heart disease by as much as eightfold. All forms of these drugs have been implicated in gastrointestinal bleeding, suicide, and an increase in the risk of cancer. Diuretics raise cholesterol, triglycerides, uric acid, and blood sugar, and may increase your risk of sudden death. ACE inhibitors have not been tested sufficiently to give us adequate knowledge of their benefits and safety. If medications must be used to lower blood pressure, my choice is usually one of the beta-blockers, which have been shown to have the fewest side effects.

You should take your blood pressure each day at home, while you are relaxed. Treatment with medication is recommended if the bottom number of your blood pressure ratio, which represents your diastolic pressure, runs over 100 mm Hg for several months. If you must take blood pressure medication, avoid overly aggressive treatment. Treatment with medication that lowers your diastolic pressure below 90 mm Hg may increase your risk of death.

HOW TO LOWER BLOOD PRESSURE SAFELY

The best way to lower blood pressure is to adopt a low-sodium, low-fat, no-cholesterol diet. Most of the patients at St. Helena Hospital go off their medication in *just one day* and soon find their blood pressure is lower than it was when they were on medication. The average drop is 6 mm Hg for the top number (systolic pressure) and 3 mm Hg for the bottom number (diastolic pressure). People initially showing blood pressures greater than 150/90 show an even greater pressure reduction. The average drop is 23 mm Hg for the top number and 14 mm Hg for the bottom number. In most cases, patients stop taking their medications on the first day of our program, unless they are on beta-blockers or large quantities of medications. Then the dosage is slowly reduced over several days (sudden discontinuation of beta-blockers can cause chest pains and possibly a heart attack).

Blood pressures of my patients fall quickly for several reasons: they're relaxed at St. Helena Hospital. They're off all caffeine and alcohol, both powerful stimulants that can raise blood pressure in sensitive people. The food is rich in potassium, which has been shown to lower blood pressure. It is also low in sodium, which elevates blood pressure. Most important, my patients experience a dramatic improvement in circulation due to the low-fat McDougall diet. They also exercise, which lowers blood pressure.

This is the only approach that I know of that will lower your blood pressure and get you off medication. Make no mistake: your goal should be to get off medication! Sick people take drugs, and the unfortunate truth is that sometimes drugs can make you even sicker.

The Connection Between Diabetes and Cardiovascular Disease

Because women are protected against developing heart disease during their reproductive years, relatively few of them suffer heart attacks or strokes—unless they suffer from diabetes. Premenopausal women with diabetes face a risk of heart attack similar to that of men of the same age. In fact, women with diabetes are three to seven times more likely to die from heart disease than are nondiabetic women.

Adult-onset diabetes affects approximately 4 percent of the U.S. population. Some ethnic groups within the United States experience much higher incidences of the disease, however. One such group is the Pima Indians of Arizona. Eighty years ago, when the Pimas lived on their traditional plant-based diet, they enjoyed excellent health and were largely free of degenerative diseases, including diabetes. All that changed when the Pimas adopted the rich, modern diet loaded with fat, cholesterol, and refined foods. Today, half the Pima Indians living in Arizona have adult-onset diabetes. They also suffer extremely high rates of obesity, heart disease, kidney failure, and gallbladder disease. Other ethnic groups who have only recently adopted the modern high-fat diet have had similar experiences.

In the 1920s, Dr. Shirley Sweeney, a renowned diabetic researcher, performed an experiment on his healthy twenty-year-old medical students. After two days of consuming a very high-fat diet, all his students tested positive for diabetes on the glucose tolerance test (values over 150 mg/dl are considered abnormal). After two days on a high-carbohydrate diet (made of half sugar and half starch) they all tested as normal. For more than seventy years, doctors have known that fat paralyzes insulin activity and contributes to diabetes. These and subsequent studies have shown that carbohydrates, even those derived from pure white sugar, make insulin work better by increasing its sensitivity to blood sugar.

Researchers at the University of Kentucky Medical School found that when they placed their adult-onset diabetic patients on a low-fat, high–complex carbohydrate diet, approximately two-thirds of them no longer needed insulin injections. Some of these people had been on insulin for fifteen years or more. Virtually all their patients were able to give up their diabetic pills when they adopted this diet. Don't get suckered into believing sugar causes diabetes! The real problem is the rich American diet, high in fat and refined and processed foods, the same diet that causes heart disease and so many other degenerative illnesses.

In my book *The McDougall Program for a Healthy Heart* (Dutton, 1996), I address all the important issues involving heart disease, medication, bypass surgery, angioplasty, angiography, and other heart tests. What I have tried to do here is give you the tools for preventing and overcoming cardiovascular disease. Many so-called experts promote programs that focus on a single aspect of the human body, claiming that this part of the body needs special foods and substances that other parts do not need. If that were the case, we would not have survived this long as a species. Diet experts, diet programs, and this week's wonder supplement are distinctly modern phenomena. Our ancestors relied on a plant-based diet to support their health. Even today, people living on plant-based diets are relatively free of the degenerative diseases that plague the modern world.

Not only is the human body marvelously consistent in its needs, but it is also miraculously resilient. Given the right conditions, the human body can heal itself, erasing the effects of even the most terrible illnesses. The McDougall Program offers people the right conditions.

Healing Yourself

In July 1996, Betty Lieberman, sixty-five years old, of Colorado, had her first attack of chest pain that ran from the center of her chest, up to her neck, jaw, teeth, and then down her left arm. "I was terrified," Betty wrote to me in December 1996. "And I knew I had to do something fast."

Chest pain was not Betty's only problem. She had documented atherosclerosis, or cholesterol plaques clogging the arteries of her heart; a cholesterol level of 240 mg/dl; asthma, allergies, and arthritis; chronic heartburn and reflux; idiopathic edema in her legs; a hot spot and chronic tingling on her right leg; and urinary incontinence. On top of all of that, she was thirty pounds overweight.

Her husband, Sam, wasn't much better off. He had had three strokes; was diabetic and needed four injections of insulin per day to control his diabetes; had high blood pressure and was on medication; had neuropathy in his legs, retinopathy in his eyes, and poor circulation in his hands. Sam's cholesterol was 260 mg/dl.

Betty realized that she had to do something so she "tried another diet program and started to feel better." Immediately after starting the new program, she and Sam went on vacation. When Betty took a walk one day, the tightness and pain in her chest resumed.

Betty wanted to know if there was more she could do for her chest pain while on vacation and decided to call a local health food store. The manager informed her that the local hospital had a nutritionist on staff who might be able to help. "When I called the nutritionist," Betty wrote, "she told me about the McDougall Program she was on and felt it was a better program than the diet I was following. The next day, I went to the library and got your new book on reversing heart disease [*The McDougall Program for a Healthy Heart*]. I practically ate it. Two days later I purchased *The McDougall Program—Twelve Days to Dynamic Health*."

Betty wanted to start the program immediately but her husband was reluctant. "Isn't your life and health worth just twelve days to see if this plan works?" she told him. Sam agreed and the two began the program.

"After eleven days on the program Sam's blood pressure was normal and he was off all blood pressure medication," Betty wrote to me. "By about two to three weeks he was down to two shots of insulin a day. The circulation in both his hands and legs had greatly improved. He also had much greater sensation in his hands.

"As for me, after eleven days I had no more chest pain and no heartburn or reflux. The fluid in my legs went away. The hot spot on my right leg was gone, and I lost twelve pounds. We both had more energy and required less sleep. My asthma and arthritis were also improved."

After three months on the McDougall diet, Betty summed up her results in a single word. "Wow! I am twenty-two pounds lighter, my asthma and arthritis are markedly improved. For twenty years, because of the edema and arthritis, I have not been able to cross my legs without hip pain—now no problem! Stairs—no problem. My chest pain is completely gone and so is my heartburn. I do not suffer from incontinence any longer. That's also gone."

Betty's cholesterol level went from 240 to 170. Sam's fell to 180. His circulation, eyesight, and retinopathy all dramatically improved. But best of all, they're feeling great!

CHAPTER 15

Surviving Is the Bottom Line

Medicine is a business dominated by men. No matter what is said about doctors today, most people want to believe that their doctor is special, that he cares about them, that he wants to give them the best possible service, that the money he makes is a distant factor in his decisions, and that he is willing to sacrifice his time, energy, and income so that his patients can be healthy. Most people want to believe that their doctor is more like a priest, minister, or rabbi than a well-trained technician who has one eye on his patient and the other on the bottom line. However, the truth is the caring doctor that so many people have in their minds is very rare.

We trust our doctors with that which is most precious to us: our health and the health of our loved ones. Health is life. We do not want to equate our lives and the lives of those we love with a business transaction. Yet your relationship with your doctor is indeed a business relationship. He performs his services for a fee. People who are not sufficiently insured or cannot cover the cost of medical services do not get the same quality of care as those who are better insured. Some people who cannot afford certain medical care are simply turned away.

This harsh reality can be not only the basis for a much more rewarding relationship with your physician but also an essential step toward better medical care.

Male Versus Female Medicine

Medicine is a profession dominated by men. Indeed, many female doctors today are so influenced by their male colleagues that they have come to accept the practice of medicine as a male-identified profession, and therefore have adopted the same kinds of behaviors as their male counterparts. A growing number of physicians, both men and women, are attempting to offer a new approach to health care, but they are still very much in the minority. You can support this trend toward a more balanced form of health care that stresses prevention and a far more gentle approach to treatment.

A doctor whose methods are overly male-identified tends to be information oriented instead of emotionally nurturing; he wants the facts, and he would like them communicated as efficiently as possible. Your concerns and fears are essentially irrelevant to his approach, and therefore largely irrelevant to your relationship with your doctor, at least insofar as he is concerned. Such a physician is very time-sensitive. There are a lot of patients waiting to see him and he would like to move as rapidly through his day as he can. He is unlikely to rush you overtly, but in subtle and effective ways he communicates the boundaries within which he would like you to remain. Tell him the physical symptoms; allow him to perform his diagnostic procedures and tests; and then follow his advice and the prescribed treatment he recommends. That is the essence of his relationship with you. It is paternalistic and sometimes even patronizing.

He is highly scientific and his approach to treatment is aggressive. When he is unsure of the origin of the illness, he acts. He doesn't wait. He sees waiting as wrong and even a bit frightening. Waiting only allows the disease to get worse. He has no faith in the body's ability to heal itself. Indeed, he hasn't got a single tool in his medical armamentarium that will encourage the body's own healing mechanisms. His approach is to fix the body. As such, he uses drugs, radiation, and surgery until the disease process is destroyed. Unfortunately, it is precisely because of this type of thinking, which on the surface seems so rational and responsible, that we have so many people taking unnecessary drugs and undergoing needless tests and operations.

In many ways, prevention of disease and the use of diet and exercise as therapy are the exact opposite approach to health care: they are gentle, yet powerful, approaches to healing. They eliminate poisons that are weakening the body, while promoting the body's own immune system and cancer-fighting mechanisms. In my view, the McDougall Program is a more balanced approach to medicine, combining the best of medical technology and science—you might say, the masculine virtues—with the gentle, supportive methods, or the more feminine characteristics.

Most patients today want a different kind of medicine, one that represents this very balance. Patients want to be cared about, listened to, and given the time needed to report their conditions in full. Let's face it, you are talking to another human being about very intimate and personal matters. You do not want to be rushed into confessing that you have symptoms that you may regard as highly personal and even a little embarrassing to talk about. Patients also want a kinder and gentler form of therapy. They realize that the more extreme the treatment, the more severe the side effects. Powerful drugs and highly invasive procedures often have life-altering side effects.

Very often, patients are frightened. They would like to be treated in ways that support their humanity and dignity; they want doctors to treat their physical disorders while being aware of their overwhelming sense of vulnerability. Many patients want the option, whenever possible, to avoid highly toxic or invasive treatments for a chance to heal themselves with diet, lifestyle, and time.

These characteristics are all associated with the feminine side of our being, a side that exists in both men and women, but that is often denied or repressed by men, especially by male doctors. You cannot deny the feminine inside yourself without denying the feminine in your patients—especially your female patients.

Throughout this book I have given you many examples of these inequities in the areas of heart disease, cancer treatments, cancer screening tests, and gynecological surgeries. Women patients are shown less respect, given more tranquilizers, more often denied lifesaving treatments, and subjected to more useless tests and treatments than are men patients. Things are unlikely to change soon.

Therefore, you must take matters into your own hands: be aware of the kind of doctor you are looking for, the kind of treatment approach he or she uses, and the kind of financial system he or she is operating under. Medicine is currently in the throes of enormous change. The old system in which you paid for services provided is giving way to managed care, and that is radically changing the kind of health care you will receive. It's your job to find a physician with the kind of character traits you are looking for, and then you must recognize and accept that, no matter how wonderful this person may be, the two of you are in a business relationship. A business relationship requires that you ask questions, evaluate the recommendations, seek other opinions, demand excellent care, do not hesitate to say no, and fire incompetent doctors. It requires that you take an active role in your care and that you accept responsibility for being the final judge of what is best for you.

In order to develop the most appropriate and rewarding relationship with your doctor, you must understand some of the most important changes occurring in medicine today.

Changing Financial Force

Like most other professions, medicine was built on the premise that the quality of your care depended, to a great extent, on how much your doctor is paid. Until recently, you paid for the services your physician provided. The more office and hospital visits you made, the more medications prescribed, the more lab tests ordered, the more money your health care providers made.

Under this pay-as-you-go, or fee-for-services system, the doctor was in control of the kinds of care and the volume of services he or she provided. The best customers were the people with generous health insurance policies, because they could afford to have the most extensive testing and treatment possible. Interestingly, this system operated under the premise that the *best* medicine was *more* medical care. The problem with this system, of course, was that it rewarded doctors for ordering every conceivable test and treatment. All too often the patient was overtested and overtreated—and, of course, overbilled.

Today, that system is changing to one that is based on exactly the opposite behavior: doctors are being rewarded today for restricting their patients' care. You would be outraged if, while you and your doctor were discussing your condition, an insurance agent came into your doctor's office and told your doctor how he could treat you. You would be even more appalled if that insurance agent actually told your doctor that he could make more money if he refused to order a test or send you to a specialist. Unfortunately, this is exactly what is happening under the new medical systems referred to as managed care.

MANAGED CARE

Runaway health care costs, which have been increasing at a rate of 8 to 13 percent annually, have finally led employers, health insurers, and the government to demand changes. The health care market has responded with efforts to manage your medical care. Managed care organizations are companies that regulate health care workers and institutions, including doctors, health clinics, and hospitals. In this system, the managed care organization places limits on what doctors and hospitals can spend on their patients. In essence, they force health care professionals to limit the costs of their services. Thus, a physician's medical approach is restricted to ensure a profit for the managed care companies. In the end, fewer tests and treatments are ordered, and fewer services are sought from specialists.

Managed care organizations are implemented in health maintenance organizations (HMOs) and preferred provider organizations (PPOs). HMOs usually hire the doctors, who are paid salaries. PPOs are organized networks of physicians who sell their services to insurance companies. Doctors can draw a salary that may be supplemented by bonuses for cost-saving care. These financial incentives cause physicians to restrict their patients' access to medical services in exchange for money. Under this system the financial risks are still borne by the insurer, which can be a private health insurance company, such as Aetna, or the self-insured HMO, such as Kaiser Permanente, your PPO, or your employer. However, the services that insurer will pay for must be approved by the managed care company first.

Many important decisions, meanwhile, are being made without the patients' knowledge. For example, patients with routine and easily solved disorders—read inexpensive patients—are steered to an HMO, but patients who are ill and likely to require expensive treatment are directed away from HMOs to fee-for-service practices like Medicare. This keeps the HMO profitable, but costs the government and ultimately the taxpayers even more money. Even though it is illegal to ask Medicare patients about their health prior to enrollment, 43 percent of HMOs ask this question.

Patients who are very ill and require extraordinary care, such as bone marrow transplants for breast cancer, will likely be denied payment for treatment under the influence of managed care plans. Experimental therapies tend to be discouraged and medical progress may be stymied.

CAPITATION CUTS CARE

Yet another way to restrict costs is to directly penalize the doctor for providing unrestricted care. Thus, a new system, called capitation, has emerged in which the doctor is paid only a certain amount of money for each of his patients. Under this method, the money is paid by the managed care organizations to the physician who is designated by the patient as his or her primary care provider. Total capitation for an internist is between $11 to $14 per patient per month. This money must cover all the doctor's charges, whether incurred in the office or hospital. Often an upper limit of liability is stipulated, so a doctor will not be seriously harmed by a catastrophic illness of one or more patients. Under the capitation system, as you can plainly see, your doctor is rewarded for holding back services.

In some systems the managed care organization pays for specialists, prescription drugs, and hospital use. Other systems pay the doctor more money up front, so that the primary care physician can pay directly for all these extra services.

As expected, these financial incentives used by managed care organizations do reduce rates of hospitalization and office visits. A recent survey conducted by the California Medical Association of 1,122 physicians found that 20 percent of doctors admitted that reimbursement or capitation "frequently" influenced their practices, and that 59.1 percent said they were "sometimes" affected by these concerns. In any case, this system has been created without concern for the patient's welfare.

Capitation places an enormous burden on the doctor, as well. The base capitation payment barely covers the doctor's office overhead. However, because he is rewarded for limiting his services, an internist with 1,500 patients may take home more than $150,000 in bonuses and incentives for saving the company money. On the other hand, he could make nothing at all if he doesn't save the company money. *The doctor's income is attached to conduct that furthers the managed care organizations' profitability—not your health.* One advantage of capitation is, however, that the decisions are the doctor's; he doesn't have to seek authorization from the insurer.

As with the old fee-for-service system, financial incentives under capitation encourage doctors to sign up more patients than they can responsibly care for; the system also encourages doctors to spend as little time as possible with each patient—in effect, to develop an "assembly line" medical practice. To conceal such conditions, managed care organizations often make contracts with doctors that prevent them from divulging their financial arrangements with insurance companies.

Under this system, the doctor has the opportunity to make a lot of money by keeping costs down. In the best case scenario, that will be done honestly by providing efficient care and avoiding unnecessary tests and treatments. But there is a real concern that costs may be reduced by avoiding sick patients, simply because they are expensive to treat. The very best physicians, such as experienced surgeons with special skills who attract very ill people, are at risk of being shut out of managed care organizations and medical groups because they incur the greatest costs. Thus, excellence in medicine is actually being discouraged.

In the end, the smartest doctors eventually will realize that in order to make this system work for both themselves and their patients, they must teach people how to be healthy.

Surviving the Medical Business

Clearly, the changes sweeping medicine today make it essential that you recognize that you are in a business relationship with your doctor and understand the financial incentives under which your doctor conducts his business. You don't want to be overtreated under a fee-for-services plan; nor do you want essential services denied you under managed care. To prevent either of these events from occurring, you should ask your doctor how he or she is paid. Also, ask how much these financial incentives influence your doctor's practice. If you feel you are receiving substandard care, discuss this with your doctor. Ask for a second opinion. Consult the administrator of the clinic or HMO and, if absolutely necessary, threaten legal action if you do not get a satisfactory response.

The best way to avoid all of these problems, of course, is to stay well and out of the system.

Ultimately, the medical system must change. The disincentives to providing the very best care must be removed. A salaried physician who receives no bonuses for saving money or encouraging more treatment is the most impartial judge, and thus in the best position to offer appropriate medical care.

In an ideal system, incentives and bonuses should be paid for *improving* the health of patients. Perhaps we should pay the doctor an extra dollar for every pound of weight lost by a patient, or every milligram reduction in cholesterol, or every millimeter decrease in blood pressure. Reward the doctor with an extra $20 for each patient he sends to a stop-smoking program—and $200 for each successful quitter. Doctors should be similarly rewarded for patients who adopt a plant-based diet and an exercise program. Patients, too, should be rewarded for improvements in their own health. Insurance companies and the government should reduce premiums for patients on healthy diets and lifestyles, just as they should pay doctors more who teach patients to adopt programs for long-term health. That is a strategy for the long-term health of individuals and our nation.

Our country's health maintenance organizations and the insurance companies who use health promotion as an advertising claim must start living up to their own self-promotion. They must start putting their money where it can really make a difference in people's lives.

CHAPTER 16

Adopting the McDougall Program Will Transform Your Health

The nucleus of the McDougall Program—and the secret to the restoration of your health—lies in making starches the centerpiece of your diet. This is where your transformation begins—with the reliance upon starches as the foundation of your diet. Among the many starch-based foods on the McDougall diet are brown rice, barley, oats, wheat, and other grains; whole-grain products, such as pastas, tortillas, breads, and puffed grains; squashes, such as acorn, buttercup, butternut, and pumpkin; many root vegetables, such as potatoes, yams, and sweet potatoes; and beans, including adzuki, black beans, chickpeas, lentils, navy beans, and pintos. Starches are the meat and potatoes of the McDougall Program.

When you were growing up and someone asked, "What's for dinner?" in all probability the response was usually "chicken," "steak," "pork chops," or "fish." Meat was the focus of the meal. When you think about it, animal foods are rather bland and tasteless, at least until you flavor them with spices, sauces, and seasonings. Plain, unsalted, and unseasoned beef or chicken are rather awful, really. There's very little flavor and, in the case of beef, you've got to chew it endlessly. To make this bland-tasting meat palatable, you've got to cover it with some kind of seasoning—for example, sweet-and-sour sauce, a barbecue sauce, or a seasoned bread crumb coating. That's the flavor people are looking for when they eat, say, a fried steak or Kentucky Fried Chicken.

Ironically, it's not the sauces and seasonings that make people fat, sick, and ugly, but the bland tasting, fat-rich animal food beneath the sauce. So, let's take a page out of the standard American cookbooks and add the sauces, seasonings, and dressings to health-promoting foods, such as pasta, potatoes, and rice. Take your favorite sauces, make them healthy by removing any oil or animal products, and then pour them over your newly chosen healthy centerpieces.

Now when someone asks, "What's for dinner?" your response will be "spaghetti," "bean burritos," "hash brown potatoes," or "spicy Spanish rice" or any one of the hundreds of McDougall recipes. Beneath so many of these new and wonderful flavors will be the new centerpiece of the meal: starch-based foods.

These starch-based plant foods are abundant sources of antioxidants, phytochemicals, vitamins, minerals, and fiber. They are also relatively low in calories, especially when compared with the high-fat animal foods that used to occupy the center of your plate. They are the basis for the restoration of your health, vitality, clarity of mind, and youthful appearance.

The diet is the most powerful of the three healing tools used in the McDougall Program. The other two are daily exercise and your willingness to eliminate some bad habits that you know deep down are making you ill and causing you much suffering. These three healing changes are more powerful medicines than anything a pharmacist, doctor, or hospital could offer you.

So let's begin right now and start to witness the miraculous transformation that awaits you. Start with the McDougall diet.

- Whole grains and whole-grain cereals, such as brown rice, barley, corn, millet, quinoa, oatmeal, bulgur wheat, and wheat berries
- Whole-grain products, such as pasta, bread, tortillas, cereals, and puffed grains
- Squashes, including acorn, buttercup, butternut, pumpkin, summer squash, and zucchini
- Roots and tubers, including potatoes, sweet potatoes, yams, carrots, rutabagas, and turnips
- Beans and other legumes, such as adzuki, black beans, black-eyed peas, chickpeas, kidney beans, lentils, navy beans, pinto beans, peas, and split peas
- Green and yellow vegetables, such as broccoli, cabbage, collard greens, kale, various kinds of lettuces, mustard greens, watercress; also celery, cauliflower, asparagus, and tomato
- Fruits, such as apples, bananas, berries, grapefruit, melons, oranges, peaches, and pears (limit servings to two to three per day)

Starches

Nothing fills us so effectively as starches, such as potatoes, rice, and beans. They completely satisfy us and that is why they are often referred to as "comfort foods." The remarkable thing about potatoes, rice, and beans is that while they fill, satisfy, and comfort, they are relatively low in calories. A three-and-a-half-ounce potato contains only 109 calories. Have two or three. Three and a half ounces of cooked brown rice contain 111 calories. Though beans vary in their calorie content, three and a half ounces of beans typically contain around 100 calories. On the other hand, a three-and-a-half-ounce portion of regular ground beef contains 289 calories, 21 grams of fat, and 8 grams of saturated fat. A couple of potatoes or six ounces or more of rice or beans—a large portion—will fill you up and satisfy you completely, yet still provide fewer than 250 calories. You'll also get an abundance of vitamins, minerals, antioxidants, and fiber. These foods contain little fat and no saturated fat. A couple of hamburgers, even without the cheese, contain nearly 600 calories (more than 600 if you eat them on refined buns) and more than 40 grams of fat, much of it saturated.

There are an endless number of ways to prepare the healthful starch-based foods to make them truly delicious and satisfying. I recommend that people start out by eating a lot of the comfort foods they were raised on. Choose recipes that contain familiar foods and your favorite spices, and whenever possible adjust the spicing to your liking. Of course, when you become more daring, you'll want to try dishes with unfamiliar vegetables and spices. Pick one or two recipes that look interesting and have ingredients and spices you have enjoyed in other recipes. Because people are rather monotonous in their eating habits, your goal is to find about a dozen dishes that you enjoy. There are more than 1,500 recipes published in the McDougall books, so finding new favorites will be an enjoyable adventure.

Changing Your Family Menu

What happens if you're excited about the McDougall Program, but the rest of the family isn't? Don't try to change them by making demands or by applying pressure. Rather, set an example for everyone. As other people in your household see you losing weight and becoming healthier, they'll want to experience the same transformation themselves. In the meantime, do not make two separate meals for the family.

Instead, make your starch-based meal and then add small amounts of the foods your family enjoys to your health-promoting foods.

For example, let's say you make bean burritos for dinner. The main dish will be "refried" beans made without oil and with whole wheat or corn tortilla shells. Put out bowls of lettuce, chopped tomatoes, onions, sprouts, and your favorite salsa sauces. To keep unconverted members happy, you might also offer a bowl of grated cheese or seasoned ground beef. Or, let's say you make spaghetti with an oil-free marinara sauce. With the spaghetti, also offer parmesan cheese and perhaps meat balls as side dishes to be added at the table. With your "fried" rice, add a plate of thinly sliced chicken that non-converted family members can add to their rice. These steps maintain family harmony, while providing healthful foods and promoting gradual change.

Make healthful meals with low-fat soy cheese, textured vegetable protein spiced with hamburger seasonings, and "meat" balls made from wheat gluten (also called seitan). You may want to use a little seitan and low-fat soy products every day to add a little richness to your dishes. In no time you will be able to conveniently forget to make the high-fat, high-cholesterol additions, and no one will protest.

Seasoning Foods

Much of a food's flavor depends on the way it is prepared and the seasonings, sauces, and dressings you use to enhance it. Use the recipes in this and other McDougall books as guidelines. Seasoning can make dishes more delicious, interesting, and enjoyable. Pick familiar spices to use in your cooking, and feel free to add more or less of a particular spice than our recipes call for. My wife, Mary, has tried to flavor the foods to satisfy the average palate. When deciding whether to use fresh herbs or dried ones, consider how long the food is going to cook. Dried herbs fare better in dishes cooked for longer times; for shorter cooking times, use fresh herbs, if available. Generally, you'll need more fresh herbs to equal the flavor of dried ones, because the dried herbs are more concentrated; however, dried herbs lose their potency and their taste when stored for too long.

People love salt and sugar for a very good reason: the tip of the tongue has taste buds that are sensitive to and satisfied by sweet and salty flavors. Nature designed us to desire sweet-tasting carbohydrates because those foods were the ones richest in nutrition and energy.

In order to get the most pleasure from salt and sugar—and do the least damage to your health—sprinkle these two condiments on the surface of the food, where your tongue can easily contact them, just before eating. When added during cooking, most of the flavor of salt or sugar is lost. Unfortunately, they still have the same effect on your body, even when you don't taste them. Which means that if you're going to use them, you might as well enjoy them.

Having the right condiment or prepared sauce on the table can make the meal palatable for family members not yet ecstatic about the new dishes. I have heard people say they would eat cardboard if it had Tabasco sprinkled on top. You can make your own condiments, or choose one of the many healthy bottled and packaged products found in your supermarket. (The most recent update of McDougall Approved Canned and Packaged Products can be found in *The McDougall Quick & Easy Cookbook*.)

HANDY TOPPINGS AND SEASONINGS

Here are some of the healthier and delicious toppings and seasonings you should have on hand to make your McDougall meals delicious.

Low-sodium, oil-free salad dressings
Lemon juice (bottled)
Vinegar (try balsamic vinegar as a salad dressing)
Low-sodium ketchup
Mustard
Salsas (oil-free)
Tabasco sauce
Hot pepper sauces
Horseradish (oil-free)
Low-sodium soy sauce
Barbecue sauces (bottled, oil-free)
Spaghetti sauce (bottled, oil-free)
Salt-free vegetable seasonings and seasoning mixes
Sugar, honey, molasses, sugar-free syrups, pure-fruit jams

Handy Snacks

Fill your kitchen cupboards with healthful snacks and treats that you enjoy and that will satisfy you without hurting your health. Here are some of my suggestions.

Rice cakes and rice crackers
Pretzels

Whole wheat crackers (oil-free)

Popcorn (spice it up by sprinkling it with garlic; chili, curry, or onion powder; poultry seasoning; or diluted Tabasco sauce; if you're not sensitive to salt, spray soy sauce on it or moisten it with water and sprinkle with table salt)

Fresh fruits and fruit snacks

Sliced raw vegetables

Seaweed

Whole-grain and sprouted wheat breads, whole wheat pitas and bagels (oil-free)

Instant oatmeal

Leftover baked potatoes (eaten cold or heated in a microwave)

Hash brown potatoes

Packaged or canned soups (for example, Dr. McDougall's Right Foods)

Canned beans

Leftovers

Fruit juice popsicles

Sorbet

Herbal teas and other noncaffeinated hot drinks

Soda water (low-sodium, flavored or unflavored) or mineral water

Cooking Tips

BROWNING VEGETABLES

Browned onions have an excellent flavor and can be used alone or mixed with other vegetables to make delicious dishes. Place 1½ cups of chopped onions in a large nonstick frying pan with 1 cup of water. Cook over medium heat, stirring occasionally, until the liquid evaporates and the onions begin to stick to the bottom of the pan. Continue to stir for a minute, then add another ½ cup of water, loosening the browned bits from the bottom of the pan. Cook until the liquid evaporates again. Repeat this procedure one or two more times, until the onions are as browned as you like. You can also use this technique to brown carrots, green peppers, garlic, potatoes, shallots, zucchini, and many other vegetables, alone or in combination.

BAKING WITHOUT OIL

Eliminating oil in baking is a real challenge because oil keeps the baked goods moist and soft. Replace the oil called for in the recipe with half the amount of another moist food, such as applesauce, mashed bananas, mashed potatoes, mashed pumpkin, tomato sauce, soft silken tofu, or soy yogurt (keep in mind that tofu and soy yogurt are high-fat foods). There are several new fat replacers on the market, for example, Wonderslim Fat and Egg Replacer and Sunsweet Lighter Bake.

Cakes and muffins made without oil usually come out a little heavier. For a lighter texture use carbonated water instead of tap water in baking recipes. Be sure to test cakes and muffins at the end of the baking time by inserting a toothpick or cake tester in the center to see if it comes out clean. Sometimes oil-less cakes and muffins may need to be baked longer than the directions advise, depending on the weather or the altitude at which you live.

SAUTÉING WITHOUT OIL

To sauté implies the use of butter or oil, but in McDougall cooking, oil is eliminated. Instead, we use other liquids to provide taste without the health hazards. Surprisingly, plain water makes an excellent sautéing liquid. It prevents foods from sticking to the pan, and still allows vegetables to brown and cook.

For additional flavor try sautéing in:

Soy sauce (tamari)
Vegetable broth
Red or white wine (alcoholic or nonalcoholic)
Sherry (alcoholic or nonalcoholic)
Rice vinegar or balsamic vinegar
Tomato juice
Lemon or lime juice
Mexican salsa
Worcestershire sauce

For even more taste, add herbs and spices, such as ginger, dry mustard, and garlic.

Shopping Tips

Before you go to the store, make a shopping list based on this week's menu. Then, pick the best market where you'll be able to find healthful grains, vegetables, beans, fruits, snacks, condiments, and supplies. During the last two decades, natural foods stores have grown as large as most supermarkets; they sell everything from dog food to toilet paper (recycled, of course). Their success has forced neighborhood super-markets to meet consumers' demands for healthier products. In-creased sales volume has brought the cost of healthful foods down in both kinds of stores.

The key to effective shopping is careful reading of labels. Ingredi-ents are supposed to be listed in descending order of amounts in the package. Manufacturers can deceive you with the present food labels. Sometimes simple sugars, such as sucrose, corn syrup, fructose, and fruit concentrate, can be listed individually, in order to move sugar from the first ingredient to further down the list. Manufacturers have found ways of hiding fats in ingredient lists by calling them mono-glycerides or diglycerides. You might recognize triglyceride as being a complex fat, but may fail to recognize the mono- and di- forms, or think they are additives unrelated to fats.

Another fat you may not recognize is lecithin. Most lecithin is made from soybeans and is no more effective at lowering blood cholesterol than any similar vegetable oil. You want to avoid fat as much as possible. Look for oils that are listed as ingredients on the label and avoid these products. The presence of dairy products in foods is often concealed

---

FIGURING PERCENT OF CALORIES

A little simple math will help you determine how much fat, pro-tein, and carbohydrate is in a labeled food or packaged product.

To calculate *percent fat*, multiply the number of grams of fat by *9 calories per gram*, divide the answer (the number of calories of fat) by the total calories, then multiply by 100 to get the percent. Your goal is less than 10% fat.

To calculate *percent protein*, multiply the number of grams of pro-tein by *4 calories per gram*, divide the answer (the number of calories of protein) by the total calories, then multiply by 100 to get the percent. Your goal is 6 to 15% protein.

To calculate *percent carbohydrate*, multiply the number of grams of carbohydrate by *4 calories per gram*, divide the answer (the number of calories of carbohydrate) by the total calories, then multiply by 100 to get the percent. Your goal is more than 75% carbohydrate.

The ideal starch-based diet is:

5 to 10% fat
6 to 15% protein
75 to 87% carbohydrate

on the ingredients list as whey, casein, and lactose. Such products should be avoided, of course.

Labels can be deceiving even when they are trying to inform. For example, very often a low-fat food lists "1 gram of fat" on the nutrition facts label, even when the food would seem to have no added fat at all. The 1 gram represents the total amount of fats found naturally in low-fat vegetable foods; don't worry about including it in your diet.

Choosing Cookware

An easy way to eliminate oil from your cooking is to use pans coated with nonstick surfaces. Acceptable materials for cookware include glass, glass coated with silicon (called Arcuisine), stainless steel, iron, nonstick-coated pans and bakeware (such as Dupont's Silverstone or Teflon), silicone-coated bakeware (such as Baker's Secret), and porcelain. A light oiling when you first get a Teflon or Silverstone implement will help to prevent sticking. Cast-iron pans and woks should be oiled before they're first used and then "seasoned" by heating.

When buying cookware, pay particular attention to the surface of the pot on which your food will be cooked. Cooking will cause your food to pick up molecules from the pot or utensil's surface, so choose your cookware carefully, and buy quality. Aluminum cookware should be avoided because of the association between aluminum ingestion and Alzheimer's disease.

Use parchment paper between the metal and your food when using cake pans, loaf pans, and baking sheets. Parchment paper also keeps food from sticking to the surface of the pans. It can be found in most grocery stores. Parchment paper can also be used under (or over) aluminum foil to prevent the aluminum from coming in contact with the food. Place a layer of parchment paper over the food in a baking dish, then cover with foil. Turn the edges of the paper and foil over the pan to hold in the steam.

If vegetables stick while cooking in a pan or baking tray, allow them to cool for five to ten minutes. Once cool, they should loosen easily. Cooling will also loosen muffins from the tins.

RECOMMENDED COOKWARE

(1) 2-quart saucepan (stainless steel)
(1) 3-quart saucepan (stainless steel)
(1) 4-quart saucepan (stainless steel)

(1) 6-quart stockpot (stainless steel)
(1) 8-quart steamer/pasta cooker (stainless steel)
(1) 12-quart stockpot (stainless steel)
(1) griddle (nonstick coating)
(1) large frying pan (nonstick coating)
(1) electric wok (nonstick coating)
(1) 9¼ × 5¼-inch loaf pan (silicone coated)
(1) 9 × 13 × 2-inch oblong baking pan (silicone coated)
(1) 8 × 8 × 2-inch square baking pan (silicone coated)
(1) muffin tin (silicone coated)
(2) baking trays (silicone coated)
(1) 2-quart covered casserole dish (glass)
(1) 3-quart covered casserole dish (glass)
(1) 6-quart square covered casserole dish (glass)
(2) 9 × 13-inch oblong uncovered baking dishes (glass)
(1) 7½ × 11¾-inch oblong uncovered baking dish (glass)

Dining Out McDougall Style

I can find a healthy, great-tasting meal for my family in eight out of ten restaurants. For breakfast, I order a whole-grain cold cereal with fruit juice, or hot oatmeal, or hash brown potatoes cooked without grease and topped with salsa or ketchup. I also request dry whole wheat toast and jelly, fresh fruit, and herbal tea for a beverage.

Lunch and dinner are usually some variation of each other. I look for a vegetarian restaurant and avoid the eggs, cheese, and oil on the menu. Chinese, Thai, and Japanese restaurants can easily make an oil-free, animal-free topping to go over rice (which is usually white rice). Indian restaurants have a tradition of vegetarian cooking. Many of their dishes are made without oil, but just before serving the chef adds ghee, or clarified butter. Tell the waiter to "hold the ghee." Chefs at most fine dining establishments consider cooking you a pure vegetarian dish with no oil a welcome challenge—if you give them notice.

You can get fast meals at salad bars—just leave out the selections with mayonnaise and olive oil. Many Mexican restaurants can put together an oil-free burrito or tostada with pinto or black beans, lettuce, tomatoes, and salsa. Pizza without the cheese is almost perfect, except for the oil in the crust and the white flour. Top with generous amounts of tomato sauce and assorted vegetables.

In Santa Rosa, California, our hometown, we have more than one hundred restaurants that list McDougall-style items on their menu.

With a little effort, you can persuade your local restaurants to provide healthful and delicious choices.

Food scientists and flavorists will tell you that the taste in the American diet flows primarily from fat, salt, and sugar. On the other hand, the great majority of the world's people have developed their traditional cuisine based on plant foods and water-based flavors. This is particularly true of the Asian cultures. If you have ever eaten in a Thai, Japanese, Chinese, or Vietnamese restaurant, you already know such foods are among the most flavorful you will ever eat. Yet, virtually all of them are plant foods and extremely low in fat.

The McDougall diet replicates this same tradition by relying on plant- and water-based flavors and the artful use of spices, seasonings, and sauces. Like traditional foods the world over, McDougall foods are bursting with flavor. Once you adopt my program and learn to prepare these foods, you'll discover their wide array of colors, flavors, textures, and aromas, and you'll realize how truly disgusting animal foods, fatty grease, and oil truly are.

Your health will change for the better—and so will your life.

Epilogue

Just for a moment, picture yourself as healthy, fit, and trim. See yourself as free of all troubling symptoms. Your appearance is more youthful, lean, and fit. You have an abundance of energy. You're joyful and focused. You look and feel great. People wonder how you look so good at your age! You have become your best self. Even you marvel at the transformation that has occurred in your life.

This is what happens to people who adopt the McDougall Program. Many of the people who achieved this condition of health—who became the best versions of themselves—had been so sick before they began the program that their doctors told them that they were beyond any hope of recovery. Despite such expressions of pessimism and doom, they overcame the odds and rediscovered their youthful vitality and beauty. In fact, they regained their lives.

The thought of becoming healthy, of becoming your best self, is so exciting and compelling that it is enough to make you want to change your diet and lifestyle this very minute. Indeed, many of you will change right now. You're already convinced and you're going to do it. I applaud you and look forward to hearing all about your miraculous experiences.

Some of you, however, are holding back. You do not believe that such wonderful things will happen to you. Or, you do not believe that you can stay on the program long enough to achieve these results.

Please understand two essential points: first, it's not as difficult to adopt the McDougall Program as you think; second, you will feel the benefits during the first few days. Yes, they may be subtle, but you will notice important and positive changes right away. You will see that your health is improving, even during the first week on the program! Remarkably, the benefits you experience will keep getting bigger and stronger the longer you maintain the McDougall regimen. After just twelve days, you will realize that not only can you regain your health, but you are already on your way. You are already losing weight; your skin is brighter and clearer. Your energy levels are improving dramatically. Your symptoms are receding and you are feeling better.

In the process, you will change fundamental beliefs about yourself and your food. Exercise will become something that you'll just want to do. You will get out and walk every day because you will see yourself as someone who exercises. You will eat a healthy breakfast, lunch, and dinner, because you are someone who is careful with her food. This is a whole new you—a healthy you—and this is what the healthy you does every day.

Recipes

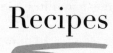

Breakfast

<u>SEASONED HASH BROWNS</u>

Contributed by Ginny Rew

Preparation Time: 5 minutes (need cooked potatoes)
Cooking Time: 10 to 15 minutes   Servings: 2 to 3

**4 to 6 medium unpeeled cooked
  potatoes
1 to 2 tablespoons
  soy sauce**

**3 to 4 tablespoons fat-free Italian
  dressing
1 tablespoon rice or balsamic
  vinegar (optional)**

Slice the potatoes thinly and place in a nonstick frying pan. Pour the soy sauce over the potatoes. Cook, turning frequently, for 2 minutes, then add the remaining ingredients. Continue to cook and turn until the potatoes are browned. The potatoes will become slightly mashed during this cooking process.

Hint: Cover the potatoes between turning to speed cooking. Add some sliced onions to the potatoes for more flavor.

BREAKFAST COUSCOUS

Preparation Time: 5 minutes   Cooking Time: 2 minutes
Resting Time: 5 minutes   Servings: 2

2 cups nonfat soy or
  rice milk
⅓ cup raisins or chopped
  dates

1 tablespoon honey or maple
  syrup
1 teaspoon vanilla
⅔ cup whole wheat couscous

Place the milk, raisins or dates, honey or maple syrup, and vanilla in a saucepan. Heat until the mixture almost boils, then remove from the heat. Stir in the couscous, cover, and let rest for 5 minutes. Stir again and serve.

MEXICANA SCRAMBLED TOFU

Preparation Time: 5 minutes
Cooking Time: 10 minutes   Servings: 2

1 12.3-ounce package extra-firm
  lite silken tofu
¼ cup vegetable broth
¼ cup chopped green bell
  pepper
2 green onions, chopped
¼ teaspoon minced fresh garlic

½ tablespoon soy sauce
⅛ teaspoon turmeric
pinch of crushed red
  pepper
⅓ cup mild or medium salsa
⅛ cup chopped fresh cilantro
dash or two of lime juice

Mash the tofu with a potato masher and set aside.

Place the broth in a nonstick frying pan and add the bell pepper, green onions, and garlic. Cook, stirring frequently, for 3 minutes. Add the mashed tofu, soy sauce, turmeric, and crushed red pepper. Cook an additional 3 minutes, stirring frequently. Add the remaining ingredients and cook another 4 minutes.

Serve rolled up in a tortilla for a delicious breakfast treat.

BEST PANCAKES EVER

Contributed by Rod and Mary Murray

Preparation Time: 15 minutes   Cooking Time: 15 minutes
Servings: Makes 12 to 15 pancakes

1 cup whole wheat flour	**¾ cup water**
¾ cup rolled oats	**3 tablespoons honey**
½ cup cornmeal	**1 tablespoon Ener-G Egg**
2 teaspoons baking powder	**Replacer mixed well with**
¾ cup soy milk	**4 tablespoons very warm water**

Mix the flour, rolled oats, cornmeal, and baking powder together in a large bowl. In a separate bowl, mix the soy milk, water, honey, and egg replacer mixture. Pour the wet mixture into the dry mixture and combine thoroughly. Let the batter rest for 5 minutes.

Heat a griddle until a drop of water will bounce on it. Ladle the batter onto the griddle. Turn the pancakes over when bubbles start to form on top and the edges are beginning to dry. Cook until lightly browned. Repeat with the remaining batter.

Serve with syrup, applesauce, or fruit spreads.

BANANA NUT BREAD

Preparation Time: 30 minutes
Cooking Time: 60 minutes   Servings: 12

¾ cup soy or rice milk	**¼ teaspoon salt**
1 tablespoon lemon juice	**⅓ cup Lighter Bake**
1¼ cups whole wheat flour	**1 cup mashed banana**
1 cup unbleached all-purpose flour	**¾ cup sugar**
1 teaspoon baking soda	**1 tablespoon egg replacer**
1 teaspoon baking powder	**¼ cup water**
1 teaspoon cinnamon	**1 teaspoon vanilla**
	⅓ cup walnut pieces

Preheat the oven to 350 degrees.

Place the milk in a cup with the lemon juice. Set aside.

Mix the flours, baking soda, baking powder, cinnamon, and salt in a large bowl.

In a separate bowl, mix the Lighter Bake, mashed banana, and sugar. Combine the egg replacer and water and beat until frothy. Add to the banana mixture along with the vanilla.

Place the walnut pieces in a small plastic bag and lightly smash with rolling pin or hammer. Add to the dry ingredients.

Add the milk mixture to the banana mixture and mix well. Add the dry ingredients and mix gently until combined. Pour into a 9 × 5-inch nonstick loaf pan. Bake for 60 minutes, or until a toothpick inserted in the center comes out clean.

Hint: Lighter Bake is a fat replacer made by Sunsweet Growers, Inc.

FRUIT SMOOTHIE

Preparation Time: 5 minutes   Servings: 2

1 banana, cut into chunks
1 cup orange juice

1½ cups assorted
frozen fruit

Combine all the ingredients in a blender jar and process until smooth.

Hint: This is delicious with many different types of frozen fruit. Chop whatever fruit is in season and freeze in resealable bags. We especially like mango, pineapple, papaya, strawberries, and/or peaches. This makes a wonderful after-school snack for children.

Salads

<u>BBQ BEAN SALAD</u>

Contributed by Joan Rice

Preparation Time: 15 minutes
Cooking Time: 10 minutes   Servings: 6 to 8

¼ cup ketchup
¼ cup cider vinegar
¼ cup vegetable broth
1 tablespoon Worcestershire
   sauce
3 tablespoons brown sugar
1 tablespoon chili powder
1 teaspoon ground cumin
¼ teaspoon black pepper
¼ teaspoon salt

¼ teaspoon Tabasco sauce
1½ tablespoons Dijon mustard
2 15-ounce cans pinto beans,
   drained and rinsed
1 red bell pepper, chopped
1 green bell pepper, chopped
1 small sweet onion, chopped
1 11-ounce can corn, drained
1½ cups crumbled fat-free
   tortilla chips

Place the ketchup, vinegar, broth, Worcestershire sauce, brown sugar, chili powder, cumin, black pepper, salt, and Tabasco sauce in a saucepan. Bring to a boil, reduce the heat, and cook over low heat for 10 minutes, stirring occasionally. Remove from the heat, stir in the mustard, and set aside.

Place the beans, bell peppers, onion, and corn in a large bowl. Pour the slightly cooled sauce over the vegetables and mix well. Stir in 1 cup of the tortilla chips. Sprinkle with the remaining chips. Serve at room temperature.

Hint: This is a wonderful dish to take to a potluck because it does not have to be served cold. If you make it ahead of time, do not add the chips until shortly before serving.

RAINBOW PASTA SALAD

Preparation Time: 20 minutes   Cooking Time: 20 minutes
Chilling Time: 2 to 3 hours   Servings: 8

2 cups orecchiette pasta
½ cup vegetable broth
3 cups chopped broccoli florets
2 cups asparagus, cut into 1-inch
    pieces
1 red bell pepper, chopped
1 bunch green onions, chopped
1 cup frozen corn kernels,
    thawed

½ teaspoon minced fresh garlic
1 15-ounce can kidney beans,
    drained and rinsed
2 tomatoes, chopped
½ cup oil-free Dijon-style
    dressing
2 tablespoons soy sauce
several twists of freshly ground
    black pepper

Cook the pasta in boiling water until just tender, 15 to 20 minutes.
Drain, rinse under cool water, and set aside.

Meanwhile, place the broth in a large nonstick frying pan. Add the
broccoli, asparagus, bell pepper, green onions, corn, and garlic to the
pan. Cook, stirring occasionally, until crisp-tender, about 5 minutes.
Place in a large bowl. Add the beans, tomatoes, and cooked pasta. Mix
well. Combine the dressing and soy sauce. Pour over the salad and toss
to mix. Season with black pepper. Refrigerate for 2 to 3 hours to blend
the flavors.

Hint: Use other small pasta shapes instead of the orecchiette for variety. Use any other canned beans in place of the kidney beans, if desired.

FIVE BEAN SALAD

Preparation Time: 15 minutes
Chilling Time: 6 to 8 hours   Servings: 12

1 14-ounce can kidney beans,
  drained and rinsed
1 14-ounce can garbanzo beans,
  drained and rinsed
1 14-ounce can green beans,
  drained and rinsed
1 14-ounce can wax beans,
  drained and rinsed
1 14-ounce can lima beans,
  drained and rinsed
1 green bell pepper, chopped

1 small red onion, sliced in half
  lengthwise, then thinly sliced
  and separated into rings
½ cup balsamic vinegar
½ cup honey
1 tablespoon soy sauce
½ teaspoon dry mustard
several twists of freshly ground
  black pepper
1 tablespoon fresh chives,
  chopped

Combine all the beans in a bowl. Add the bell pepper and onion and mix well. Combine the vinegar, honey, soy sauce, mustard, and black pepper in a jar. Shake well to mix. Pour over the vegetables and toss to mix. Sprinkle with the chives and mix again. Cover and refrigerate for 6 to 8 hours to allow the flavors to blend, stirring occasionally if possible.

QUINOA GARDEN SALAD

Preparation Time: 15 minutes   Cooking Time: 15 minutes
Chilling Time: 2 hours   Servings: 6 to 8

2 cups water
1 cup quinoa, well rinsed
1 cup chopped red bell
  pepper
¾ cup chopped green bell
  pepper
¼ cup chopped yellow bell
  pepper
1 cup chopped tomatoes
1 cup chopped green onions

1 14.5-ounce can garbanzo beans,
  drained and rinsed
½ cup chopped fresh parsley
¼ cup chopped fresh mint
½ cup fresh lemon juice
1 tablespoon soy sauce
several dashes of Tabasco
  sauce
several twists of freshly ground
  black pepper

Place the water and quinoa in a saucepan. Bring to a boil, reduce the heat, cover, and cook for about 15 minutes, until the water is absorbed. Remove from the heat and set aside.

Meanwhile, combine the bell peppers, tomatoes, green onions, garbanzos, parsley, and mint in a large bowl. Add the cooked quinoa and mix well. Add the remaining ingredients and mix again. Cover and refrigerate for at least 2 hours to blend the flavors.

CHINESE PASTA SALAD

Preparation Time: 20 minutes   Cooking Time: 8 to 10 minutes
Chilling Time: 2 hours   Servings: 6

16 ounces linguine
1 cup vegetable broth
½ cup soy sauce
½ cup rice vinegar
1 tablespoon sherry
1 tablespoon sugar
1 tablespoon cornstarch
1½ teaspoons minced fresh
   ginger
½ teaspoon crushed red
   pepper
dash of dark sesame oil

1 red bell pepper, thinly sliced
   into 1-inch strips
1 green bell pepper, thinly sliced
   into 1-inch strips
1 8-ounce box frozen baby pea
   pods, thawed
2 6.5-ounce packages smoked
   tofu, cubed
1 bunch green onions, chopped
⅓ cup chopped fresh cilantro
several twists of freshly ground
   black pepper (optional)

Bring a large pot of water to a boil. Drop in the linguine and cook until just tender, 8 to 10 minutes. Drain and rinse under cool water. Set aside.

Combine ½ cup of the broth with the soy sauce, rice vinegar, sherry, sugar, cornstarch, ginger, crushed red pepper, and sesame oil. Set aside.

Place the remaining ½ cup of broth in a large nonstick frying pan. Add the bell peppers and cook, stirring frequently, for 2 to 3 minutes. Add the peas and cook another minute. Add the tofu, cooked linguine, and the liquid mixture. Cook, stirring constantly, until the mixture boils and thickens. Stir in the green onions and cilantro. Mix well. Place in a covered bowl and refrigerate at least 2 hours before serving. Check the seasoning before serving and add a little more soy sauce and some black pepper, if desired.

VEGETABLE TABBOULEH

Preparation Time: 15 minutes   Resting Time: 30 minutes
Chilling Time: 2 to 3 hours   Servings: 8

1 cup uncooked bulgur
2 cups boiling water
3 tomatoes, chopped
1 cucumber, chopped
1 green bell pepper, chopped

6 green onions, chopped
1 cup chopped fresh parsley
½ cup chopped fresh mint
½ cup lemon juice
freshly ground black pepper

Place the bulgur in a bowl and pour the boiling water over it. Cover and let rest for 30 minutes. Transfer to a strainer to cool and drain.

Meanwhile, prepare the vegetables and herbs and place them in a separate large bowl.

Combine the drained bulgur and vegetables. Add the lemon juice and black pepper to taste. Mix well and chill 2 to 3 hours before serving.

Hint: A 15-ounce can of any kind of cooked beans, drained and rinsed, makes a nice addition to this salad. Try garbanzo, kidney, black, or white beans.

GAZPACHO SALAD

Preparation Time: 15 minutes
Chilling Time: 1 to 2 hours   Servings: 4

2 tomatoes, coarsely chopped
1 cucumber, coarsely chopped
1 yellow bell pepper, coarsely
  chopped
1 stalk celery, chopped

¼ cup chopped red onion
½ cup V-8 juice or Spicy V-8 juice
½ teaspoon Tabasco sauce
2 tablespoons chopped fresh
  cilantro

Place the vegetables in a bowl. Combine the V-8 juice and Tabasco sauce and pour over the vegetables. Refrigerate for 1 to 2 hours, stirring occasionally. Stir in the cilantro just before serving. Serve in a bowl with a small amount of the juice spooned over the vegetables.

GARBANZO-SPINACH SALAD

Preparation Time: 15 minutes
Chilling Time: 1 to 2 hours   Servings: 4 to 6

3 15-ounce cans garbanzo beans,
   drained and rinsed
2 cups loosely packed chopped
   fresh spinach
½ cup chopped red bell
   pepper

½ cup chopped yellow bell
   pepper
3 green onions, finely chopped
½ cup oil-free Italian dressing
several twists of freshly ground
   black pepper

Combine the beans and vegetables in a bowl. Pour the dressing over and toss to mix. Season with black pepper. Refrigerate for 1 to 2 hours for the best flavor.

Hint: This is one of my favorite salads; very often I eat it right after putting it together. This salad keeps well in the refrigerator for several days.

RAINBOW SALAD

Preparation Time: 15 minutes (need cooked rice)
Chilling Time: 2 hours   Servings: 6 to 8

3 cups cooked brown rice
1 15-ounce can kidney beans,
   drained and rinsed
1 15-ounce can garbanzo beans,
   drained and rinsed
1 15-ounce can black beans,
   drained and rinsed
1 cup frozen corn kernels,
   thawed
1 cup frozen green peas, thawed

¼ cup chopped red onion
¼ cup chopped pimiento
2 tablespoons chopped black
   olives
2 tablespoons chopped fresh
   cilantro
¾ cup oil-free Dijon-style
   dressing
2 tablespoons soy sauce
½ teaspoon Tabasco sauce

Place the rice in a large bowl. Add the beans, corn, peas, onion, pimiento, olives, and cilantro. Mix well. Combine the dressing, soy sauce, and Tabasco sauce in a jar. Cover and shake well to mix. Pour over the salad and mix well. Refrigerate for 2 hours before serving.

Hint: This colorful, delicious salad is excellent to take to a potluck or picnic because everyone loves it. To thaw corn and peas, place in a colander and run cold water over the vegetables until thawed.

PINEAPPLE RICE SALAD

Preparation Time: 20 minutes (need cooked rice)
Chilling Time: 1 to 2 hours   Servings: 6 to 8

4 cups cooked brown rice
1 6-ounce bag baby spinach, chopped
1 bunch green onions, chopped
1 20-ounce can pineapple chunks, drained

½ pound fresh mushrooms, sliced
1 cup oil-free Dijon-style dressing
3 tablespoons soy sauce
½ teaspoon dried dill weed
freshly ground black pepper

Place the cooked rice in a bowl. Add the spinach, green onions, pineapple, and mushrooms. Mix well.

Combine the dressing, soy sauce, and dill weed in a jar and mix well. Pour over the salad and toss well to mix. Season with black pepper to taste. Chill 1 to 2 hours before serving.

SANTA FE RICE SALAD

Preparation Time: 10 minutes (need cooked rice)
Servings: 4

2½ cups cooked brown rice
1 15-ounce can black beans, drained and rinsed
1 cup frozen corn kernels, thawed
1 tomato, chopped
4 green onions, chopped

2 tablespoons chopped fresh cilantro
½ cup salsa
¼ cup Tofu Mayonnaise (page 321) or fat-free mayonnaise

Place the rice, beans, corn, tomato, green onions, and cilantro in a bowl and mix well. Combine the salsa and mayonnaise and pour over the salad. Toss well to mix. Serve at once or refrigerate until serving time.

Hint: There is an excellent fat-free mayonnaise made by Nasoya Foods, Inc., called Nayonaise, available at most natural foods stores.

WINTER VEGETABLE COUSCOUS SALAD

Preparation Time: 15 minutes (need cold cooked couscous)
Cooking Time: 5 minutes   Servings: 6

2 cups broccoli florets
2 cups cauliflower florets
¾ cup oil-free Dijon-style dressing
2 tablespoons soy sauce
1 15-ounce can black beans,
  drained and rinsed

¼ cup chopped green onions
1 4-ounce jar chopped
  pimientos
4 cups chilled cooked couscous
freshly ground black pepper

Place the broccoli and cauliflower in water to cover. Bring to a boil and cook for 5 minutes. Drain. Place in a bowl filled with ice water. Drain again and set aside.

Combine the dressing and soy sauce. Set aside.

Mix the beans, green onions, pimientos, and couscous together. Add the broccoli, cauliflower, and dressing mixture. Mix well. Season with black pepper to taste. Serve cold.

Hint: Make this salad with other kinds of beans, such as kidney, garbanzo, or pinto.

Soups and Stews

BROCCOLI BISQUE

Preparation Time: 15 minutes
Cooking Time: 18 minutes   Servings: 6

4 cups broccoli florets
2½ cups vegetable broth
2 cups frozen chopped hash
  brown potatoes
1 small onion, chopped

1 teaspoon dried dill weed
2½ cups fat-free soy or
  rice milk
1 tablespoon Dijon mustard
Pinch of white pepper

Place the broccoli, broth, potatoes, onion, and dill weed in a medium pot. Bring to a boil, reduce the heat, cover, and cook for 15 minutes. Process in batches in a blender, adding some of the milk to each batch. Pour the processed soup into a pan, add the mustard and pepper, and heat through. Serve at once.

CREAMY POTATO CHOWDER

Preparation Time: 5 minutes
Cooking Time: 60 minutes   Servings: 8 to 10

1 32-ounce bag frozen
  chopped hash brown
  potatoes
3 leeks, white part only, sliced
4 cups vegetable broth
4 cups water

2 cups frozen corn kernels
1 tablespoon soy sauce
½ teaspoon dried dill weed
½ teaspoon paprika
pinch of cayenne
1 cup soy or rice milk (optional)

Place the potatoes, leeks, broth, and water in a large pot. Bring to a boil, reduce the heat, cover, and cook for 30 minutes. Add the remaining ingredients and cook an additional 30 minutes, stirring once or twice.

ASPARAGUS CREAM SOUP

Preparation Time: 10 minutes
Cooking Time: 10 minutes   Servings: 4

2 cups vegetable broth
2 cups chopped asparagus stalks
1½ cups frozen chopped hash
  brown potatoes

1 cup water
1 cup asparagus tips
1 cup soy milk
freshly ground black pepper

Place the broth, asparagus stalks, and potatoes in a medium pan. Bring to a boil, reduce the heat, cover, and cook for 5 minutes, or until the asparagus is just barely tender. Remove from the heat, pour into a blender jar, and process until very smooth. Return to the pan.

Meanwhile, place the water and asparagus tips in a small saucepan.

Bring to a boil, reduce the heat, and cook for 5 minutes, or until crisp-tender. Drain and add to the pureed soup. Stir in the milk and season with black pepper to taste. Heat through and serve at once.

Variation: Do not add the asparagus tips to the pureed soup. Instead, add the milk and pepper and heat through. Ladle a portion into individual serving bowls and place an equal amount of the tips on the surface of each bowl before serving.

MISO SOUP

Preparation Time: 10 minutes   Cooking Time: 5 minutes
Resting Time: 2 minutes   Servings: 6 to 8

8 cups water
½ cup mellow white miso
1 or 2 12.3-ounce packages extra-firm lite silken tofu, cubed

¼ cup soy sauce
1 bunch green onions, chopped

Place the water in a pot and bring to a boil. Remove about 1 cup of the hot broth and mix into the miso until it is very smooth. Stir this into the broth in the pot, along with the remaining ingredients. Turn off the heat and let rest for 2 minutes. Serve at once.

VEGETABLE UDON SOUP

Preparation Time: 20 minutes
Cooking Time: 10 minutes   Servings: 8

8 cups vegetable broth
¼ cup soy sauce
1 teaspoon crushed fresh garlic
1 teaspoon minced fresh ginger
1 bunch green onions, sliced into 1-inch pieces
8 fresh shiitake mushrooms, stems removed, then thinly sliced

2 cups sliced bok choy leaves
1 cup snow peas
1 2-inch piece daikon, peeled and sliced
½ cup julienned red bell pepper
1 14-ounce package fresh udon noodles
1 12.3-ounce package firm lite silken tofu, cubed (optional)

Place the broth, soy sauce, garlic, and ginger in a large pot. Bring to a boil. Add the green onions, mushrooms, bok choy, snow peas, daikon, and red pepper. Cook for 3 minutes. Add the udon and the tofu, if using. Cook for another 3 to 4 minutes until the noodles are tender.

Hint: If you cannot find fresh udon noodles, use dried noodles and add them when you add the vegetables. Add the tofu just a couple of minutes before serving.

JACK'S ITALIAN SPINACH SOUP

Contributed by Jack Dixon

Preparation Time: 10 minutes
Cooking Time: 10 minutes   Servings: 6 to 8

2 cups vegetable broth
1 10-ounce package frozen
  chopped spinach
½ cup frozen chopped onions
1 15-ounce can white beans,
  drained and rinsed
1 15-ounce can tomato sauce
1½ cups water
1 8-ounce can mushrooms,
  drained

1 cup small uncooked pasta shells
1 tablespoon soy sauce
1 teaspoon dried minced onion
1 teaspoon dried basil
⅛ teaspoon Italian seasoning
  blend
⅛ teaspoon dried minced garlic
⅛ teaspoon crushed red pepper
freshly ground black pepper
  to taste

Combine all the ingredients in a large soup pot. Bring to a boil, cover, and cook over medium heat for 10 minutes, stirring occasionally.

IN A FLASH BLACK BEAN SOUP

Preparation Time: 5 minutes
Cooking Time: 10 minutes   Servings: 4

3 15-ounce cans black beans,
  drained and rinsed
1¾ cups vegetable broth
1 cup fresh salsa

¼ teaspoon ground oregano
¼ teaspoon chili powder
several dashes of Tabasco sauce

Drain the beans and place 1¼ cups aside in a separate bowl. Place the remaining beans, the broth, and the salsa in a blender jar and process until fairly smooth. Pour into a saucepan. Mash the remaining beans with a bean/potato masher and add to the pan with the remaining ingredients. Cook over medium heat for 10 minutes, stirring occasionally.

Hint: Serve with a loaf of fresh bread to dunk in this soup. This quick soup is so delicious you'll want to make it again and again.

THAI CURRIED LENTIL SOUP

Preparation Time: 5 minutes
Cooking Time: 30 minutes   Servings: 6

6½ cups water
1 onion, chopped
1 cup red lentils
1 14.5-ounce can chopped
　tomatoes

2 tablespoons chopped
　fresh basil
1 tablespoon green curry paste
freshly ground black pepper
　to taste

Place ½ cup of the water in a medium pot. Add the onion and cook, stirring occasionally, for 5 minutes. Add the remaining water and the lentils. Bring to a boil and cook over low heat for 15 minutes. Add the tomatoes and mix well. Remove 4 cups of the soup to a blender jar and puree. Return to the pot. Add the remaining ingredients and cook for 10 more minutes.

Hint: Green curry paste is a mixture of chiles, garlic, lemongrass, and ginger. It is sold in Asian markets and at Trader Joe's.

HOT AND SOUR SOUP

Preparation Time: 30 minutes   Cooking Time: 17 minutes
Resting Time: 2 minutes   Servings: 6 to 8

1 quart water
1 quart vegetable broth
1 red bell pepper, chopped
1 onion, sliced
1½ cups sliced fresh
  mushrooms
½ cup sliced carrots
1 teaspoon minced fresh ginger
½ teaspoon minced fresh garlic
1½ cups thinly sliced Napa
  cabbage
1½ cups snow peas, cut in half

1 12.3-ounce package extra-firm
  lite silken tofu, cubed
½ cup cornstarch
¼ cup rice vinegar
¼ cup soy sauce
¼ teaspoon black pepper
⅛ teaspoon white pepper
⅛ teaspoon crushed red pepper
dash of sesame oil
4 green onions, sliced
2 tablespoons chopped fresh
  cilantro

Place the water, broth, bell pepper, onion, mushrooms, carrots, ginger, and garlic in a large pot. Bring to a boil, cover, and cook over medium heat for 15 minutes. Add the cabbage, snow peas, and tofu. Cook for 5 minutes longer.

Meanwhile, mix the remaining ingredients, except the green onions and cilantro, in a bowl. Add to the soup, stirring constantly until thickened and clear. Add the green onions and cilantro. Mix well. Remove from the heat and let rest for 2 minutes before serving.

HEARTY VEGETABLE BEAN SOUP

Preparation Time: 20 minutes
Cooking Time: 50 minutes   Servings: 6 to 8

½ cup water
2 leeks, sliced (white part only)
½ pound cremini mushrooms, chopped
1 red bell pepper, chopped
1 green bell pepper, chopped
6 cups vegetable broth
1 14.5-ounce can chopped tomatoes
1 15-ounce can garbanzo beans, drained and rinsed
1 15-ounce can kidney beans, drained and rinsed

1 15-ounce can cannellini beans, drained and rinsed
1 cup frozen corn kernels
2 tablespoons soy sauce
¼ cup chopped fresh parsley
2 teaspoons chopped fresh basil
1 teaspoon chili powder
several twists of freshly ground black pepper
½ cup uncooked orzo pasta

Place the water, leeks, mushrooms, and bell peppers in a large soup pot. Cook over medium heat, stirring frequently, for 10 minutes. Add the remaining ingredients, except the pasta, bring to a boil, reduce the heat, cover, and cook for 30 minutes. Remove the cover, stir in the orzo, and cook for 10 more minutes.

MOROCCAN BEAN SOUP

Preparation Time: 25 minutes
Cooking Time: 40 minutes   Servings: 8

3½ cups water
1 onion, chopped
1 green bell pepper, chopped
4 medium carrots, chopped
2 celery stalks, chopped
1 teaspoon minced fresh garlic
2 teaspoons grated fresh ginger
2 teaspoons ground cumin
½ teaspoon dried thyme
½ teaspoon turmeric
¼ teaspoon ground coriander
Dash of ground cloves

1 cup red lentils
2 cups vegetable broth
1 14.5-ounce can chopped
   tomatoes
1 bay leaf
several twists of freshly ground
   black pepper
1 15-ounce can garbanzo beans,
   drained and rinsed
2 cups cauliflower florets
½ cup raisins
¼ cup chopped fresh cilantro

Place ½ cup of the water in a large pot. Add the onion, bell pepper, carrots, celery, garlic, and ginger. Cook, stirring occasionally, for 5 minutes. Add the cumin, thyme, turmeric, coriander, and cloves. Mix well. Add the lentils, the remaining water, the broth, tomatoes, bay leaf, and black pepper. Bring to a boil, cover, reduce the heat, and simmer for 20 minutes. Add the garbanzo beans, cauliflower, and raisins. Cook an additional 12 minutes. Stir in the cilantro just before serving.

CURRIED POTATO SOUP

Preparation Time: 15 minutes
Cooking Time: 55 minutes   Servings: 8

½ cup water
2 onions, chopped
1 teaspoon minced fresh garlic
1 green bell pepper, chopped
4 cups frozen chopped hash
   brown potatoes
1½ teaspoons curry powder
¼ cup chopped fresh parsley

6 cups vegetable broth
1 bay leaf
1½ cups frozen corn kernels
2 tablespoons chutney
1½ cups rice or soy milk
2 tablespoons unbleached
   all-purpose flour
freshly ground black pepper

Place the water, onions, and garlic in a large pot. Cook, stirring frequently, for 2 minutes. Add the bell pepper and continue to cook for 2 minutes. Add the potatoes, curry powder, and parsley. Mix well, then add the broth and bay leaf. Bring to a boil, cover, and cook over low heat for 30 minutes. Add the corn and chutney and cook for 10 more minutes. Mix the milk and flour in a bowl, add to the soup, and cook, stirring frequently, for 10 more minutes. Season to taste with black pepper.

POLISH SWEET POTATO SOUP

Preparation Time: 15 minutes
Cooking Time: 33 minutes   Servings: 6

2 leeks, white part only, thinly
  sliced
1 teaspoon minced fresh garlic
5½ cups vegetable broth
2 large sweet potatoes, peeled
  and thinly sliced

2 cups chopped kale
⅛ teaspoon crushed red
  pepper
4 non-fat, non-meat sausages,
  thinly sliced

Place the leeks and garlic in a large pot with ½ cup of the broth. Cook, stirring frequently, for 2 minutes. Add the remaining broth and the sweet potatoes. Bring to a boil, cover, and cook over low heat for 15 minutes. Remove from the heat. Mash with a potato masher while still in the pot until only a few small chunks remain. Return to the heat. Add the kale and crushed red pepper. Cook for 10 minutes. Add the sausages and cook an additional 5 minutes. Serve at once.

Hint: This is most attractive when made with the bright orange sweet potatoes, sometimes referred to as yams.

ITALIAN CAULIFLOWER MINESTRONE

Preparation Time: 15 minutes
Cooking Time: 20 minutes   Servings: 6

1 onion, sliced
1 teaspoon minced fresh garlic
5¼ cups vegetable broth
1 14.5-ounce can chopped
   tomatoes
1 potato, scrubbed and chopped

2 cups cauliflower florets
1 15-ounce can kidney beans,
   drained and rinsed
1 cup small uncooked pasta
freshly ground black pepper
   to taste

Place the onion and garlic in a large pot with ¼ cup of the broth. Cook, stirring frequently, for 2 minutes. Add the remaining broth, the tomatoes, and the potato. Bring to a boil, cover, and cook for 3 minutes. Add the remaining ingredients, cover, and cook over low heat for 15 minutes, stirring occasionally.

FAST HEARTY VEGETABLE SOUP

Preparation Time: 10 minutes
Cooking Time: 47 minutes   Servings: 8

1 onion, chopped
2 stalks celery, sliced
1 16-ounce bag frozen broccoli,
   cauliflower, and carrots
1 cup frozen cut green beans
1 cup frozen corn kernels
2 quarts vegetable broth

1 15-ounce can chopped tomatoes
1 8-ounce can tomato sauce
2 tablespoons soy sauce
1 tablespoon parsley flakes
½ teaspoon Tabasco sauce
⅓ cup cornstarch mixed in
   ½ cup water

Place all the ingredients, except the cornstarch mixture, in a large soup pot. Bring to a boil, reduce the heat, and cook over medium-low heat for 45 minutes, or until the vegetables are very soft. Add the cornstarch mixture, cook, and stir for 2 minutes.

HEAVENLY VEGETABLE SOUP

Preparation Time: 20 minutes
Cooking Time: 62 minutes   Servings: 8

½ cup water
1 onion, chopped
2 stalks celery, chopped
2 carrots, sliced
1 cup green beans, cut into 1-inch
    pieces
1 cup sliced mushrooms
1 cup broccoli florets
1 cup cauliflower florets
1 15-ounce can chopped tomatoes
2 quarts vegetable broth

1 cup frozen corn kernels
1 8-ounce can tomato sauce
2 tablespoons parsley flakes
2 teaspoons dried basil
2 tablespoons soy sauce
½ teaspoon Tabasco sauce
¼ teaspoon chili powder
several twists of freshly ground
    black pepper
⅓ cup cornstarch mixed in ½ cup
    cold water

Place the water, onion, celery, carrots, and green beans in a large soup pot. Cook, stirring frequently, for 10 minutes. Add the remaining ingredients, except the cornstarch mixture, and cook over low heat for 50 minutes. Add the cornstarch mixture while stirring. Cook and stir for 2 minutes. Serve at once.

Variation: Add ½ cup uncooked small pasta about 15 minutes before the end of cooking time. Eliminate the cornstarch mixture.

MEXICAN VEGETABLE SOUP
WITH CILANTRO PESTO

Preparation Time: 30 minutes
Cooking Time: 40 minutes   Servings: 8

½ cup water
1 onion, chopped
1 red bell pepper, chopped
2 leeks, white part only, thinly
   sliced
1 teaspoon minced fresh garlic
8 cups vegetable broth
1 14.5-ounce can Mexican-style
   stewed tomatoes
1 4-ounce can chopped green
   chiles
1 8-ounce can tomato sauce
1 whole dried chipotle chile

1 teaspoon chili powder
1 teaspoon ground oregano
½ teaspoon Tabasco sauce, or
   to taste
2 zucchini, chopped
1 cup Savoy cabbage, chopped
1½ cups chopped kale
1½ cups frozen corn kernels
2 15-ounce cans pinto beans,
   drained and rinsed
1 cup small uncooked pasta, such
   as orzo
Cilantro Pesto (page 278)

Place the water in a large pot with the onion, bell pepper, leeks, and garlic. Cook, stirring frequently, for 7 minutes. Add the broth, tomatoes, green chiles, tomato sauce, chipotle chile, chili powder, oregano, and Tabasco sauce. Bring to a boil, cover, reduce the heat, and cook over low heat for 10 minutes. Add the vegetables and beans. Cook for 10 minutes. Add the pasta and cook for an additional 4 to 8 minutes, until the pasta is tender. Remove the whole chipotle before serving. Stir 1 to 2 teaspoons of Cilantro Pesto into each bowl before eating.

CILANTRO PESTO

Preparation Time: 10 minutes   Yield: 1 cup

1 cup packed cilantro leaves
1 tablespoon raw cashews
½ teaspoon minced fresh garlic

1 teaspoon lime juice
2 teaspoons water

Place the cilantro in a blender or food processor and process until chopped. Add the remaining ingredients and process until well mixed.

Use this pesto to add more flavor to soups and stews. It's also delicious spread on bread.

SUNSHINE STEW

Preparation Time: 15 minutes
Cooking Time: 30 minutes   Servings: 6

6 cups water
1½ cups split mung beans
2 tomatoes, chopped
1 onion, chopped
2 cups chopped, peeled sweet
    potato
1 teaspoon minced fresh garlic

2 tablespoons parsley flakes
1 teaspoon dried dill weed
2 cups small broccoli florets
1 tablespoon soy sauce
freshly ground black pepper
several dashes of Tabasco
    sauce

Place 4 cups of the water in a medium saucepan. Add the mung beans and tomatoes. Bring to a boil, reduce the heat, cover, and cook for 30 minutes, stirring frequently. Meanwhile, place the remaining water in another saucepan. Add the onion, sweet potato, garlic, parsley, and dill. Bring to a boil, reduce the heat, cover, and cook for 15 minutes. Add the broccoli and cook for 5 minutes longer. Add the cooked mung bean mixture to the vegetables and mix well. Season to taste with soy sauce, black pepper, and Tabasco sauce.

FESTIVE PUMPKIN STEW

Preparation Time: 60 minutes
Cooking Time: 1 hour, 22 minutes   Servings: 6 to 8

2 cups vegetable broth
1 onion, chopped
1 red or green bell pepper,
  coarsely chopped
1 teaspoon minced garlic
2 teaspoons chili powder
1½ teaspoons ground oregano
2 bay leaves
several twists of freshly ground
  black pepper
3 carrots, scrubbed and cut into
  1-inch pieces
2 ears corn, cut into 1-inch pieces

2 yams, peeled and cut into large
  chunks
2 russet potatoes, peeled and cut
  into large chunks
1 10-ounce bag frozen petite
  whole onions
1 4-ounce can chopped green
  chiles
8 ounces seitan, cut into bite-sized
  pieces
1 pumpkin, 4 to 5 pounds
2 tablespoons pure maple
  syrup

Place ¼ cup of the broth in a large pot. Add the onion, bell pepper, and garlic. Cook and stir until softened, about 5 minutes. Add the chili powder, oregano, bay leaves, and black pepper. Cook and stir for 2 more minutes. Add the remaining broth, the carrots, corn, yams, potatoes, frozen onions, canned chiles, and seitan. Cook, covered, over low heat for 30 minutes.

Preheat the oven to 350 degrees.

While the stew is cooking, prepare the pumpkin by cutting off the top, as if you were going to make a jack-o'-lantern. Set the top aside. Clean out the seeds and stringy portion. Brush the inside with the maple syrup. Put the top back on. Place in a 9 × 12-inch baking dish with ½ inch water in the bottom. Bake for 30 minutes. Remove from the oven. Ladle the stew into the pumpkin, cover with the pumpkin top, and bake for 45 minutes.

Serve from the pumpkin, scooping out bits of pumpkin with the stew.

Hint: This stew may seem like a lot of work, but it is very festive and it is delicious. It makes a wonderful holiday centerpiece.

MEDITERRANEAN VEGETABLE STEW

Preparation Time: 20 minutes
Cooking Time: 55 minutes   Servings: 6 to 8

1¾ cups tomato or V-8 juice
10 ounces pearl onions, cleaned
  and left whole
3 yellow Finn potatoes, cut into
  chunks
12 peeled baby carrots
2 stalks celery, thickly sliced
½ pound mushrooms,
  cut in half
2 zucchini, cut into chunks
1 6-ounce package baked tofu,
  cut into cubes
5 baby turnips, peeled and cut
  into chunks

2 cups vegetable broth
1 14.5-ounce can chopped
  tomatoes
1 8-ounce can tomato sauce
2 tablespoons soy sauce
1 tablespoon parsley flakes
1 teaspoon basil
½ teaspoon paprika
several twists of freshly ground
  black pepper
¼ cup cornstarch mixed in ½ cup
  cold water

Place the juice in a large pot with the onions, potatoes, carrots, and celery. Bring to a boil, reduce the heat, cover, and cook for 15 minutes. Add the remaining ingredients, except the cornstarch mixture. Bring to a boil again, reduce the heat, cover, and cook for 40 minutes. Stir in the cornstarch mixture and cook, stirring constantly, until thickened.

Serve over couscous.

Bean Entrées

BRAZILIAN FEIJOADA

Preparation Time: 60 minutes (need cooked rice)
Cooking Time: 42 minutes   Servings: 6 to 8

ONIONS

¼ cup water
1 onion, sliced

2 tablespoons lemon juice
½ teaspoon Tabasco sauce

VEGETABLE TOPPING

½ cup water
2 sweet potatoes, peeled and
   chopped
2 leeks, white part only, sliced
1 cup red bell pepper, chopped
1 cup green bell pepper, chopped
1 cup yellow bell pepper,
   chopped

1 onion, cut in half lengthwise,
   then sliced
1 tablespoon lime juice
1 teaspoon ground cumin
½ teaspoon Tabasco sauce
½ teaspoon ground coriander
1 tomato, cut in half and sliced
   lengthwise

BEANS

4 15-ounce cans black beans,
   drained and rinsed

1 10-ounce can Rotel chopped
   tomatoes and green chiles

GREENS

⅓ cup water
1 onion, chopped

1 bunch kale, chopped
1 tablespoon lemon juice

1 to 2 cups salsa

4 cups hot cooked brown rice

To prepare the onion, place the water and onion in a small pan. Cook over low heat for 5 minutes. Drain. Place in a bowl and add the lemon juice and Tabasco sauce. Mix well. Refrigerate.

To prepare the vegetable topping, place the water in a large pot with the sweet potatoes, leeks, bell peppers, and onion. Cook, stirring frequently, for 10 minutes. Add the lime juice, cumin, Tabasco sauce, and coriander and cook an additional 10 minutes until the potatoes are tender. Add the tomato and cook for 2 more minutes.

While the vegetable mixture is cooking, place the beans and tomatoes in a pan. Cook over low heat for 5 to 10 minutes until the beans are heated through.

To prepare the greens, place the water, onion, and kale in a large pot. Cover and steam for 10 minutes, stirring occasionally. Remove from the heat and sprinkle with the lemon juice.

When ready to serve, place all the ingredients in bowls, including the salsa: put a layer of rice on the bottom of each person's bowl, followed by a layer of beans, then the vegetable topping, some greens, a few onions, and top with the salsa.

Hint: Don't let the long list of ingredients scare you off. This festive dish has been a family favorite for many years. You can also serve it without the rice, but I never omit the greens, onions, or salsa. They really add a special touch to the meal.

BLACK BEAN AND CORN CHILI

Preparation Time: 15 minutes
Cooking Time: 25 minutes   Servings: 6 to 8

½ cup water
1 onion, chopped
1 large red bell pepper, chopped
1 medium green bell pepper,
   chopped
1 teaspoon minced fresh garlic
3 15-ounce cans black beans,
   drained and rinsed
2 14.5-ounce cans diced tomatoes
   with jalapeños

1 cup salsa
2 teaspoons chili powder
1 teaspoon ground cumin
2 cups frozen corn kernels
dash or two of Tabasco sauce
   (optional)
¼ cup chopped fresh cilantro for
   garnish (optional)

Place the water in a large pot with the onion, bell peppers, and garlic. Cook, stirring occasionally, for 10 minutes. Add the beans, tomatoes, salsa, chili powder, and cumin. Cook over low heat for 10 minutes. Stir in the corn and cook for 5 minutes. If desired, season with Tabasco sauce and garnish with cilantro before serving.

Serve over whole grains or potatoes.

COWPOKE CHILI

Preparation Time: 15 minutes
Cooking Time: 33 minutes   Servings: 8

¼ cup water
1 onion, chopped
2 14.5-ounce cans chopped
   tomatoes
1 15-ounce can kidney beans
1 15-ounce can pinquitos
   (seasoned red beans),
   undrained
1 15-ounce can tomato sauce
2⅔ cups vegetarian burger bits
   (see Hint)

1 4-ounce can chopped green
   chiles
1½ tablespoons chili powder
1 tablespoon canned diced
   jalapeños
2 teaspoons ground cumin
2 teaspoons brown sugar
2 teaspoons Wonderslim cocoa
   powder
1½ teaspoons ground oregano
½ teaspoon ground cinnamon

Place the water and onion in a large pot. Cook, stirring occasionally, for 3 minutes. Add the remaining ingredients and cook, uncovered, over low heat for 30 minutes.

Serve over rice or baked potatoes, or in a bowl by itself.

Hint: Several manufacturers make vegetarian burger bits. Morningstar Farms Ground Meatless and Green Giant Harvest Burgers for Recipes can both be found in the freezer section of your supermarket. They are fat free and are fully cooked so you just need to thaw them and use in place of ground beef in recipes. Yves Veggie Cuisine makes a similar product called Veggie Ground Round.

BISTRO BEANS

Preparation Time: 20 minutes
Cooking Time: 70 minutes   Servings: 6

⅓ cup water
1 large onion, chopped
2 teaspoons minced fresh garlic
½ cup nonalcoholic red wine
2 bay leaves
1 teaspoon crushed rosemary
½ teaspoon dried marjoram
½ teaspoon dried thyme
1 cup chopped potatoes
1 cup chopped carrots
1 cup chopped celery

1 cup chopped tomatoes
1 cup chopped Yves Veggie
    Pepperoni
1 tablespoon blackstrap molasses
1 tablespoon Dijon mustard
1 15-ounce can kidney beans,
    drained and rinsed
1 15-ounce can cannellini beans,
    drained and rinsed
freshly ground black pepper
    to taste

Preheat the oven to 350 degrees.

Place the water in a large pot with the onion and garlic. Cook, stirring occasionally, for 2 minutes. Add the wine, bay leaves, rosemary, marjoram, and thyme. Cook, covered, for 3 more minutes. Add the potatoes, carrots, celery, and tomatoes. Cover and cook for 10 minutes, stirring occasionally. Add the remaining ingredients and cook for 5 more minutes. Pour into a covered casserole dish and bake for 50 minutes.

Hint: Yves Veggie Pepperoni is a fat-free vegetarian product that tastes remarkably similar to pepperoni. It is made by Yves Veggie Cuisine, Inc.

RED BEAN GUMBO

Preparation Time: 20 minutes (need cooked rice)
Cooking Time: 30 minutes   Servings: 6 to 8

½ cup water
1 onion, chopped
1 green bell pepper, chopped
1 stalk celery, chopped
1 teaspoon minced fresh
  garlic
6 cups vegetable broth
1 14.5-ounce can Cajun-style
  stewed tomatoes
1 8-ounce can tomato sauce
1½ teaspoons ground oregano
1 bay leaf

¼ teaspoon crushed red pepper
several twists of freshly ground
  black pepper
1 15-ounce can kidney beans,
  drained and rinsed
1 15-ounce can red beans,
  drained and rinsed
4 cups chopped greens, such as
  kale, chard, or spinach
¼ cup chopped fresh parsley
2 to 4 cups hot cooked brown
  basmati or jasmine rice

Place the water, onion, bell pepper, celery, and garlic in a large pot. Cook, stirring occasionally, for 5 minutes. Add the broth, tomatoes, tomato sauce, and seasonings. Bring to a boil, cover, and cook over low heat for 15 minutes. Add the beans and greens and cook an additional 10 minutes. Stir in the parsley.

To serve, place ½ cup of the rice in the bottom of a soup bowl. Ladle the gumbo over the rice and mix well before eating.

SEITAN CHILI

Preparation Time: 25 minutes
Cooking Time: 33 minutes   Servings: 6 to 8

½ cup water
1 onion, chopped
1 teaspoon minced fresh garlic
1 12-ounce package chicken-style
seitan, cut into bite-sized pieces
1 tablespoon chili powder
½ tablespoon ground cumin
2 teaspoons ground oregano
3 cups vegetable broth
1 14.5-ounce can chopped
tomatoes

1 4-ounce can chopped green
chiles
1 15-ounce can kidney beans,
drained and rinsed
1 15-ounce can red beans,
drained and rinsed
1 15-ounce can black beans,
drained and rinsed
½ cup chopped fresh cilantro
(optional)

Place the water, onion, and garlic in a large pot. Cook, stirring frequently, for 3 minutes. Add the seitan, chili powder, cumin, and oregano. Stir to mix well. Add the broth, tomatoes, and chiles. Bring to a boil, then add the beans and mix well. Cover and cook for 15 minutes over low heat. Uncover and cook for 15 minutes longer to thicken the chili. Garnish with chopped cilantro before serving, if desired.

COSTA RICAN GALLO PINTO

Preparation Time: 20 minutes (need cooked rice)
Cooking Time: 4 hours, 15 minutes   Servings: 8 to 10

BEAN MIXTURE

2 cups dried black beans
6 cups water
1 onion, chopped
2 stalks celery, chopped

1 teaspoon crushed fresh
garlic
2 bay leaves
1 teaspoon dried oregano

VEGETABLE MIXTURE

⅓ cup water
1 onion, chopped
1 stalk celery, chopped
1 tomato, chopped

¼ cup chopped fresh cilantro
4 cups cooked long-grain brown
  rice
Tabasco or another hot sauce

Place all the ingredients for the bean mixture in a large pot. Bring to a boil, reduce the heat, cover, and cook over low heat for 4 hours, or until the beans are tender. Remove from the heat and set aside.

To prepare the vegetable mixture, about 15 minutes before serving, place the water, onion, and celery in a large frying pan or stockpot. Cook, stirring frequently, for 5 minutes. Add the tomato and cilantro and continue to cook for 5 minutes. Add the cooked rice and the bean mixture. Mix well and heat through. Season to taste with Tabasco or another hot sauce.

Serve topped with Pico de Gallo (page 319), in a bowl or rolled up in a tortilla.

CAJUN PEAS WITH MUSTARD GREENS

Preparation Time: 15 minutes
Cooking Time: 25 minutes   Servings: 6 to 8

½ cup water
1 onion, chopped
1 stalk celery, chopped
1 green bell pepper, chopped
4 green onions, chopped
1 teaspoon minced fresh
  garlic

2 15-ounce cans Cajun-style
  stewed tomatoes
½ teaspoon crushed red pepper
2 15-ounce cans black-eyed peas,
  drained and rinsed
1 bunch mustard greens, chopped
several dashes of Tabasco sauce

Place the water in a large pot with the onion, celery, bell pepper, green onions, and garlic. Cook, stirring occasionally, for 5 minutes. Add the tomatoes and red pepper. Mix well and cook for 15 minutes, breaking up the tomatoes as they cook. Add the black-eyed peas, mustard greens, and Tabasco sauce, mix well, and cook for 5 minutes.

MARDI GRAS BEANS

Preparation Time: 25 minutes
Cooking Time: 30 minutes   Servings: 8

½ cup water
1 large onion, chopped
2 stalks celery, chopped
2 carrots, chopped
1 green bell pepper, chopped
1 teaspoon minced fresh garlic
½ pound sliced fresh
   mushrooms
2 15-ounce cans kidney beans,
   drained and rinsed

2 14.5-ounce cans chopped
   tomatoes
1 teaspoon dried oregano
1 teaspoon dried basil
1 teaspoon dried marjoram
¼ teaspoon crushed red pepper
1 tablespoon brown sugar
1 tablespoon Dijon mustard
1 cup chopped Swiss chard
1 cup chopped green onions

Place the water in a large pot with the onion, celery, carrots, bell pepper, and garlic. Cook, stirring occasionally, for 10 minutes. Add the mushrooms and cook for 5 minutes. Add the beans, tomatoes, oregano, basil, marjoram, and red pepper. Cook for 10 minutes, then add the brown sugar and mustard. Mix well, add the Swiss chard, and cook for 5 minutes longer.

Top with green onions and serve over brown rice.

TAMALES

Preparation Time: 2 hours
Cooking Time: 60 minutes   Servings: Makes 40 to 50 tamales

WRAP

Banana leaves or corn husks
   (see Hint)

FILLING

⅓ cup water
1 small onion, finely chopped
½ teaspoon minced fresh garlic
1 15-ounce can black beans,
   drained and rinsed

½ cup roasted red pepper,
   chopped
1 small fresh jalapeño, seeded
   and finely chopped

DOUGH

5 cups fine masa flour, plus extra for kneading as necessary
4 cups water at room temperature

6 cups mashed potatoes
½ teaspoon salt
several twists of freshly ground black pepper

Thaw the banana leaves or soak the corn husks in warm water until soft. Separate the husks to make softening easier. Rinse both to make sure they are clean.

Place the water for the filling in a small saucepan. Add the onion and garlic and cook for 5 minutes, stirring occasionally. Add the remaining filling ingredients and cook over low heat for an additional 5 minutes. Set aside.

To make the dough, place the masa flour in a large bowl. Add the water and mix with a spoon until it sticks together and starts to come away from the sides of the bowl. Sprinkle a couple of tablespoons of the masa flour on the counter or kneading surface. Remove the dough from the bowl, place it on the masa flour, and knead for 10 minutes, until the dough is smooth and stretchy, adding more flour as necessary to keep it from sticking to the counter. Place the ball of dough in a very large clean bowl. Add the mashed potatoes and mix together well using your hands. Season with salt and pepper.

Cut the banana leaves into pieces approximately 7 to 8 inches by 12 to 14 inches. Keep the corn husks covered with a damp paper towel while filling.

Spread ⅛ to ¼ cup of the potato-masa mixture in the center of either a banana leaf or corn husk. Make a small indentation in the center of the mixture and fill with 1 teaspoon of the filling mixture. Fold the wrap over lengthwise to cover the mixture and fold again lengthwise. Fold both ends under and set aside with the folded ends down. The filling should be completely enclosed. Repeat until all the mixture is gone. Put the completed tamales under damp paper towels until all are assembled.

Arrange the tamales in loose layers in a steamer. Steam over boiling water for 1 hour, adding more water as necessary.

To serve, remove the wrapper and discard. Season with salsa before eating, if desired.

Hint: Dried corn husks are sold in the specialty food section of most supermarkets. You can also find them at Mexican markets. Banana leaves will probably be more difficult to find. Mexican markets or specialty stores sometimes carry them. They are usually sold frozen. The taste is the same no matter which one you use. Banana leaves are larger, so they hold a greater amount of the dough. A less authentic, but effective, way to wrap the tamales is to use parchment paper and aluminum foil. Place filling in parchment paper and fold over to enclose completely. Then wrap in foil.

Tamales are a lot of work, but they are delicious. They freeze well and are easy to reheat in a steamer basket. Other fillings to try include mango salsa, mashed pinto or black beans, and seasoned rice or vegetables. You can also wrap them up with no filling at all.

Grain Entrées

VEGETABLES AND BARLEY

Preparation Time: 20 minutes
Cooking Time: 1 hour, 15 minutes   Servings: 4 to 6

6 cups vegetable broth
1 onion, chopped
1 stalk celery, chopped
1 medium red bell pepper, chopped
½ teaspoon fresh minced garlic
1 cup barley
1 zucchini, cut in half lengthwise, then sliced

½ cup frozen corn kernels, thawed
1 cup packed coarsely chopped fresh spinach
2 tablespoons soy sauce
freshly ground black pepper to taste
dash or two of Tabasco sauce (optional)

Place ½ cup of the broth in a large pot. Add the onion, celery, bell pepper, and garlic. Cook, stirring occasionally, for 5 minutes. Add the remaining broth and the barley. Bring to a boil, cover, reduce the heat, and cook for 60 minutes, stirring occasionally. (Add a little more broth if the barley begins to stick to the bottom of the pot.) Add the remaining ingredients and cook an additional 10 minutes, stirring frequently. Serve hot.

THAI CURRIED RICE

Preparation Time: 20 minutes (need cooked rice)
Cooking Time: 12 minutes   Servings: 4 to 6

⅓ cup water
1 onion, chopped
1 red bell pepper, chopped
1 yellow bell pepper, chopped
½ teaspoon minced fresh garlic
1 to 2 tablespoons green
    curry paste
2 cups chopped Napa cabbage
1 cup small broccoli florets

1 bunch green onions, chopped
½ cup soy sauce
4 cups cooked brown rice
1 tomato, chopped
1 cup mung bean sprouts
1 tablespoon chopped fresh
    basil
1 tablespoon chopped fresh
    cilantro

Place the water, onion, bell peppers, and garlic in a pot. Cook, stirring occasionally, for 5 minutes. Stir in the curry paste. Add the cabbage, broccoli, green onions, and soy sauce. Mix well, cover, and cook over medium heat for 5 minutes. Add the remaining ingredients and cook until heated through, 2 to 3 minutes.

Hint: If you don't like spicy foods, use only 1 tablespoon of curry paste. In our family we like to use 2 tablespoons of the curry paste, and I know people who like really spicy foods that use 3 tablespoons. Green curry paste is sold in Asian markets and at Trader Joe's.

HERBED RICE CASSEROLE

Preparation Time: 15 minutes (need cooked rice)
Cooking Time: 45 minutes   Servings: 4 to 6

½ cup water
1 onion, chopped
1 green bell pepper, chopped
2 stalks celery, chopped
½ pound sliced fresh mushrooms
2 tablespoons soy sauce
¼ teaspoon dried sage
¼ teaspoon dried marjoram
¼ teaspoon dried thyme

¼ teaspoon dried rosemary
¼ teaspoon poultry seasoning
3 cups cooked brown rice
½ cup chopped green onions
1 15-ounce can kidney beans,
    drained and rinsed
1 2.5-ounce can sliced black
    olives, drained
¼ cup grated fat-free soy cheese

Preheat the oven to 350 degrees.

Place the water, onion, bell pepper, and celery in a large pot. Cook, stirring frequently, for 5 minutes. Add the mushrooms and seasonings. Cook for 10 more minutes. Stir in the rice, green onions, kidney beans, and black olives. Mix well. Transfer to a covered casserole dish, sprinkle with the grated cheese, and bake for 30 minutes.

CARIBBEAN RICE SURPRISE

Preparation Time: 15 minutes   Cooking Time: 57 minutes
Resting Time: 10 minutes   Servings: 6 to 8

⅓ cup water
1 onion, chopped
1 teaspoon minced fresh
   garlic
1 4-ounce can chopped green
   chiles
3 cups peeled, chopped
   butternut squash
2 teaspoons curry powder
1 teaspoon ground coriander

½ teaspoon ground cumin
several twists of freshly ground
   black pepper
3½ cups water
1 cup long-grain brown rice
½ cup wild rice
1 15-ounce can kidney beans,
   drained and rinsed
1 cup chopped Swiss chard
¾ cup chopped green onions

Place the ⅓ cup water in a large pot with the onion, garlic, and chiles. Cook, stirring occasionally, for 5 minutes. Add the squash, curry powder, coriander, cumin, and black pepper. Mix well and cook for 2 minutes. Add the 3½ cups water and both kinds of rice. Bring to a boil, cover, reduce the heat to low, and cook for 45 minutes. Add the beans and heat through, about 5 minutes. Stir in the chard and green onions, remove from the heat, and let rest for 10 minutes.

MOROCCAN VEGETABLES WITH COUSCOUS

Preparation Time: 30 minutes
Cooking Time: 45 minutes   Servings: 8

2½ cups water
1¾ cups uncooked couscous
8 small red potatoes, quartered
3 carrots, sliced lengthwise, then
  cut into 1-inch pieces
1 turnip, peeled and cut into
  chunks
2 cups green beans, cut into
  1-inch pieces
4 medium plum tomatoes, cut
  into 1-inch chunks
2 zucchini, sliced 1 inch thick
1 green bell pepper, cut into
  1-inch pieces

2½ cups cauliflower florets
¼ cup raisins
2¾ cups vegetable broth
⅓ cup unbleached white flour
½ teaspoon crushed fresh
  garlic
¼ teaspoon cinnamon
¼ teaspoon allspice
¼ teaspoon ground coriander
¼ teaspoon ground cumin
¼ teaspoon tumeric
⅛ teaspoon crushed red pepper
1 15-ounce can garbanzo beans,
  drained and rinsed

Place the water in a saucepan and bring to a boil. Add the couscous, stir, and return to a boil. Cover, remove from the heat, and let rest.

Place all the vegetables and the raisins in a large pot in the order given. Place the broth and flour in a bowl and whisk to blend. Add the garlic and all the seasonings and mix well. Pour over the vegetables. Bring to a boil, cover, reduce the heat to medium, and cook for 10 minutes. Stir and continue to cook for another 30 minutes, stirring occasionally. Add the garbanzo beans and cook for 5 more minutes.

Fluff the couscous with a fork and serve the vegetables over the couscous.

Hint: The vegetables may also be made in a slow cooker. Layer the vegetables as directed and pour the liquid over them. Cook on high for 4 to 4½ hours or on low for 8 to 9 hours. Stir a couple of times while cooking, if possible. Otherwise, stir well when you add the garbanzo beans and a few more times while you are waiting for the couscous to absorb the water, about 5 minutes.

WILD HASH

Preparation Time: 20 minutes   Cooking Time: 45 minutes
Resting Time: 10 minutes   Servings: 6

1 cup Lundberg Wild Blend
2⅓ cups water
1 onion, chopped
1 red bell pepper, chopped
½ pound mushrooms, sliced
1 stalk celery, chopped
1¾ cups vegetable broth
2 tablespoons cornstarch
2 tablespoons soy sauce
1 tablespoon parsley flakes

1 teaspoon dried basil
1 teaspoon dried oregano
½ teaspoon dried sage
½ teaspoon dried marjoram
¼ teaspoon dried rosemary
several twists of freshly ground
    black pepper
1 12-ounce package Yves Veggie
    Ground Round

Place the rice blend in a saucepan with 2 cups of the water. Bring to a boil, reduce the heat, cover, and cook for 45 minutes. Let rest for 10 minutes.

Meanwhile, place the remaining water in a large nonstick frying pan. Add the onion, bell pepper, mushrooms, and celery. Cook, stirring occasionally, for 5 minutes.

Mix the broth, cornstarch, soy sauce, and seasonings in a separate bowl. Add to the vegetable mixture while stirring. Cook and stir until the mixture boils and thickens. Add the Ground Round and cooked rice mixture. Cook, stirring occasionally, for 5 minutes.

Hint: To cut down on cooking time, use leftover cooked rice, preferably a combination of wild rice and brown rice. Yves Veggie Ground Round is a meatless burger substitute found in natural foods stores and some supermarkets.

Soy Entrées

ÉTOUFFÉE

Preparation Time: 30 minutes
Cooking Time: 25 minutes   Servings: 4 to 6

⅓ cup water
1 onion, chopped
1 green bell pepper, chopped
1 stalk celery, chopped
1 bunch green onions, chopped
1 fresh jalapeño, seeded and
  chopped
2 teaspoons minced fresh garlic
1 teaspoon Cajun Dust seasoning
1 teaspoon paprika
⅛ teaspoon cayenne

several twists of freshly ground
  black pepper
1 15-ounce can chopped tomatoes
1½ cups vegetable broth
2 teaspoons Worcestershire
  sauce
4 tablespoons cornstarch mixed
  in ½ cup cold water
13 to 14 ounces smoked tofu,
  sliced
⅓ cup chopped fresh parsley

Place the water, onion, bell pepper, celery, green onions, jalapeño, garlic, Cajun Dust, paprika, cayenne, and black pepper in a large pot. Cook, stirring frequently, for 10 minutes. Add the tomatoes, broth, and Worcestershire sauce. Bring to a boil, reduce the heat, stir in the cornstarch mixture, and continue to stir until thickened. Add the tofu and cook over low heat for 10 minutes, stirring frequently. Stir in the parsley and serve at once over rice.

Hint: Cajun Dust seasoning is manufactured by Cajun Dust in Phoenix, Arizona. It is sold in natural foods stores. If you are unable to find it, look for any other Cajun-style seasoning mixture.

GRILLED SKEWERED TOFU

Preparation Time: 5 minutes   Marinating Time: 2 to 3 hours
Grilling Time: 12 minutes   Servings: 2

1 12-ounce package firm Soy-Deli
  LowFat Nigari Tofu
Bamboo skewers

1½ cups fat-free marinating
  sauce, such as barbecue,
  teriyaki, garlic, or jerk

Cut the tofu in half lengthwise. Cut each half into 4 pieces crosswise, then cut those pieces in half. You should have 16 pieces of tofu, approximately ½ × ½ × 1 inch.

Soak the bamboo skewers in water for at least 1 hour.

Place half of the sauce in the bottom of a medium oblong pan. Lay the pieces of tofu in the sauce and pour the remaining sauce over the tofu. Cover and refrigerate for 2 to 3 hours, turning occasionally, if possible.

Thread the tofu on the skewers and grill over medium coals, brushing with marinade and turning until brown on both sides, about 12 minutes.

Hint: Grilling tofu makes it very flavorful and it's easy. We also like to use thawed frozen tofu, which changes the texture completely. Place the tofu in its unopened package in the freezer. Freeze for at least 24 hours or up to 3 months. (Do not freeze aseptically packaged tofu.) To thaw, place the package in boiling water, changing the water several times until the tofu is completely thawed. Press out excess water by following the directions on page 297. Then proceed as directed above. If you are not able to find this particular brand of tofu, you will have to follow the directions for removing excess water on page 297.

GRILLED TOFU-VEGETABLE KABOBS

Preparation Time: 45 minutes   Marinating Time: 60 minutes
Grilling Time: 15 minutes   Servings: 4

MARINADE

2 cups water	1 teaspoon minced fresh ginger
½ cup soy sauce	½ teaspoon minced fresh garlic
2 tablespoons sherry	several dashes of Tabasco sauce

20 bamboo skewers	2 long eggplant
2 12-ounce packages firm Soy Deli LowFat Nigari Tofu	2 yellow crookneck squash
	1 15-ounce can pineapple chunks, drained
¾ pound mushrooms	20 large cherry tomatoes
10 ounces pearl onions	2 tablespoons cornstarch

Mix the marinade ingredients together in a bowl. Set aside.

Soak the bamboo skewers in water until ready to use. Cut the tofu into cubes. Clean the mushrooms and onions and leave whole. Place the onions in a saucepan with water to cover. Bring to a boil and cook over low heat for 5 minutes. Drain. Slice the eggplant and squash into ½-inch slices.

Place the tofu, mushrooms, onions, eggplant, and squash into a large bowl. Pour the marinade over the vegetables and mix well. Let rest in the marinade for at least 1 hour, mixing occasionally to distribute the marinade.

Skewer the tofu, marinated vegetables, pineapple chunks, and tomatoes in any order you choose. Pour the remaining marinade into a small saucepan and add the cornstarch, mixing well. Cook, stirring constantly, until the mixture boils and thickens. Remove from the heat.

Place the skewers on a grill over medium coals, brushing with the thickened marinade. Turn and brush with additional marinade until the tofu is browned and the vegetables are tender, about 15 minutes. Serve with the remaining marinade to dunk the vegetables.

Hint: Soy Deli LowFat Nigari Tofu is very firm; it doesn't contain a lot of extra water. If you cannot find this kind of tofu, you will have to press the tofu between 2 heavy surfaces to remove excess water. Place the tofu in a baking sheet and cover with 2 or 3 paper towels. Place another baking sheet over the tofu and set some heavy books on the second baking sheet to press the water out. This will take about 30 minutes.

I use a baster to evenly distribute the marinade over the vegetables. Squeeze up some of the marinade into the baster, then squirt it over the vegetables.

If you would like to prepare this recipe ahead of time and let the vegetables soak for a longer period of time, cover the dish and place it in the refrigerator. Stir or baste occasionally to make sure all the vegetables are evenly coated with the marinade.

FRITTATA FLORENTINE

Preparation Time: 25 minutes   Cooking Time: 70 minutes
Resting Time: 10 minutes   Servings: 8

1 cup water
1 onion, chopped
1 leek, sliced
½ pound mushrooms, sliced
½ teaspoon minced fresh garlic
4 cups chopped fresh spinach
2 12.3-ounce packages extra-firm
   lite silken tofu
½ cup unbleached all-purpose
   flour plus 2 tablespoons
2½ tablespoons cornstarch

1½ tablespoon soy sauce
1 teaspoon nutritional yeast
½ teaspoon dried basil
¼ teaspoon turmeric
¼ teaspoon salt (optional)
⅛ teaspoon cayenne
several twists of freshly ground
   black pepper
1 2.25-ounce can sliced
   black olives, drained
   (optional)

Preheat the oven to 350 degrees.

Place ½ cup of the water in a large nonstick frying pan. Add the onion, leek, mushrooms, and garlic. Cook, stirring frequently, for 8 minutes. Add the spinach. Cook and stir for 2 minutes longer. Remove from the heat and drain.

Meanwhile, place the tofu, the remaining ½ cup of water, the flour, cornstarch, soy sauce, nutritional yeast, basil, turmeric, salt, if using, the cayenne, and black pepper in a food processor. Process until smooth. Set aside.

Combine the drained vegetables and the tofu mixture. Stir in the olives, if desired. Pour into a 10-inch round nonstick pie plate. Bake for 60 minutes. Let rest for 10 minutes before cutting.

SOY SLOPPY BARBECUE

Preparation Time: 5 minutes   Resting Time: 30 minutes
Cooking Time: 30 minutes   Servings: 12

3 cups soy strips or textured
   vegetable protein (TVP)
   chunks
4 cups boiling water
1 onion, chopped

1 green bell pepper, chopped
1 teaspoon crushed fresh garlic
⅓ cup water
3 18-ounce jars fat-free barbecue
   sauce

Place the soy strips or TVP chunks in a large bowl. Pour the boiling water over them to rehydrate and let rest for 30 minutes, stirring occasionally. Drain off excess water.

Meanwhile, place the onion, bell pepper, garlic, and water in a large pot. Cook, stirring occasionally, for 5 minutes, until softened. Add the soy strips and the barbecue sauce. Cook over low heat for 30 minutes, stirring occasionally.

Serve on whole wheat buns.

Hint: The longer this cooks, the better it tastes. You can use a slow cooker and cook on low for 5 hours. It also reheats well and freezes well. For a little extra zest, I sometimes add 2 to 3 tablespoons of prepared mustard with the barbecue sauce.

LASAGNA

Preparation Time: 30 minutes   Cooking Time: 60 minutes
Resting Time: 10 minutes   Servings: 12 to 15

2 12-ounce packages LowFat Nigari Tofu
1 teaspoon onion powder
¼ teaspoon garlic powder
1 10-ounce package frozen chopped spinach, thawed and squeezed dry

4 26-ounce jars fat-free pasta sauce
1 16-ounce package lasagna noodles
1 16-ounce package fat-free soy mozzarella cheese, thinly sliced
Soy parmesan cheese (optional)

Preheat the oven to 350 degrees.

Crumble the tofu into a bowl. Mix in the onion and garlic powders. Stir in the spinach and mix well.

Pour 1 jar of the pasta sauce in the bottom of a deep 11½ × 14-inch baking dish. Lay 6 of the uncooked lasagna noodles over the sauce. Take half of the tofu mixture and spread it over the noodles, then pour another jar of the pasta sauce over the tofu mixture and spread to cover well. Lay half of the sliced soy mozzarella over the sauce, then follow with another layer of noodles, tofu mixture, sauce, and soy mozzarella. Finish with a layer of noodles, another jar of sauce, and sprinkle with soy parmesan, if desired. Cover with parchment paper and then cover tightly with foil. Bake for 60 minutes. Remove from the oven, uncover, and let rest for 10 minutes before serving.

Hint: This recipe makes a large amount of lasagna. It freezes well after baking, so you may want to make it in 2 pans and save one for later use. The recipe can easily be cut in half to make a smaller amount. Use your favorite brand of fat-free pasta sauce, egg-free lasagna noodles, soy cheese, and fresh tofu. Do not use aseptically packaged tofu in this recipe.

Vegetable Entrées

MEDITERRANEAN PIZZA

Preparation Time: 15 minutes
Cooking Time: 12 minutes   Servings: 8

1¼ cups fat-free hummus
1 large fat-free prepared pizza crust
¼ cup chopped yellow bell pepper
¼ cup chopped canned roasted red pepper

10 thin slices Japanese eggplant
2 slices sweet onion, separated into rings
2 tablespoons chopped fresh basil
2 tablespoons sliced black olives (optional)

Preheat the oven to 450 degrees.

Spread the hummus evenly over the pizza crust. Layer the remaining ingredients over the hummus. Bake for 12 minutes.

Hint: Kabuli Pizza Crust is a delicious fat-free prepared pizza crust made by Dallas Gourmet Bakery. It may be ordered directly from the manufacturer by calling (972) 247-9835. It is also sold in natural foods stores.

STUFFED BELL PEPPERS WITH TOMATO-LEEK SAUCE

Preparation Time: 30 minutes
(need cooked rice and Tomato-Leek Sauce)
Cooking Time: 57 minutes   Servings: 8 to 10

8 to 10 medium green or red bell peppers
1 onion, chopped
1 stalk celery, chopped
1 pound fresh mushrooms, chopped
½ cup water
1 tomato, chopped
1 8-ounce can tomato sauce

4 cups cooked brown rice
2 tablespoons soy sauce
1 teaspoon dried basil
½ teaspoon dried thyme
freshly ground black pepper to taste
2 cups Tomato-Leek Sauce (page 313)

Preheat the oven to 350 degrees.

Wash the bell peppers and cut a thin slice off the tops. Clean out the peppers and set aside. Chop the tops of the peppers and set aside.

Place the onion, celery, mushrooms, and reserved chopped pepper tops in a large pot with the water. Cook, stirring occasionally, for 5 minutes. Add the tomato and cook another 2 minutes. Stir in the remaining ingredients, except the Tomato-Leek Sauce, and heat through, about 5 minutes. Spoon the rice mixture into the bell peppers.

Place about 2 cups of Tomato-Leek Sauce in the bottom of a 9 × 12-inch baking dish. Set the peppers on top of the sauce and spoon the remaining sauce over the peppers. Place a sheet of parchment paper over the peppers, then cover with foil. Bake for 45 minutes.

Hint: Store leftovers in individual serving bowls. These reheat well in the microwave.

GARBANZO-CAULIFLOWER CURRY

Preparation Time: 25 minutes
Cooking Time: 20 minutes   Servings: 6 to 8

⅓ cup water
1 onion, chopped
1 green bell pepper, chopped
½ cup chopped red bell pepper
1 cup sliced fresh mushrooms
1 cup cut green beans
1 teaspoon minced fresh garlic
1 teaspoon minced fresh ginger
1 tablespoon curry powder
1 14.5-ounce can chopped
  tomatoes

1 14.5-ounce can garbanzo beans,
  drained and rinsed
½ cup regular or spicy
  V-8 juice
2 cups cauliflower florets
2 cups tightly packed baby
  spinach leaves
2 tablespoons cornstarch mixed
  in ¼ cup cold water
freshly ground black pepper

Place the water in a large pot with the onion, bell peppers, mushrooms, green beans, garlic, and ginger. Cook, stirring occasionally, for 5 minutes. Add the curry powder and mix in well. Add the tomatoes, garbanzo beans, and V-8 juice. Bring to a boil. Stir in the cauliflower and cook for 10 minutes. Add the spinach and cook an additional 5 minutes. Add the cornstarch mixture and cook and stir until thickened. Season to taste with black pepper.

CHILI-STUFFED BELL PEPPERS

Preparation Time: 15 minutes
Cooking Time: 40 minutes   Servings: 4 to 6

4 medium bell peppers, halved
  lengthwise, seeds and
  membranes removed
2 tablespoons water
1½ cups reconstituted textured
  vegetable protein (TVP)
1 teaspoon chili powder

½ teaspoon ground cinnamon
½ cup quick-cooking barley
1½ cups tomato salsa (mild,
  medium, or hot)
1 cup water
¼ cup raisins

Heat the broiler.

Place the peppers cut side down on a nonstick baking sheet. Broil 4 inches from the heat for 4 minutes. Turn over and broil for an additional 4 minutes. Remove from the broiler and set aside. Set the oven to 375 degrees.

Meanwhile, place the water, TVP, chili powder, and cinnamon in a nonstick frying pan. Stir until well mixed. Add the remaining ingredients, mix well, bring to a boil, reduce the heat, and cook for 15 minutes. Spoon into the pepper halves on the baking sheet. Cover first with parchment paper, then with foil. Bake for 25 minutes.

Hint: Use dried TVP reconstituted in water. Or use thawed Morningstar Farms Ground Meatless or Green Giant Harvest Burgers for Recipes in this recipe.

SEITAN À LA KING

Preparation Time: 20 minutes
Cooking Time: 20 minutes   Servings: 4

½ cup water
1 onion, chopped
1 green bell pepper, chopped
½ pound sliced fresh mushrooms
½ cup unbleached all-
  purpose flour
1¾ cups vegetable broth

2 cups rice milk
1½ cups diced chicken-style
  seitan
1 4-ounce jar chopped
  pimiento
several twists of freshly ground
  black pepper

Place the water in a large pot with the onion, bell pepper, and mushrooms. Cook, stirring occasionally, for 10 minutes. Stir in the flour and cook for 2 minutes, stirring constantly. Slowly stir in the broth. Cook over medium heat, stirring almost constantly, until the mixture boils. Add the rice milk, seitan, pimiento, and black pepper. Cook over low heat, stirring occasionally, for 8 minutes.

Serve over whole wheat toast, muffins, potatoes, or grains.

FAJITAS

Preparation Time: 20 minutes
Cooking Time: 15 minutes   Servings: 6 to 8

⅔ cup water

1 onion, cut in half lengthwise, then thickly sliced

1 red bell pepper, cut into strips

1 green bell pepper, cut into strips

1 teaspoon minced fresh garlic

2 tablespoons chopped green chiles

¼ cup mild or medium salsa

½ teaspoon chili powder

½ teaspoon ground cumin

1 8-ounce package seitan, sliced into strips

6 to 8 flour tortillas

Place ⅓ cup of the water, the onion, bell peppers, garlic, and chiles in a large nonstick frying pan. Cook, stirring frequently, for 5 minutes. Add the remaining water, the salsa, chili powder, and cumin. Cook an additional 5 minutes. Add the seitan and cook 5 minutes longer.

Serve rolled up in a tortilla garnished with tomatoes, onions, lettuce, and additional salsa, if desired.

MEXICAN NOT-BEEF NOODLES

Preparation Time: 10 minutes
Cooking Time: 10 minutes   Servings: 4

1 12-ounce package Yves Veggie Ground Round

1 cup frozen corn kernels

1 cup chopped green onions

2 8-ounce cans tomato sauce

1 cup water

½ cup chunky salsa

2 cups uncooked GardenTime Fancy Ribbons

Combine all the ingredients in a large nonstick frying pan. Bring to a boil, reduce the heat, cover, and cook over low heat, stirring occasionally, 6 to 8 minutes, or until the noodles are tender.

Hint: Other types of uncooked pasta may be used; adjust the cooking time.

GNOCCHI WITH HERBED TOMATO SAUCE

Preparation Time: 10 minutes
Cooking Time: 30 minutes   Servings: 6

2 leeks, white part only, thinly sliced	1 tablespoon parsley flakes
½ cup vegetable broth	1 teaspoon dried oregano
1 teaspoon minced fresh garlic	1 teaspoon dried basil
1 28-ounce can crushed tomatoes	freshly ground black pepper to taste
1 15-ounce can tomato sauce	2 1.1-pound packages gnocchi
	soy parmesan cheese (optional)

Place the leeks and broth in a large frying pan. Add the garlic and cook, stirring occasionally, for 3 minutes. Add the remaining ingredients, except the gnocchi and parmesan cheese. Cook, uncovered, stirring occasionally, for 25 minutes.

Shortly before serving time, bring a large pot of water to a boil. Drop in the gnocchi and boil for 2 to 3 minutes, or according to the package directions. Drain and place in a serving bowl. Pour the sauce over the gnocchi and sprinkle with soy parmesan cheese, if desired.

Hint: This delicious simple meal is almost always a favorite with kids. If you want to make this with fresh herbs, use ¼ cup chopped fresh parsley and 1 tablespoon each of fresh oregano and basil.

PASTA JUMBLE

Preparation Time: 15 minutes
Cooking Time: 20 minutes   Servings: 6 to 8

¼ cup vegetable broth
1 onion, chopped
½ teaspoon minced fresh
  garlic
1 teaspoon dried basil
1 teaspoon dried oregano
⅛ teaspoon crushed red
  pepper
1 14.5-ounce can chopped
  tomatoes
1 14.5-ounce can pasta-style
  tomatoes

2 cups uncooked medium-
  shaped pasta
1 15-ounce can black beans,
  drained and rinsed
1 4.5-ounce jar sliced mushrooms,
  drained and rinsed
1 14-ounce can water-packed
  artichokes, drained and cut
  into quarters
⅛ cup soy parmesan cheese
  (optional)
freshly ground black pepper

Put a large pot of water on to boil.

Place the broth, onion, and garlic in a medium sauce pot. Cook, stirring frequently, for about 5 minutes. Add the basil, oregano, red pepper, and both kinds of tomatoes. Bring to a boil, cover, reduce the heat, and cook for 8 minutes.

Drop the pasta in the boiling water and cook until tender, 5 to 8 minutes. Drain.

Add the beans and mushrooms to the tomato sauce and cook an additional 5 minutes, stirring occasionally. Add the artichokes and cook for 2 minutes. Remove from the heat.

Place the pasta in a large bowl. Pour the tomato mixture over the pasta and mix well. Sprinkle with the parmesan cheese, if desired, and season to taste with black pepper. Toss again to mix and serve at once.

Hint: You can use a 26- to 28-ounce jar of fat-free pasta sauce in place of the tomatoes. Eliminate the seasoning or reduce it by half. Reduce the cooking time for the tomatoes to 5 minutes. The total cooking time is only 15 minutes.

PASTA PRIMAVERA

Preparation Time: 20 minutes
Cooking Time: 15 minutes   Servings: 6

12 ounces penne pasta
½ cup vegetable broth
1 sweet onion, cut in half
   lengthwise, then thinly sliced
½ teaspoon minced fresh garlic
¼ cup slivered fresh basil leaves
1½ cups sliced fresh mushrooms
1 cup thinly sliced red bell pepper
1 cup thinly sliced green bell pepper

1 cup snow pea pods, cut in half
1 cup asparagus, sliced into
   1-inch pieces
2 cups plum tomatoes, cut into
   large chunks
freshly ground black pepper
   to taste
soy parmesan cheese
   (optional)

Put a large pot of water on to boil. Drop the pasta into the boiling water and cook according to package directions. Drain.

Place the broth, onion, garlic, and basil in a large frying pan. Cook, stirring occasionally, for 3 minutes. Add the mushrooms and bell peppers and cook an additional 3 minutes. Add the remaining vegetables and cook, stirring occasionally, for about 8 minutes. Season to taste with black pepper.

Toss the pasta and vegetables together and sprinkle with soy parmesan cheese, if desired.

Hint: You can vary this recipe by changing the vegetables to take advantage of fresh vegetables in season. Some excellent additions are zucchini, fresh peas, broccoli, or cauliflower.

MEXICAN RAVIOLI

Preparation Time: 5 minutes
Cooking Time: 8 minutes   Servings: 3 to 4

2 packages Putney Sweet Red
   Pepper Ravioli

1½ cups Verde Sauce
   (page 316)

Cook the ravioli according to the package directions. Heat the Verde Sauce in a separate pan.

Drain the ravioli and place in a serving dish. Pour the Verde Sauce over the ravioli and serve at once.

Hint: Sweet Red Pepper Ravioli is made by Putney Pasta of Chester, Vermont. You should be able to find it in your natural foods store. Filled with black beans and chiles, it is dairy and fat free.

Side Dishes

ROASTED GARLIC MASHED POTATOES

Preparation Time: 20 minutes
Cooking Time: 1½ hours for garlic; 20 minutes for potatoes
Servings: 2 to 3

1 whole garlic head	3 cups water
2 tablespoons vegetable broth	½ cup soy milk
4 cups peeled and quartered Yellow Finn or Yukon Gold potatoes	dash of salt freshly ground black pepper

Preheat the oven to 350 degrees.

Peel some of the loose papery skin from the garlic head, leaving the whole garlic head intact. Slice a thin strip off the top of the garlic so that most of the cloves are exposed.

Tear off an 8-inch strip of aluminum foil and place on a counter. Place a 4-inch square of parchment paper in the center of the foil. Place the garlic head, cut side up, in the center of the parchment paper and fold up the foil partially around it to cup the garlic head.

Spoon the broth over the cut top of the garlic. Fold the parchment paper over it and then continue to fold up the foil so the garlic head is completely enclosed. Bake for 1½ hours. Remove from the oven and cool.

To extract the garlic, remove the head from the foil and paper, turn it over so that the cut side is down, then squeeze well to remove all pulp. Set aside. You should have about ⅛ cup.

Place the potatoes and water in a pan. Bring to a boil, reduce the heat, cover, and cook for 15 to 20 minutes until soft. Drain and place in a mixing bowl. Add the milk to the potatoes and beat with an electric mixer until smooth. Add the garlic pulp and mix again. Season to taste with salt and pepper.

Hint: Yellow Finn and Yukon Gold potatoes have a beautiful yellow color and buttery taste. For an interesting variation, stir in ½ cup of finely chopped green onions after mashing.

SAVORY MASHED SWEET POTATOES

Preparation Time: 15 minutes
Cooking Time: 25 minutes   Servings: 4

2½ cups vegetable broth
1 onion, chopped
6 medium sweet potatoes, peeled
  and cut into chunks

2 tablespoons honey
2 tablespoons Dijon mustard
several twists of freshly ground
  black pepper

Place ½ cup of the broth in a large pot with the onion and sweet potatoes. Cook, stirring frequently, for 5 minutes. Add the remaining broth and the honey and mustard. Mix well, bring to a boil, cover, reduce the heat, and cook for about 20 minutes, until the sweet potatoes are tender. Mash with a potato masher, electric beater, or food processor. Season to taste with black pepper.

Serve plain or with a sauce or gravy. Try Jamaican Pumpkin Sauce (page 315) or Mixed Mushroom Sauce (page 314).

ROASTED PEPPERS AND POTATOES

Preparation Time: 30 minutes
Cooking Time: 1½ hours   Servings: 6 to 8

¾ cup vegetable broth
¼ cup lemon juice
1 tablespoon soy sauce
1 teaspoon minced fresh garlic
1 teaspoon paprika
½ teaspoon ground coriander
½ teaspoon ground cumin
¼ teaspoon crushed red pepper
4 medium to large Yellow Finn
  potatoes, sliced
1 medium red bell pepper, cut
  into chunks

1 medium green bell pepper, cut
  into chunks
1 medium yellow bell pepper, cut
  into chunks
1 medium onion, cut into wedges
3 stalks celery, cut into chunks
2 medium tomatoes, cut into wedges
¼ cup chopped fresh parsley
2 tablespoons chopped fresh
  cilantro
1 tablespoon cornstarch mixed in
  ¼ cup cold water

Preheat the oven to 350 degrees.

Combine the broth, lemon juice, soy sauce, garlic, paprika, coriander, cumin, and crushed red pepper in a bowl. Set aside.

Combine the vegetables in a large oblong baking dish and mix well. Sprinkle with the parsley and cilantro. Pour the sauce over the vegetables. Cover with parchment paper and follow with aluminum foil. Bake for 1 hour. Remove the covering. Baste the vegetables with some of the sauce and return to the oven. Bake, uncovered, for 30 minutes longer, basting occasionally. Remove from the oven and remove as much sauce as possible from the baking dish. (This is easy to do by tipping the dish and then using the baster to remove the liquid.)

Place the sauce in a small saucepan. Place on a burner over low heat. Gradually add the cornstarch mixture while stirring. Cook and stir until thickened. Pour over the vegetables and serve at once.

GRILLED GOLDEN POTATOES

Preparation Time: 5 minutes   Cooking Time: 13 to 15 minutes
Grilling Time: 10 minutes   Servings: 4

**6 medium Yukon Gold
  potatoes**

**½ cup fat-free sauce, such as
  barbecue, teriyaki, Cajun**

Wash the potatoes and prick them all over with a fork. Place on a paper towel in the microwave. Microwave on high for 13 to 15 minutes, turning several times, until a fork easily pierces them, but they are not too soft. Remove from the microwave and cool slightly.

Cut the potatoes in half lengthwise. Cut a thin slice off the opposite side so that there are two peeled, flat surfaces. Brush the potatoes with the sauce and grill over medium heat, turning and brushing with sauce until they are golden brown, about 10 minutes.

Hint: You can use other potatoes in this recipe; pick medium, thin-skinned, firm potatoes and follow the directions above.

ALL-WRAPPED-UP POTATOES

Preparation Time: 10 minutes
Cooking Time: 1½ hours   Servings: 4 to 6

8 medium thin-skinned white
  potatoes, thinly sliced
1 onion, sliced and separated
  into rings

3 tablespoons soy sauce
⅛ teaspoon paprika
several twists of freshly ground
  black pepper

Preheat the oven to 350 degrees.

Place a large sheet of heavy-duty aluminum foil over a 15 × 10-inch baking tray. Place an identical layer of parchment paper over the foil. Layer the potatoes and onion rings on the parchment paper in the center of the baking tray. Drizzle the soy sauce over the potatoes and onions, then sprinkle with paprika and pepper. Fold over the parchment paper to enclose the vegetables, then wrap securely in the foil. Bake on the baking tray for 1½ hours.

Hint: This is an easy, delicious way to cook potatoes and there is no pan to clean up afterward. To cook on a grill, just put the foil on the grill rack and cook until the potatoes are done. If you use fewer potatoes, you will have fewer layers and this will shorten the cooking time to about 1 hour.

STEWED POTATOES AND GREENS

Preparation Time: 20 minutes
Cooking Time: 50 minutes   Servings: 6

⅓ cup water
1 onion, sliced
½ pound mushrooms, sliced
½ teaspoon minced garlic
1 pound small red potatoes,
  cut into quarters
1 14.5-ounce can stewed tomatoes
  (Italian, Mexican, or Cajun)

1 15-ounce can garbanzo beans,
  undrained
1 tablespoon soy sauce
4 cups coarsely chopped Swiss
  chard or kale
freshly ground black
  pepper

Place the water, onion, mushrooms, and garlic in a large pot. Cook, stirring occasionally, for 5 minutes. Add the potatoes, tomatoes, beans, and soy sauce. Cover and cook over medium heat for 35 minutes, stirring occasionally. Add the greens and the black pepper to taste. Cook an additional 10 minutes.

STUFFED MUSHROOMS

Preparation Time: 30 minutes   Cooking Time: 20 minutes
Servings: makes 20 to 40 stuffed mushrooms

40 medium to large mushrooms or 20 extra-large mushrooms
1 12.3-ounce package lite silken tofu

1 10-ounce package frozen chopped spinach, thawed and squeezed dry
1 package dehydrated onion soup mix

Preheat the oven to 350 degrees.

Clean the mushrooms and remove the stems. Place the tofu in a food processor and process until smooth. Place in a large bowl and add the spinach and onion soup mix. Mix well. Fill the mushroom caps with the tofu mixture and place filled-side up on a nonstick baking sheet. Cover with parchment paper, then cover and seal the edges with aluminum foil. Bake for about 20 minutes, depending on the size of the mushrooms.

Serve warm as an appetizer.

Hint: Check the mushrooms several times while baking to make sure that they do not get too soft. Smaller mushrooms cook faster than larger ones. Mushrooms should be fork-tender when done, but not mushy.

COSTA RICAN GRILLED VEGETABLES

Preparation Time: 10 minutes
Cooking Time: 15 minutes   Servings: 2

1 large onion, cut in half
  lengthwise, then sliced and
  separated into half-rings
1 zucchini, sliced
1 yellow summer squash, sliced

1 thin eggplant, sliced
1 to 2 large portobello mushrooms,
  thickly sliced (optional)
¼ cup soy sauce
¼ cup water

Mix all the vegetables together. Set aside.

Mix the soy sauce and water together.

Heat the grill to medium. Place the vegetables in a flat grilling basket. Brush with the soy sauce mixture. Cover the grill for a few minutes. Continue to flip and baste the vegetables until they are tender and browned; cover the grill between bastings.

Hint: Mango Salsa (page 319) goes well with these vegetables.

CAJUN-DUSTED CHARD

Preparation Time: 20 minutes
Cooking Time: 12 minutes   Servings: 6

⅓ cup water
1 small onion, chopped
½ pound sliced fresh mushrooms
1 teaspoon minced fresh garlic

2 teaspoons Cajun Dust
  seasoning
2 bunches chard, red or green
1 tomato, chopped

Place the water in a large nonstick frying pan. Add the onion, mushrooms, and garlic. Cook, stirring occasionally, for 5 minutes. Add the Cajun Dust and chard. Cook, stirring frequently, until the chard is tender, about 5 minutes. Add the tomato and cook another 2 minutes.

Serve as a side dish or over whole grains or potatoes.

Hint: Cajun Dust seasoning is manufactured by Cajun Dust in Phoenix, Arizona (see page 295).

ARTICHOKES

Preparation Time: 10 minutes
Cooking Time: 45 minutes   Servings: 4

3 quarts water
3 tablespoons lemon juice

1 teaspoon black peppercorns
4 medium to large artichokes

Place the water in a large pot with the lemon juice and peppercorns. Bring to a boil.

While the water is coming to a boil, trim the artichokes by cutting the tips off each leaf with scissors. When you get near the top of the artichoke, slice off about ½ inch with a sharp knife, so the top is flat. Pull off the small lower leaves and slice off the stem so that the bottom is flush with the leaves. Add the artichokes to the boiling water. Cover and cook over medium heat for 45 minutes, until the bottoms pierce easily with a fork. Drain.

Serve hot or cold with Artichoke Dipping Sauces (page 316).

Sauces

TOMATO-LEEK SAUCE

Preparation Time: 10 minutes
Cooking Time: 10 minutes   Servings: makes about 4 cups

⅓ cup water
2 leeks, white part only, thinly
   sliced
½ pound mushrooms, chopped
½ teaspoon minced fresh garlic

1 15-ounce can crushed
   tomatoes
1 8-ounce can tomato sauce
½ teaspoon chili powder
several dashes of Tabasco sauce

Place the water, leeks, mushrooms, and garlic in a medium saucepan. Cook, stirring frequently, for 5 minutes. Add the remaining ingredients and cook for an additional 5 minutes.

COSTA RICAN TOMATO SAUCE

Preparation Time: 20 minutes
Cooking Time: 2 hours, 10 minutes   Servings: makes 1½ quarts

½ cup water
1 onion, cut in half lengthwise,
   then thinly sliced into half-rings
1 stalk celery, thinly sliced
½ pound fresh mushrooms, sliced

5 tomatoes, pureed in a blender
   or food processor
5 tomatoes, chopped
1 cup ketchup
2 tablespoons fennel seeds

Place the water, onion, celery, and mushrooms in a large pot. Cook, stirring occasionally, for 10 minutes. Add the remaining ingredients and cook, uncovered, over low heat for 2 hours.

Serve over pasta, potatoes, or whole grains.

MIXED MUSHROOM SAUCE

Preparation Time: 30 minutes
Cooking Time: 20 minutes   Servings: 6

1 ounce dried porcini mushrooms
1 cup hot water
2 cups sliced leeks
4¾ cups vegetable broth
4 cups mixed sliced fresh
   mushrooms (white button,
   shiitake, cremini, oyster,
   chanterelle)

¼ cup dry white wine
¼ cup minced fresh parsley
2 tablespoons minced fresh dill
several twists of freshly ground
   black pepper
3 tablespoons cornstarch mixed
   in ¼ cup cold water
½ cup fat-free soy milk

Place the porcini mushrooms and hot water in a small bowl. Set aside for 30 minutes. Drain, reserving the soaking liquid. Slice the mushrooms and set aside.

Place the leeks in a large nonstick frying pan with ¾ cup of the broth. Cook, stirring occasionally, for 5 minutes. Add the remaining broth, all the mushrooms, the wine, reserved mushroom broth, parsley, dill, and black pepper. Bring to a boil, reduce the heat, and cook for 15 minutes, stirring occasionally. Add the cornstarch mixture and cook and stir until thickened. Stir in the soy milk and serve at once over pasta or potatoes.

SPICY SWEET GARBANZO SAUCE

Preparation Time: 5 minutes
Cooking Time: 20 minutes   Servings: 4 to 6

⅓ cup water
1 large onion, chopped
1 16-ounce can chopped tomatoes
1 16-ounce can crushed tomatoes
2 16-ounce cans garbanzo beans,
  drained and rinsed
2 tablespoons soy sauce
1 tablespoon lemon juice

1 teaspoon ground coriander
½ teaspoon ground cumin
2 teaspoons pure prepared
  horseradish
several dashes of Tabasco
  sauce
2 cups packed chopped fresh
  spinach

Place the water in a large pot with the onion. Cook, stirring occasionally, for 3 minutes. Add the remaining ingredients, except the spinach. Cook for 15 minutes. Add the spinach and cook for 2 minutes longer.
Serve over rice.

Hint: Try other leafy greens, such as kale or chard; remember to adjust the cooking time for the greens.

JAMAICAN PUMPKIN SAUCE

Preparation Time: 15 minutes
Cooking Time: 25 minutes   Servings: 4

⅓ cup water
1 onion, chopped
1 red bell pepper, chopped
½ teaspoon minced fresh garlic
1 fresh jalapeño, seeded and
  minced
2 cups vegetable broth
1 15-ounce can pumpkin
1 6.5- to 7-ounce package smoked
  tofu, sliced

½ cup frozen corn kernels
1½ teaspoons curry powder
½ teaspoon ground coriander
several twists of freshly ground
  black pepper
1 cup fat-free soy milk
2 tablespoons cornstarch mixed
  in ¼ cup cold water
¼ cup chopped fresh
  parsley

Place the water in a medium saucepan with the onion, bell pepper, garlic, and jalapeño. Cook, stirring occasionally, for 5 minutes. Add the broth, pumpkin, tofu, corn, and seasonings. Bring to a boil, reduce the heat, and cook for 15 minutes, stirring occasionally. Add the milk and cornstarch mixture. Cook and stir until thickened. Stir in the parsley and serve at once over whole grains, pasta, or potatoes.

VERDE SAUCE

Preparation Time: 10 minutes
Cooking Time: 12 minutes   Servings: makes 1 quart

1 cup Mexican green salsa
  (see Hint)
4 cups water
½ cup chopped green onions
1 tablespoon soy sauce

2 tablespoons chopped fresh
  cilantro
⅓ cup cornstarch mixed in ½ cup
  cold water

Place the salsa, water, green onions, and soy sauce in a saucepan. Bring to a boil and cook over medium heat for 10 minutes. Stir in the cilantro and cornstarch mixture. Cook, stirring constantly, for 2 minutes, until thickened.

Serve as a warm sauce for Mexican-style foods.

Hint: You can find many varieties of Mexican green sauce in most supermarkets. Look in the Mexican food section and choose one that is mild or medium and contains no oil. This sauce keeps well in the refrigerator.

ARTICHOKE DIPPING SAUCES

Preparation Time: 5 minutes
Chilling Time: 1 to 2 hours   Servings: makes about 1 cup

about ¾ cup silken tofu
  (half of a 10.5-ounce package)
2 tablespoons lemon juice

1 tablespoon rice vinegar
½ teaspoon dry mustard
dash of salt and white pepper

Place all the ingredients in a blender jar and process until very smooth. Refrigerate for at least 1 hour to allow the flavors to blend.

Variations: Make the basic sauce first, then add one of the following ingredients for each variation. These sauces also make delicious dips for vegetables and crackers.

½ cup lightly packed watercress

½ cup lightly packed fresh cilantro

¼ cup roasted red peppers

½ teaspoon minced fresh garlic

½ teaspoon curry powder and 2 teaspoons parsley flakes

½ teaspoon Dijon mustard, ½ teaspoon prepared horseradish, ¼ teaspoon dill weed, and ¼ teaspoon soy sauce

HEARTY VEGETABLE SAUCE

Preparation Time: 20 minutes
Cooking Time: 20 minutes   Servings: 6 to 8

½ cup water

1 onion, chopped

1 red or green bell pepper, chopped

½ pound fresh mushrooms, sliced

1 8-ounce package seasoned seitan, cut into bite-sized pieces

1 cup frozen peas

5 cups vegetable broth

⅓ cup soy sauce

1 4-ounce jar diced pimientos

1 tablespoon chopped fresh basil

several twists of freshly ground black pepper

5 tablespoons cornstarch mixed in ½ cup cold water

Place the water in a pot with the onion, bell pepper, and mushrooms. Cook, stirring occasionally, for 5 minutes. Add the seitan and peas. Cook for another 5 minutes. Add the remaining ingredients except the cornstarch mixture. Bring to a boil, reduce the heat, and simmer for 5 minutes. Add the cornstarch mixture and cook, stirring constantly, until the sauce thickens.

Serve over whole wheat toast, potatoes, or whole grains.

SAVORY BEAN TOPPING

Preparation Time: 10 minutes
Cooking Time: 20 minutes   Servings: 6 to 8

¼ cup water
1 onion, chopped
1 15-ounce can stewed
   tomatoes (Italian, Mexican,
   or Cajun)
2 15-ounce cans vegetarian baked
   beans

1 15-ounce can small red beans,
   drained and rinsed
⅓ cup barbecue sauce
¼ cup packed brown sugar
2 tablespoons prepared mustard
several twists of freshly ground
   black pepper

Place the water and onion in a medium pot. Cook, stirring occasionally, for 5 minutes. Add the remaining ingredients and cook for 15 minutes.

Serve over baked potatoes, whole grains, or whole wheat toast or muffins.

Dips, Spreads, and Dressings

DIJON HORSERADISH DIP

Preparation Time: 5 minutes
Chilling Time: 1 to 2 hours   Servings: makes 2 cups

1 12.3-ounce package lite silken
   tofu
1½ tablespoons soy sauce
3 teaspoons Dijon mustard
1½ teaspoons pure prepared
   horseradish

½ teaspoon minced fresh
   garlic
¾ teaspoon dried dill weed
½ teaspoon onion powder
⅛ cup chopped fresh
   cilantro

Place the tofu in a food processor and blend until fairly smooth. Add the remaining ingredients, except the cilantro, and process until very smooth. Add the cilantro and process briefly, until the cilantro is mixed in well.

Serve over baked potatoes, use as a dip for artichokes or asparagus, spread on crackers or bagels, or use as a dip for assorted raw vegetables.

MANGO SALSA

Preparation Time: 15 minutes
Chilling Time: 1 hour   Servings: makes 3 cups

2 cups peeled, chopped, ripe
mango
½ cup finely chopped onion
½ cup finely chopped red bell
pepper
1 whole fresh jalapeño, seeded
and finely chopped

¼ teaspoon minced fresh
garlic
1 tablespoon cider vinegar
1 tablespoon warm water
several twists of freshly ground
black pepper
dash of salt

Combine all the ingredients in a bowl and mix well. Cover and chill for 1 hour before serving.

Hint: Be sure to wear rubber gloves when seeding and chopping the jalapeño.

PICO DE GALLO

Preparation Time: 15 minutes
Chilling Time: 1 hour   Servings: makes 2 cups

2 cups chopped tomato
½ cup finely chopped
onion
½ cup finely chopped green bell
pepper

1 whole fresh jalapeño, seeded
and finely chopped
2 tablespoons chopped fresh
cilantro
dash of salt

Combine all the ingredients in a tightly covered bowl. Refrigerate at least 1 hour, turning the container over several times, to allow the flavors to blend.

Serve over Costa Rican Gallo Pinto (page 286), or as a dip for tortillas.

Hint: Be sure to wear rubber gloves when seeding and chopping the jalapeño.

GARBANZO SPREAD

Contributed by Diane Church

Preparation Time: 8 minutes   Servings: makes 1½ cups

1 15-ounce can garbanzo beans,
   drained; reserve ⅓ cup liquid
1 green onion, chopped
1 garlic clove

3 sprigs fresh parsley
Pinch of oregano
1 tablespoon fresh lemon juice
dash of Tabasco sauce (optional)

Place all the ingredients, including the reserved garbanzo liquid, in a food processor and process until smooth and creamy.

Use as a spread on bread, crackers, or pita bread.

HERBED LENTIL SPREAD

Preparation Time: 15 minutes
Cooking Time: 45 minutes   Servings: makes 4 cups

1 cup dried lentils
4 cups water
½ cup vegetable broth
1 onion, chopped
½ pound sliced fresh
   mushrooms
½ teaspoon minced fresh
   garlic
1 tablespoon parsley flakes
1 teaspoon dried basil
1 teaspoon dried marjoram

1 teaspoon dried rosemary
1 teaspoon dried sage
1 teaspoon dried thyme
1 teaspoon dry mustard
½ teaspoon cayenne
¼ teaspoon black pepper
¼ teaspoon allspice
¼ teaspoon ground ginger
1 bay leaf
2 tablespoons soy sauce
1 tablespoon sherry

Place the lentils in a saucepan with the water, bring to a boil, reduce the heat, cover, and cook for about 40 minutes, until tender. Drain and set aside.

Meanwhile, place the broth in another saucepan, add the onion and mushrooms, and cook, stirring frequently, for about 8 minutes. Add the remaining ingredients, except the soy sauce and sherry. Cook for an additional 10 minutes, stirring occasionally, adding more broth if necessary to keep the mixture from sticking to the pan. Add the soy sauce, sherry, and drained lentils. Cook until all liquid is absorbed, about 5 minutes. Remove from the heat and remove the bay leaf. Process in a food processor until smooth. Serve warm or cold.

Hint: This is an excellent spread for crackers or bread. Use presliced mushrooms to save time.

TOFU MAYONNAISE

Preparation Time: 5 minutes
Servings: makes about 1¼ cups

1 12.3-ounce package lite silken tofu
1 tablespoon cider vinegar
1 tablespoon lemon juice

1 to 2 teaspoons Dijon mustard (optional)
dash of salt

Combine all the ingredients in a food processor or blender and process until smooth. Place in a jar and store in the refrigerator.

Hint: This will keep for about a week in the refrigerator. It makes an excellent sandwich spread. Omit the mustard for a milder mayonnaise.

PEA PÂTÉ

Preparation Time: 5 minutes   Cooking Time: 45 minutes
Chilling Time: 2 hours   Servings: makes 2 cups

3 cups vegetable broth
1 cup dried yellow split peas
½ cup chopped onion
½ teaspoon minced fresh garlic

1 tablespoon fresh lemon juice
1 tablespoon soy sauce
freshly ground black pepper
2 tablespoons chopped fresh cilantro, parsley, or dill

Place the broth, peas, onion, and garlic in a saucepan. Bring to a boil, reduce the heat, cover, and cook over low heat for 30 minutes. Remove the cover and cook for about 15 more minutes until the mixture is very thick. Remove from the heat and let cool slightly.

Place the mixture in a food processor and add the lemon juice and soy sauce. Process until smooth. Transfer to a bowl. Add the black pepper to taste and stir in the fresh herb of your choice.

Use as a spread on crackers or bread.

TEMPTRESS ISLAND DRESSING

Preparation Time: 10 minutes
Chilling Time: 2 hours   Servings: makes 2 cups

1 12.3-ounce package lite silken tofu
5 tablespoons water
5 tablespoons ketchup
1 tablespoon lemon juice
2 tablespoons sweet pickle relish
1 tablespoon minced red onion

1 teaspoon soy sauce
1 teaspoon parsley flakes
1 teaspoon minced capers
½ teaspoon onion powder
2 dashes of Tabasco sauce
freshly ground black pepper to taste

Place the tofu, water, ketchup, and lemon juice in a food processor and process until smooth. Pour into a covered container and stir in the remaining ingredients. Cover and refrigerate for 2 hours to blend the flavors.

Desserts

ALMOST HEAVEN SORBET

Preparation Time: 5 minutes (need frozen bananas)
Servings: 4

2 frozen bananas, cut into chunks
1 cup frozen blueberries

1 6-ounce can frozen apple juice concentrate

Place the bananas in a food processor and process until smooth. Add the blueberries slowly through the feed tube and continue to process. Add the apple juice concentrate and process until very smooth. Serve immediately.

Hint: Use other frozen fruit, like strawberries or raspberries, in place of the blueberries. To freeze bananas, peel and cut into chunks, freeze on a baking sheet, then store in a covered container in the freezer until ready to use.

PINEAPPLE-LEMON PUDDING

Contributed by Robert Siegel

Preparation Time: 5 minutes   Cooking Time: 5 minutes
Chilling Time: 2 hours   Servings: 6 to 8

3 cups pineapple juice
½ cup orange juice concentrate
½ cup arrowroot

½ cup sugar
⅓ cup fresh lemon juice
1 tablespoon lemon zest

Combine all the ingredients in a blender jar and process until smooth. Pour into a medium saucepan and cook, stirring constantly, until thickened and clear, about 5 minutes.

Transfer to a covered glass container and refrigerate for 2 hours until well chilled.

Hint: You can also put the pudding in individual serving bowls for chilling. Cover each one with plastic wrap before placing in the refrigerator.

RAISIN-CARROT CAKE

Preparation Time: 45 minutes
Cooking Time: 55 minutes   Servings: 12

1¾ cups water
1 cup raisins
1 cup grated carrots
½ cup honey
¼ cup chopped dates
1 teaspoon cinnamon
1 teaspoon allspice

½ teaspoon nutmeg
¼ teaspoon ground cloves
1½ cups whole wheat flour
½ cup bran
1 teaspoon baking soda
¼ cup chopped walnuts
(optional)

Preheat the oven to 350 degrees.

Place the water in a large saucepan. Add the raisins, carrots, honey, dates, and all the spices. Bring to a boil, reduce the heat, cover, and cook for 10 minutes. Remove from the heat and cool slightly.

Meanwhile, combine the flour, bran, baking soda, and walnuts, if using. Add the cooled raisin-carrot mixture and mix well. Pour into a nonstick 9 × 9-inch baking dish. Bake for 45 minutes.

Serve warm or cold.

Appendix A:
Major Medical
Indications for the
McDougall Approach

The health problems most people suffer from today flow directly from their diets and lifestyles. That is why dietary change brings about such dramatic results. The common disorders and illnesses listed below show the underlying dietary causes of disease. For more information about these individual problems, please see my other books, including: *The McDougall Program—Twelve Days to Dynamic Health, The McDougall Program for Maximum Weight Loss,* and *The McDougall Program for a Healthy Heart.* I also encourage you to consult the scientific research cited at the end of each book.

ACNE Oily skin and acne can be dramatically improved by a very-low-fat diet. Even small amounts of fats and oils can make for serious complexion problems.

ALLERGIC DISEASES Food allergies are cured when the offending food is removed from the diet. Pinpoint which food is triggering the problem by keeping a food diary, or start eliminating suspect foods from your diet.

ARTHRITIS Gout is well recognized as a disease caused by rich food and cured by eating a starch-based diet. Inflammatory arthritis, rheumatoid arthritis, lupus, psoriasis, and ankylosing spondylitis are also dramatically improved and often cured by switching to a starch-based diet without animal products.

ATHEROSCLEROSIS A low-fat vegetarian diet has been documented to reverse coronary artery disease. The frequency of chest pain episodes (angina) is reduced by more than 90 percent in less than three weeks with this diet. Improvement in walking time for persons who suffer with intermittent claudication begins in about five days.

CANCER Most authorities accept that diet plays a major, not to mention controllable, part in causing major cancers, including breast, colon, and prostate cancers. Alcohol and tobacco are also known to cause cancer. The benefits of a dietary change for people already suffering with cancer are still unknown. Studies are under way to determine how much benefit a good diet can be for cancer victims.

CHOLESTEROL Average reductions of 29 mg/dl are seen in eleven days on the McDougall diet, and the reductions usually continue for about six to eight weeks.

COLITIS Irritable bowel syndrome (spastic colon) and nonspecific colitis are quickly resolved by changing the contents of the colon. Most Crohn's disease and ulcerative colitis patients are dramatically benefited by a change in diet. Frequency decreases in two days after removal of all extra fats, and the disease can reverse over the next few weeks or months.

COLON POLYPS These polyps are the result of constant irritation of the colon mucosa from the unhealthy remnants of the Western diet. Adding fiber to the diet of people with chronic polyposis has been shown to inhibit polyp formation.

CONSTIPATION Almost everyone experiences excellent bowel function after two days of a healthy high-fiber vegetable diet. Straining from constipation causes hemorrhoids, varicose veins, and hiatus hernia. These structural changes are not reversed with a good diet, but the symptoms can at least be improved with better eating.

DIABETES Juvenile diabetes is caused in most cases by an autoimmune reaction to cow's milk in young children. The pancreas is destroyed and function will not return with a better diet. Adult-onset diabetes is caused by the high-fat Western diet in susceptible people. In almost every case, diabetic pills can be stopped and in most cases (50 to 75 percent) insulin can be stopped. Both kinds of diabetes cause rapid deterioration of the patient's health and lead to blindness, heart attacks, and kidney failure. A starch-based diet can prevent these common consequences.

DIVERTICULAR DISEASE Diverticulosis is caused by the high bowel pressures required to move the tiny Western stool through the colon. Bleeding and painful symptoms of diverticulitis are relieved with a healthy diet. Diverticula are permanent structural changes, but eating a high-fiber vegetable diet may prevent the formation of new ones.

GALLBLADDER DISEASE More than 90 percent of gallstones are made principally of cholesterol. Diets high in polyunsaturated fats seem to promote the development of gallbladder disease. The time-honored treatment for gallbladder pain is a low-fat diet. Once formed, gallstones will not dissolve with a low-fat diet, but they almost always stop hurting. Asymptomatic gallstones are best left untreated.

HEADACHES Most nonspecific headaches are alleviated with a diet change. More than 70 percent of migraines are believed to be due to food allergies and can be relieved with a change in diet.

HIATUS HERNIA Indigestion associated with a hiatus hernia is usually relieved with a healthy diet. Raising the head of the bed four to six inches helps, too.

HORMONE-DEPENDENT DISEASES

- *Heavy periods:* With a change in diet, menstrual bleeding becomes lighter, periods are shorter, and the time between periods becomes longer.
- *Abnormal uterine bleeding (AUB):* Generally, this problem is due to a high-fat diet, and menstrual bleeding becomes less with a diet change.
- *Fibrocystic breast disease:* In most cases, breast pain is relieved and in 60 percent of cases, lumps disappear in six months.
- *Fibroids of the uterus:* They are caused by the elevated hormone levels of a high-fat diet, but I've never seen them disappear with a change in diet. Symptoms of bleeding and pain do seem to improve.
- *Polycystic ovary disease:* Cysts will disappear, and the associated problems of infertility and excess body hair may also improve with a change in diet and accompanying weight loss.
- *Premenstrual syndrome* (PMS): Fluid retention, tender breasts, bloating, and mood swings improve soon after changing to low-fat, low-sodium foods.
- *Hair loss* (male-pattern baldness): This occurs in some women because of high testosterone levels due to the effects of a rich diet. Hair regrowth should not be expected.

HYPERTENSION Blood pressure usually drops precipitately after a diet change, exercise, and stopping caffeine.

KIDNEY DISEASE A high-protein diet encourages the progression of kidney failure from almost all causes, and a low-protein starch-based diet can slow and often stop the progression of kidney failure, thereby keeping many patients off dialysis.

Nephritis (glomerulonephritis) is an auto immune disease often caused by animal protein. Eliminating cow's milk, beef, pork, and other animal proteins from your diet can often cure the disease.

KIDNEY STONES Both calcium and uric acid stones are caused by the high-protein Western diet rich in animal products. A change in diet can prevent recurrence. Once formed, the stones do not dissolve with a change in diet.

LIVER FAILURE A low-protein diet is fundamental in patients with symptoms of liver failure. Vegetable protein is much better tolerated than animal protein.

MULTIPLE SCLEROSIS Forty-five years of research on more than 4,500 patients demonstrates how a low-fat diet will stop the progression of MS in more than 95 percent of cases. All other therapies have proved to be dismal failures, with half the patients wheelchair bound, bedridden, or dead in ten years.

OBESITY Changing to a low-fat, high-carbohydrate diet means that you can lose weight while never being hungry. For maximum weight loss, eliminate flour products, including breads, bagels, and pastas, and instead focus on beans, corn, potatoes, rice, and green and yellow vegetables. Exercise also helps a lot.

OSTEOPOROSIS The acidic, high-protein animal foods of the Western diet, such as meat, poultry, fish, and eggs are a primary cause of osteoporosis. Other contributing factors are lack of exercise, excessive sodium intake, and caffeine. A low-protein starch-based diet and exercise should reverse the disease.

UPPER INTESTINAL DISTRESS Esophagitis, gastritis, and indigestion are caused by putting the wrong things into the stomach! A starch-based diet is an effective cure for most people. Some vegetable foods can prove irritating, such as raw vegetables (especially onions, green peppers, radishes, and cucumbers), fruit juice, tomato sauces, and hot spicy foods like chiles. Helicobacter pylori has been blamed for indigestion and ulcers, and eradication with antibiotics has been helpful. However, these bacteria are more likely to grow when the wrong foods are in your stomach.

Scientific references supporting the use of diet in the above diseases can be found in previous McDougall books—especially valuable for this are *The McDougall Program—Twelve Days to Dynamic Health* and *McDougall's Medicine—A Challenging Second Opinion.*

APPENDIX B:
EARLY DETECTION TESTS

Consider this: The National Cancer Institute estimates that a 30 percent reduction in tobacco use would yield a 10 percent reduction in cancer deaths, whereas widespread screening for breast and cervical cancer would yield only a 3 percent reduction. *Prevention* is where we need to focus our efforts as individuals, and in devising a national health policy.

Here's my observation of the behavioral bottom line: When people believe they will be saved by early detection and treatment, they are simply less likely to take steps toward prevention. Consider the change in sexual practices. In the 1970s, gonorrhea and syphilis were treated easily with a shot of penicillin, and many people embraced "free love." In the 1990s, incurable herpes and AIDS have seriously changed people's behavior. An understanding of the lethal course of cancer, which is unchecked by treatment in most cases, and that early detection at best offers only very limited benefits, will propel more of us toward adopting preventive diets and lifestyles.

When medical scientists disagree about the effectiveness of early detection tests, it means that *whatever effect there may be is small, and there must be significant costs and side effects associated with the tests.* Many top researchers who are not influenced by political pressures to conform to the business side of cancer have come to conclusions considerably different than those commonly advertised by the Cancer Society and most practicing doctors. You need to have hard information about this controversy in order to decide whether to choose cancer early detection tests.

Breast Cancer

An estimated 184,300 new cases of invasive breast cancer will have been diagnosed in women in 1996, with an expected 44,300 deaths.

PHYSICAL EXAMINATION

The American Cancer Society recommends monthly breast self-examination after the age of twenty. Clinical (by a professional) examination every three years between ages twenty and thirty-nine, and yearly for age forty and over. More than 90 percent of cancers are found by women, not their doctors.

Another Opinion

There is *no* evidence that a doctor's physical examination of your breasts, your own breast self-examination, or breast ultrasound will reduce your chance of dying from breast cancer. Studies fail to support survival benefits of breast self-examination. For example, a study showed that 63,636 women between ages forty-five and sixty-four in England who were offered breast self-examination education had a higher death rate from breast cancer than a comparison group of 127,117 *not* offered class instruction. Another study found a higher risk of developing advanced breast cancer in women who reported they performed breast self-examination than in those who did not. The most recent study, published in 1997 in the *Journal of the National Cancer Institute*, assigned more than 250,000 Chinese women who worked in a textile factory to either a breast self-examination or a control group. The instruction group received intensive training, two reinforcement sessions, and multiple reminders. Compliance was high (83.6 percent). There was no difference in survival or in stage or size of tumors for women who performed routine breast self-examination when compared with the control group. Knowing the natural history of breast cancer development will make it easy for you to understand why survival cannot be improved by physical examination of the breasts; however, self-examination *will* find smaller tumors that can be removed more often by a nondeforming lumpectomy.

MAMMOGRAPHY

The American Cancer Society recommends mammography for women ages forty to forty-nine every one to two years; yearly after age fifty.

Another Opinion

Studies show limited survival benefits only for women between fifty and sixty-nine years as discussed in chapter 7.

Colorectal Cancer

Cancer of the colon and rectum (colorectal cancer) is the second leading cause of death due to cancer, with 55,000 deaths and 135,000 new cases in 1996.

DIGITAL RECTAL EXAM

The American Cancer Society recommends digital rectal exam (DRE) yearly after age forty, stool blood tests yearly after age fifty, and sigmoidoscopy every three to five years after age fifty.

Another Opinion

Like most physical examination procedures, DRE has not been tested in properly designed studies. Since colorectal cancer will be at least ten years old by the time it is discovered, little benefit can be expected.

OCCULT BLOOD TEST

This is one of the most controversial areas of screening. Bleeding usually begins in the late stages of cancer, when cure is unlikely. Authors of an article in the 1993 issue of *The Journal of the American Medical Association* concluded: "Based on our observations in the screening setting, fecal blood appears to be a poor marker for colorectal neoplasia. Most cancers and the vast majority of polyps will be missed. Hemoccult and HemoQuant are similarly insensitive." Fecal blood screening has failed to date to detect 70 percent of colorectal cancers and more than 90 percent of polyps.

SIGMOIDOSCOPY EXAMS

In one oft-cited study, sigmoidoscopy examination once every ten years reduced the risk of dying from colorectal cancer by 50 percent. More frequent screening gave no better results.

Polyp Removal

Cancer begins with a small symptomless polyp, or projecting growth. Studies support survival benefit for detection of precancerous polyps; but no survival benefit for detection of actual colorectal cancers. The National Polyp Study of more than 1,418 patients who had complete colonoscopy with one or more polyps removed, had an incidence of colon cancer 76 percent to 90 percent lower than expected. The same study showed that screening every three years proved as beneficial as annual screening.

Since 90 percent of cancer occurs after the age of fifty-five and the time required for transition from a normal colon to cancer is between ten and thirty-five years, an effective way to screen would be to do one exam between the ages of fifty-five and sixty. This would find most of the cancers already beginning as polyps. If no disease were present at this time, future examinations would be unlikely to benefit the person since it takes so many years for a cancer to develop, and finally to kill.

Colonoscopy examination with a long flexible tube is most often recommended for evaluation of the colon and rectum; however, my preferred alternative, because of much lower costs and fewer complications, is a double-contrast barium enema and a flexible sigmoidoscope. Colonoscopy examinations, performed by experienced specialists, miss finding polyps 24 percent of the time, and they are much more dangerous than a barium enema and a sigmoidoscope exam.

Cervical Cancer

There are estimated to be 15,700 new cases of cervical cancer with 4,900 deaths in 1996.

Pap Smears

The American Cancer Society recommends a Pap test be performed annually on women who are eighteen years old, or sexually active. After three or more consecutive annual exams with normal findings, the Pap test can be performed less frequently at the discretion of the physician.

Another Opinion

Many studies have shown a fall in death rate from cervical cancer at the time of introduction of Pap smears. However, some investigators feel this change is due to factors other than the Pap smears, and that mass screening may be doing more harm than good. They point out that death rates were declining before screening began, and by the time 80 percent of the coverage was achieved in 1972, almost half the reduction in mortality rate had occurred.

One recent study of screening in Bristol, England, of 225,974 women found that during each five-year screening period, 15,000 healthy women were being incorrectly told that they were "at risk," and more than 5,500 were being investigated for disease that would never have troubled them. Those women were left with problems that included lasting worries about cancer, difficulties in obtaining life insurance, and worries concerning the effects of treatment on their future reproductive abilities. Yet, the effect on death rate was too small to detect. "The limitations of screening stem not only from the fact that abnormal cells can be found in the smears of numerous women never destined to get cervical cancer, but also from the fact that local treatment of CIN (carcinoma) does not ensure the prevention of invasive disease in every case."

Many health organizations recommend discontinuation of smears after the ages of sixty to sixty-five, for healthy women with normal Pap smears. One large study in Scotland found 798 cases of cervical cancer over a three-year period. Almost all cases (711) were in women under forty-six. Of the twenty-six cases in women diagnosed over the age of fifty, none had participated in an adequate screening program. The authors concluded: "Cervical intraepithelial neoplasia (cancer) typically occurs in younger women. All women over 50 with an adequate history of negative results on smear testing every three years may be safely discharged from further screening if these findings are confirmed in other populations."

After a hysterectomy, Pap smears should be stopped. After analyzing studies published between 1966 and 1995, a recent article in the *Journal of the American Medical Association* found "there is insufficient evidence to recommend routine vaginal smear screening in women after total hysterectomy."

Uterine (Endometrial) Cancer

There are estimated to be 34,000 new cases of uterine cancer with 6,000 deaths in 1996.

Pap Smear

The American Cancer Society says a Pap smear is only partially effective. Women at high risk should have an endometrial tissue sampling (biopsy) at menopause.

Another Opinion

The Canadian Task Force was unable to recommend any screening techniques for endometrial cancer and the American College of Physicians agrees.

Ovarian Cancer

Ovarian cancer is the fifth most common cancer of women, and the leading cause of death from gynecologic malignancies. An estimated 26,700 new cases will have been diagnosed and 14,800 women will have died of this disease in 1996. The overall prognosis is poor, with 65 to 75 percent of cases appearing in an advanced stage of disease.

Pelvic Exams, Transvaginal Ultrasound, and CA 125

The American Cancer Society says periodic pelvic exams are important. Transvaginal ultrasound and a tumor marker, CA 125, may assist in diagnosis.

Another Opinion

Pelvic examination is not effective and bimanual examination should not be performed as a routine screening in asymptomatic women. According to the authors of a 1995 article in the *Journal of the American Medical Association*, "there is no evidence available yet that the current screening modalities of CA 125 and transvaginal ultrasonography can be effectively used for widespread screening to reduce the mortality from ovarian cancer nor that their use will result in decreased rather than increased morbidity and mortality."

Lung Cancer

The American Cancer Society says early detection is difficult.

Another Opinion

Lung cancer is so advanced by the time of diagnosis with chest X ray or tests of sputum that there is little hope of helping patients.

Skin Cancer

SKIN SELF-EXAM

The American Cancer Society says early detection is critical. Adults should practice skin self-exam once a month, and any suspicious lesions should be evaluated by a physician.

Another Opinion

Many precancerous and early cancers of the skin can be simply and effectively treated. An occasional look is safe and costs nothing.

McDougall's Recommendations

The aim of early detection techniques is to find the disease when it is small, before it has had a chance to spread to other parts of the body (metastasize). Early detection tests that have the potential to make the biggest difference rely on finding cells before they have actually turned into cancer (precancerous cells). These precancerous changes can sometimes be seen under a microscope and treated before actual cancer develops and spreads to other parts of the body. This search can be successful for precancerous lesions found in the mouth (leukoplakia), on the uterine cervix (cervical dysplasia), on the skin (dysplastic nevi), and in the large intestine (colon polyps).

Based on my understanding of cancer and on findings in the current scientific literature I can make the following *general* screening recommendations for otherwise healthy people:

Breast Cancer

No breast self- or clinical examination
No mammography under fifty and over sixty-nine
No definite recommendation for women fifty to sixty-nine—the bene-
    fits are limited at best (consider the evidence before deciding)

Colorectal Cancer

No DRE or occult blood tests
One sigmoidoscopy exam combined with a double-contrast barium
    enema at ages fifty-five to sixty

Cervical Cancer

Pap smears every three years after two consecutive normal annual
    smears between ages eighteen (or sexually active) and fifty; no Pap
    smears after age sixty or after a hysterectomy

Skin Cancer

Periodic examination of the skin for lesions

Screening Not Recommended

uterine cancer
ovarian cancer
lung cancer

Though many early detection screening programs are of questionable benefit, there is no doubt they're capable of definite harm: cost,
inconvenience, unnecessary procedures, and accidental complications, to say nothing of the anxiety, distress, and discrimination experienced by cancer victims. Before a screening program is unleashed on
the unsuspecting public, the medical profession must prove that the
testing will be of benefit. To date the proof of benefit is either lacking
or quite small for most of the early detection screening recommended.
Yet doctors encourage healthy people to partake in costly and potentially harmful medical testing.

APPENDIX C:
THE LOW-FAT FOOD
TRADE-OFF

B ack in the 1980s, food manufacturers realized that people all over the country wanted to improve their health by lowering the fat and cholesterol in their diets. The food industry's response to this new consumer demand was interesting. Many companies did, indeed, produce a variety of "low-fat" and "fat-free" foods. Natural foods supermarkets sprang up around the country to provide delicious and healthful natural foods that were low in fat and cholesterol, and rich in nutrition. Many truly creative and health-conscious food companies were formed to offer a wide variety of natural, organic, and healthy products. This, you might say, was the light side of the transformation we have witnessed during the last ten to twenty years.

But there was also the dark side of the picture. Many companies saw the opportunity to make enormous amounts of money by misleading consumers with their advertising. Many foods that contained significant amounts of fat were advertised as "low in fat," while other foods that were advertised as "fat-free," in fact, contained fat. Vegetable oils and processed, plant-based foods that were rich in hydrogenated vegetable oils were routinely advertised as having "no cholesterol." Since plants contain no cholesterol, the claim of "no cholesterol" was merely the food industry's way of misleading consumers into thinking these foods were healthy, when in fact they were essentially fat bombs that could blow up your arteries and your heart, and even contribute to some cancers.

But fat was not the only concern. Many foods advertised as low in fat were loaded with processed carbohydrates, such as sugar and white flour, which made these foods rich in calories and lacking in nutrition. The biggest increase in calories during the past fifteen years has been from processed carbohydrates, which are rapidly absorbed by the body and contribute to weight gain and obesity. Processed foods have not only harmed people's health, but also confused people about the nature of carbohydrates. Many people today do not realize the difference between a processed or simple carbohydrate, such as sugar or flour, and the kinds of complex carbohydrates that are bound up in fiber- and nutrition-rich foods, such as brown rice, barley, whole wheat, corn, millet, and oats.

Hence, many foods that were being advertised as "no cholesterol" were actually "high in fat," "low-fat" foods were in fact "devoid of nutritional value," and "fat-free" might mean they were "loaded with animal protein." Of course, advertisers are not going to tell people the truth; their job is to sell products.

Nature created foods to be whole and balanced. Each plant food contains its own unique blend of natural carbohydrates, fat, protein, vitamins, minerals, phytochemicals, and fiber. But strange things happen to a food when you take one or more of these individual constituents out of it during processing. For example, when food manufacturers remove the fat from a food, the relative contributions of animal protein and/ or refined carbohydrate increase, causing other problems. My greatest concerns are about the milk and egg proteins. These two are the first and second leading causes of food allergy, a problem for as many as 60 percent of people. Excess animal protein overloads the kidneys, causing a consequential loss of calcium that results in osteoporosis. The calcium spilling into the urine provides an excellent environment for crystallization, or the formation of calcium kidney stones. Animal protein causes a greater rise in cholesterol than vegetable protein and will be a factor in the development of atherosclerosis. Excess protein overworks the liver and kidneys, aggravating serious disease in people with previous damage to these organs.

In other low-fat products, sugar replaces the fat, which leads to sugar-related problems such as high triglycerides in sensitive people, difficulty in losing weight, and tooth decay. The carbohydrate in milk, known as lactose, causes diarrhea, stomach cramps, and gas, especially in nonwhite people.

The impact of misleading advertising and the ill effects of foods that were advertised as "healthy" but had no positive effect on health have been devastating to many people who formerly believed they could improve their health by improving their diets. People became cynical about the relationship between diet and disease, and then surrendered to their own worst instincts. Many people were so put off by the manipulation of the food industry and by the contradictory reports sometimes published by scientists that they simply threw up their hands and said, "Pass the steak and cigars."

The irony is that the underlying truth about diet and health has not changed one bit. The right diet is as powerful today at healing our illnesses as it has always been. My program is having the same results on people today as it did ten years ago. If anything, it's having a bigger impact on health than it had a decade ago because I know so much more about helping people make changes, and Mary has been working hard to improve the quality of our foods and recipes so that the McDougall diet will be the most delicious and health-promoting regimen you will find. Virtually anyone can eat the McDougall diet and, with a little time for adaptation, become completely and exceedingly happy with this food—and a whole lot healthier.

Still, I understand why people are angry and cynical. After all, your trust has been violated. But rather than give up on the dream of good health, you should instead become better informed. That's the job we face today. In an effort to help you distinguish foods that are healthful and good for you from those that are merely advertised as such, I offer this guide to better eating through knowing the meaning behind food labels.

Disguising Fat in Packaged Foods

Sometimes the ingredients list misrepresents the actual fat content by using names many people do not recognize as fat. For example, two varieties of fats, monoglycerides and diglycerides, are commonly found in ingredients lists. You may fail to identify these as fat unless you connect the similarity of their names to a better-known fat, triglycerides.

Lecithin is another ingredient that few people recognize as fat. Furthermore, there is nothing magic about lecithin when it comes to cholesterol. Scientific research shows that lecithin's cholesterol-lowering effects are only the result of the polyunsaturated content (especially the linoleic acid content) of the lecithin; in fact, it lowers cholesterol no better than any other vegetable oil.

FAT-FREE AND FAT-REDUCED

To qualify as "fat-free" a product must contain less than ½ gram of fat per serving. In this case the fat content in the nutritional information section of the label can be listed as 0 (zero). However, when the actual ingredients are examined you may find lard or a vegetable oil prominently listed. This is accomplished by keeping the serving size small enough to meet the definition of less than ½ gram per serving. Kraft Foods, Inc., markets a line of salad dressings called, "FREE" Fat-Free Dressing." But they're not free of fat. For example, the Free Catalina dressing lists soybean oil as the seventh ingredient. A serving size is 2 tablespoons and contains 35 calories. The definition for fat-free is less than ½ gram of fat per serving, which means up to 4.5 calories per serving can be fat (9 calories per gram times ½ gram).

"Fat-reduced" refers to a reduction in fat compared to the content of fat usually expected in this product. There is no rule on how much reduction is required to claim that a product is fat-reduced. Fat-reduced may still mean half or more of the calories are from fat. For example, Reduced Fat Monterey Jack Cheese (Kraft Foods, Inc.), a brand of fat-reduced cheese, is 63 percent fat compared with regular Monterey Jack Cheese, which is 73 percent fat. Mocha Mix Lite Nondairy Creamer (Presto Food Products, Inc.) claims on the front label, "50% less fat than regular nondairy creamers." But the ingredients say 75 percent of the calories are from fat. Outrageously offensive is Cool Whip FREE (Kraft Foods, Inc.) made from water, corn syrup, and hydrogenated coconut and palm kernel oils. These two oils are the two most saturated fats found in nature, and to make them even more saturated the manufacturer hydrogenates them. (Saturated fat raises cholesterol, which causes heart disease.)

FAT SUBSTITUTES

A fat substitute is simply an ingredient that replaces the fat in a product with a substance with the smooth taste, texture, and characteristics of fat. When used in packaged foods, fat substitutes may account for 30 to 40 percent of the ingredients. (Most other food additives account for 1 to 2 percent of a food.) Therefore, they have the potential to be consumed in large quantities and have a significant impact on your health.

Fat substitute classification is based on their derivation from fats, proteins, and carbohydrates of natural and synthetic origin.

Protein-based

These substitutes are made by whipping milk and/or egg proteins into polymers that simulate the feel of fat. This high-shear, cooking, and blending process is called microparticulation. The products contain about 1.3 calories/gram.

They are used in dairy products such as ice cream, sour cream, cheese, yogurt, frozen desserts, and baked goods. They cannot be used for frying, but can be used in many high-temperature products, such as pizza, lasagna, and cheesecake.

Examples are Simplesse, Simplesse 100, Trailblazer, Ultra-Bake, Ultra-Freeze.

My concerns are that egg and dairy proteins cause food allergy. Excess protein leads to osteoporosis, kidney stones, and burdens on the liver and kidneys.

Fat-based

These substitutes are made from vegetable fats (monoglycerides and diglycerides), milk fat or nonfat dried milk base, modified food starch, and/or guar gum mixed with water to dilute the fat. Some of the fats are only partially absorbed, which reduces their effective calorie content from 9 calories/gram to 5 calories/gram.

They are used in cake mixes, cookies, icings, and dairy products. Many calorie-reduced margarines are made by mixing water and oil. Examples are Ceprenin, Duro-Lo, N-Flate, Veri-Lo.

Because this is still 100 percent fat, just diluted with water or less able to be digested, all the adverse effects from fat, including obesity, are expected from this class of fat substitutes.

Olestra is a nonabsorbable fat used in some chips, but will soon appear in other products. Diarrhea and loss of nutrients are two common side effects.

Carbohydrate-based

These substitutes are made from extracts of plant parts, such as corn, oats, potatoes, kelp, wood fiber, and dextrose. They include dextrins, modified food starches, polydextrose, and gums. They provide 0 to 4 calories/gram. Modified starch refers to the alteration of natural starches to make them easier to digest or to increase their thickening and gelling properties.

They are used in sauces, frozen desserts, spreads, margarines, cereals, snacks, and salad dressings to modify texture and add body, and are mixed with processed meats and ground beef to reduce fat content. They are heat stable and can be used in baking; however, because they do not melt they cannot be used in frying. Examples are:

Cellulose: made from wood pulp; noncaloric; Avicel, Cellulose Gel
Gums: plant extracts; xanthan, guar, locust bean, gum Arabic, carrageenan
Dextrins: bland, nonsweet, fully digestible, made from hydrolyzed starches; N-Oil (tapioca), Oatrim (oat fiber), Leanesse
Modified Food Starch (STA-SLIM 143)
Multodextrins: Lycadex, Maltrin (corn), Paselli SA2 (potato), Star-Dri
Polydextrose (Litesse)

This is the safest kind of fat alternative. Cellulose and gums are natural dietary fibers. Gums have been shown to reduce cholesterol and lower blood sugar. However, other carbohydrate-based fat substitutes are synthetic polymers of simple sugars that lack the beneficial properties of natural dietary fiber.

Fat-Free Dairy Products

New fat-free products enter the market daily. You must read the ingredients list carefully to determine if you want to include them in your diet. *None of these foods are recommended,* because of the high animal protein contained in most of them.

Cheeses: These cheeses are made from cheese cultures, salt, and enzymes. Other dairy products such as cheese, skim milk, whey, and buttermilk may be present. Sugars like corn syrup and maltodextrin and salt are added. Examples are:

Borden Fat Free American Nonfat Process Cheese Product (Borden)
Kraft Free Singles (Kraft Foods)
Kraft Free Fat Free Cheddar Cheese (Kraft Foods)
Alpine Lace FAT FREE Singles (Alpine Lace Brands, Inc.)
Alpine Lace FAT FREE Shredded (Alpine Lace Brands, Inc.)
Healthy Choice Fat Free Cheese (Con-Agra)
Lifetime Fat Free Cheese (Lifetime)
Precious Fat Free Cheese (Sorrento Cheese Co.)

Cottage Cheese: These products are made from nonfat milk, sugar (dextrin), and modified food starch. Examples are Knudsen Free Nonfat Cottage Cheese (Kraft Foods), Alta Dena Low-fat Cottage Cheese (Alta Dena), and Nancy's Lowfat Cottage Cheese (Springfield Creamery).

Sour Cream: These products are made from nonfat milk, modified food starch, and sugar. Examples are Knudsen Free Fat Free Sour Cream (Kraft Foods) and Land-O-Lakes No Fat Sour Cream (Land-O-Lakes).

Ice Cream: These products are made from skim milk, sugars, and ice cream flavorings. Some contain fruit, milk protein, Simplesse, artificial sweeteners, whole milk, salt, flavorings, and additives. Examples are:

Breyer's Fat Free Ice Cream (Good Humor–Breyer's Ice Cream)
Dreyer's Fat Free Ice Cream (Dreyer's)
SnackWells Low Fat Ice Cream (Nabisco)
Healthy Choice Low Fat Ice Cream (Con-Agra)
Healthy Temptations Low Fat Snack Sandwiches (Betty Crocker)

Cream Cheese: These products are made from skim milk, cultures, and sugar. Examples are Healthy Choice Fat Free Nonfat Cream Cheese (Con-Agra) and Kraft Philadelphia Free Fat Free Cream Cheese (Kraft Foods).

Yogurt: These products are made from skim milk, cornstarch, whey, and pectin or gelatin. Many contain fruits and sweeteners. Some contain aspartame. Examples are:

Dannon Fat Free Yogurt (Dannon)
Dannon Light Yogurt (Dannon)
Yoplait Light Fat Free Yogurt (Yoplait)
Mello Bros. Fat Free Yogurt (Mello Bros.)
Alta Dena Non-fat Yogurt (Alta Dena)

Puddings: These products are made primarily from nonfat milk, sugar, and starch. Examples are Hunts Fat Free Snack Pack (Hunt-Wesson) and Jell-O Free Fat Free Pudding Snacks (Kraft Foods).

Egg Substitutes

Packaged frozen egg substitutes using mostly egg whites are found in the market. Most are fat free, containing egg whites, additives, and usually nonfat milk. If you use these products, you face the problems of food allergy and calcium loss from excess animal protein. The list of additives is formidable. Examples are Eggbeaters (Nabisco), Second Nature Eggs (M Star, Inc.), and Morningstar Farms Fat Free Scramblers (Worthington Foods).

Snack Foods

FAT-FREE CAKES, COOKIES, BARS, AND MUFFINS

Prominent ingredients in these products are sugar, white flour, nonfat milk, egg whites, and whey. Other kinds of simple sugars may also appear in the ingredients list, such as corn syrup, brown sugar, dextrose, polydextrose, dextrin, and maltodextrin. Fats like hydrogenated vegetable (soybean) oils, monoglycerides, diglycerides, and lecithin are commonly found in "fat-free" desserts. Examples are:

Entenmann's Light Fat Free Twists (Entenmann's)
Entenmann's Light Fat Free Golden Loaf (Entenmann's)
Entenmann's Fat Free Oatmeal Raisin Cookies (Entenmann's)
Entenmann's Fat Free Cholesterol Free Creme Filled Chocolate Cupcakes (Entenmann's)
Entenmann's Low Fat Multi Grain Cereal Bars (Entenmann's)
Sara Lee Fat Free Golden Loaf Cake (Sara Lee Corp.)
Sara Lee Fat Free Oatmeal Raisin Cookies (Sara Lee Corp.)
Bakery Wagon Fat Free Cobblers (M.C. Cookie Co.)
Newton's Fat Free Cobblers (Nabisco)
Greenfield Fat Free Apple Spice Blondie (Greenfield Healthy Foods Co.)
Greenfield Fat Free Brownies (Greenfield Healthy Foods Co.)
SnackWells Toaster Pasteries (Nabisco)
SnackWells Snack Bars (Nabisco)
SnackWells Brownie Bars (Nabisco)
SnackWells Fat Free Cereal Bars (Nabisco)
SnackWells Creme Sandwich Cookies (Nabisco)
SnackWells Fat Free Devil's Food Cookie Cakes (Nabisco)
SnackWells Fudge Brownie Mix (Pillsbury)

SnackWells Blueberry Muffin Mix (Pillsbury)
Sweet Rewards Fat Free Snack Bars (Betty Crocker)
Sweet Rewards Fat Free Snack Cake Mix (Betty Crocker)
Sweet Rewards Fat Free Muffin Mix (Betty Crocker)
Krusteaz Fat Free Muffin Mix (Continental Mills)

Spreads

MAYONNAISE-TYPE SPREADS

The prominent ingredients in these products include simple carbohydrates, such as corn syrup and sugar, and modified food starch. Dairy proteins and egg whites are present with a multitude of chemical additives. Examples are Weight Watchers Fat-Free Mayonnaise Dressing (Weight Watchers), Kraft Mayo Fat Free Mayonnaise Dressing (Kraft Foods), and Smart Beat Non Fat Mayonnaise Dressing (Heart Beat Foods).

Butter Substitutes

SPREADS

These products are made from water, starch, mono- and diglycerides, and milk products such as lactose or skim milk. Examples are:

Fleischmann's Fat Free 5 Calorie Spread (Nabisco)
Fleischmann's Fat Free Healthy 15 Calorie Spread (Nabisco)
Promise Ultra Fat Free Nonfat Margarine (Van Den Bergh Foods)
Smart Beat Fat Free Nonfat Margarine (Heart Beat Foods)

SPRINKLES

These products are made from maltodextrins, salt, butter, and lecithin or oil. Spray-dried butter, found in Butter Buds, contributes about 20 mg of cholesterol per 100 grams of dry mixture. Significant amounts of sodium are present. Examples are Butter Buds Sprinkles (Cumberland Packaging Corp.) and Molly McButter Fat Free (Alberto Culver).

Sour Cream Substitutes

These products are made from water, coconut oil, and whey, plus additives. Examples are Sour Cream Substitute (Dean Foods) and IMO Sour Cream Substitute (Rod's Food Products).

Cooking Sprays

These products are made from oil, alcohol, and additives. Examples are PAM No Stick Cooking Spray (American Home Foods) and Wesson Lite No-Stick Cooking Spray (Hunt-Wesson).

Healthy Use of Fat-Free Products

With the exception of products using natural gums, such as low-fat salad dressings, most low-fat packaged products cannot be placed on the McDougall-Approved List. However, you may decide to use some of these foods, especially if your primary health concern is your weight. Keep in mind that some problems like food allergies, arthritis, osteoporosis, kidney stones, liver failure, kidney failure, and high triglycerides may be made *worse* by eating commercial low-fat products. Even so, for most people, the lower-fat products will be a considerable improvement over the original high-fat formulas. But don't fool yourself: they will never come close to providing the excellent nutrition from natural low-fat starches, vegetables, and fruits.

SCIENTIFIC REFERENCES

Introduction

The evidence supporting the comparable benefits of lumpectomy had been available for almost thirty years:
Smith, S. Cancer of the breast in Rockford, Illinois. *Am J Surgery* 98:653, 1959.

More than 65 percent of women still undergoing breast amputation:
Nattinger, A. The effect of legislative requirements on the use of breast-conserving surgery. *N Engl J Med* 335:1035, 1996.

Dr. McDougall's 1984 publication on the low-fat dietary treatment for breast cancer:
McDougall, J. Preliminary study of diet as an adjunct therapy for breast cancer. *Breast* 10:18, 1984.

Chapter 1. Solving the Mystery of Women's Diseases

By the fourth grade, 40 percent of girls have begun dieting:
Schreiber, G. Weight modification efforts by black and white preadolescent girls: National Heart, Lung, and Blood Institute Growth and Health Study. *Pediatrics* 98:63, 1996.

Oily skin and acne are directly related to the kinds of foods women eat:
Ito, A. A novel enzymatic assay for the quantification of skin surface lipids. *J Int Med Res* 24:69, 1996.
Rosenberg, E. Acne diet reconsidered. *Arch Dermatol* 117:193, 1981.
Pochi, P. Sebum production, casual sebum levels, titratable acidity of sebum, and urinary fractional 17-ketosteroid excretion in males with acne. *J Invest Dermatol* 43:383, 1964.

Wilkinson, D. Psoriasis and dietary fat: the fatty acid composition of surface and scale (ether-soluble) lipids. *J Invest Dermatol* 47:185, 1966.

Rasmussen, J. Diet and acne (review). *Int J Dermatol* 16:488, 1977.

More than 65 percent of these women will undergo mastectomies:

Nattinger, A. The effect of legislative requirements on the use of breast-conserving surgery. *N Engl J Med* 335:1035, 1996.

Two hundred thousand women are diagnosed with breast cancer and approximately 46,000 die:

Landis, S. Cancer statistics, 1998. *CA Cancer J Clin* 48:6, 1998.

Overweight women are more prone to many diseases:

Lean, M. Impairment of health and quality of life in people with large waist circumference. *Lancet* 351:853, 1998.

Manson, J. Body weight and mortality among women. *N Engl J Med* 333:677, 1995.

One-third of Americans are affected by such chronic illnesses:

Hoffman, C. Persons with chronic conditions. Their prevalence and costs. *JAMA* 276:1473, 1996.

The Surgeon General's report:

The Surgeon General's report on nutrition and health. U.S. Department of Health and Human Services. Public Health Service. GPO Stock Number 017-001-00465-1.

High-fat, low-fiber diets elevate estrogen and prolactin levels:

Adlercreutz, H. Estrogen metabolism and excretion in Oriental and Caucasian women. *J Natl Cancer Inst* 86:1076, 1994.

Woods, M. Hormone levels during dietary changes in premenopausal African-American women. *J Natl Cancer Inst* 88:1369, 1996.

Adlercreutz, H. Diet and plasma androgens in postmenopausal vegetarian and omnivorous women and postmenopausal women with breast cancer. *Am J Clin Nutr* 49:433, 1989.

Woods, M. Low-fat, high-fiber diet and serum estrone sulfate in premenopausal women. *Am J Clin Nutr* 49:1179, 1989.

Rose, D. Effect of a low-fat diet on hormone levels in women with cystic breast disease. I. Serum steroids and gonadotropins. *J Natl Cancer Inst* 78:623, 1987.

Rose, D. Effect of a low-fat diet on hormone levels in women with cystic breast disease. II. Serum radioimmunoassayable prolactin and growth hormone and bioactive lactogenic hormones. *J Natl Cancer Inst* 78:627, 1987.

Howie, B. Dietary and hormonal interrelationships among vegetarian Seventh-Day Adventists and nonvegetarian men. *Am J Clin Nutr* 42:127, 1985.

Hill, P. Plasma hormones and lipids in men at different risk of coronary artery disease. *Am J Clin Nutr* 33:1010, 1980.

Hill, P. Diet, lifestyle, and menstrual activity. *Am J Clin Nutr* 33:1192, 1980.

Hill, P. Diet and prolactin release. *Lancet* 2:806, 1976.

Hamalainen, E. Diet and serum sex hormones in healthy men. *J Steroid Biochem* 20:459, 1984.

Ingram, D. Effect of low-fat diet on female sex hormone levels. *J Natl Cancer Inst* 79:1225, 1987.

Gorbach, S. Estrogens, breast cancer, and intestinal flora. *Rev Infect Dis* 6 (suppl 1):S85, 1984.

Goldin, B. Estrogen excretion patterns and plasma levels in vegetarian and omnivorous women. *N Engl J Med* 307:1542, 1982.

Goldin, B. Effect of diet on excretion of estrogens in pre- and post-menopausal women. *Cancer Res* 41:3771, 1981.

Goldin, B. The effect of dietary fat and fiber on serum estrogen concentrations in premenopausal women under controlled dietary conditions. *Cancer* 74:1125, 1994.

Insulin-dependent diabetes is caused by cow's milk fed to susceptible young children:

Fava, D. Relationship between dairy product consumption and incidence of IDDM in childhood in Italy. *Diabetes Care* 17:1488, 1994.

Work Group on Cow's Milk Protein and Diabetes Mellitus. Infant feeding practices and their possible relationship to the etiology of diabetes mellitus. *Pediatrics* 94:752, 1994.

Cavallo, M. Cell-mediated immune response to B casein in recent-onset insulin-dependent diabetes: implications for disease pathogenesis. *Lancet* 348:926, 1996.

Karjalainen, J. A bovine albumin peptide as a possible trigger of insulin-dependent diabetes. *N Engl J Med* 327:302, 1992.

Milk and meat infected with bovine immunodeficiency viruses (BIV) and bovine leukemia viruses (BLV):

Ferrer, J. Milk of dairy cows frequently contains a leukemogenic virus. *Science* 213:1014, 1981.

Gonda, M. Bovine immunodeficiency virus (editorial review). *AIDS* 6:759, 1992.

Jacobs, R. Detection of multiple retroviral infections in cattle and cross-reactivity of bovine immunodeficiency-like virus and human immunodeficiency virus type 1 proteins using bovine and human sera in a western blot assay. *Can J Vet Res* 56:353, 1992.

Free radicals contribute to more than sixty major illnesses:

Brody, J. Natural chemicals now called major cause of disease. *New York Times,* April 26, 1988.

Meat, which includes all muscle foods (beef, chicken, fish, lobster, etc.), and eggs are acidic:

Breslau, N. Relationship of animal protein–rich diet to kidney stone formation and calcium metabolism. *J Clin Endocrinol Metab* 66:140, 1988.

Animal proteins, rich in sulfur-containing amino acids, break down in the body into powerful sulfuric acids:

Trilok, G. Sources of protein-induced endogenous acid production and excretion by human adults. *Calcif Tissue Int* 44:335, 1989.

Acidification from animal protein dissolves the bones—plants are alkaline by nature:
Sebastian, A. Improved mineral balance and skeletal metabolism in postmenopausal women treated with potassium bicarbonate. *N Engl J Med* 330: 1776, 1994.
Sebastian, A. Improved mineral balance and skeletal metabolism in postmenopausal women treated with potassium bicarbonate (letter). *N Engl J Med* 331:279, 1994.

Animal protein causes calcium losses in people in natural living conditions:
Hu, J. Dietary intakes and urinary excretion of calcium and acids: a cross-sectional study of women in China. *Am J Clin Nutr* 58:398, 1993.
Itoh, R. Dietary protein intake and urinary excretion of calcium: a cross-sectional study in healthy Japanese population. *Am J Clin Nutr* 67:438, 1998.

Chapter 2. Eating Your Way to Health

Vegetable oils, including olive oil, promote obesity:
Calle-Pascual, A. Changes in nutritional pattern, insulin sensitivity, and glucose tolerance during weight loss in obese patients from a Mediterranean area. *Horm Metab Res* 27:499, 1995.

Vegetable oils of all types promote cancer under certain conditions:
Ip, C. Review of the effects of trans fatty acids, oleic acid, n-3 polyunsaturated fatty acids, and conjugated linoleic acid on mammary carcinogenesis in animals. *Am J Clin Nutr* 66 (6 suppl):1523S, 1997.
Welch, C. Relationship between dietary fat and experimental mammary tumorigenesis: a review and critique. *Cancer Res* 52:2040S, 1992.

Some vegetable oils, including olive oil, promote heart disease:
Blankenhorn, D. The influence of diet on the appearance of new lesions in human coronary arteries. *JAMA* 263:1646, 1990.
Rudel, L. Compared with dietary monounsaturated and saturated fat, polyunsaturated fat protects African green monkeys from coronary artery atherosclerosis. *Arterioscler Thromb Vasc Biol* 15:2101, 1995.
Felton, C. Dietary polyunsaturated fatty acids and plaque composition of human aortic plaque. *Lancet* 344:1195, 1994.
Hennig, B. Linoleic acid and linolenic acid: effect on permeability properties of cultured endothelial cell monolayers. *Am J Clin Nutr* 49:301, 1989.
Larsen, L. Effects of dietary fat quality and quantity on postprandial activation of blood coagulation factor VII. *Arterioscler Thromb Vasc Biol* 17:2904, 1997.

Calories from refined flours are rapidly absorbed calories, raising insulin levels:
Jenkins, D. Wholemeal versus wholegrain breads: proportion of whole or cracked grain and the glycaemic response. *BMJ* 297:958, 1988.

O'Dea, K. Physical factors influencing postprandial glucose and insulin responses to starch. *Am J Clin Nutr* 33:760, 1980.

O'Dea, K. The rate of starch hydrolysis in vitro as a predictor of metabolic responses to complex carbohydrate in vivo. *Am J Clin Nutr* 34:1991, 1981.

Snow, P. Factors affecting the rate of hydrolysis of starch in food. *Am J Clin Nutr* 34:2721, 1981.

Published outcomes of the McDougall Program at St. Helena Hospital:

McDougall, J. Rapid reduction of serum cholesterol and blood pressure by a twelve-day, very low fat, strictly vegetarian diet. *J Am Coll Nutr* 14:491, 1995.

B₁₂ can be stored in your tissues for up to twenty to thirty years:

Herbert, V. Vitamin B-12: plant sources, requirements, and assay. *Am J Clin Nutr* 48:852, 1988.

In fact, a dietary origin of calcium deficiency is unknown in human beings:

Prentice, A. Maternal calcium requirements during pregnancy and lactation. *Am J Clin Nutr* 59 (2 suppl):477S, 1994.

Walker, A. The human calcium requirement: should low intakes be supplemented. *Am J Clin Nutr* 25:518, 1972.

Symposium on human calcium requirements. *JAMA* 185:588, 1963.

Goodhart and Shils. *Modern nutrition in health and disease (dietotherapy)*, 5th ed. (Philadelphia: Lea and Febiger, 1973), 274.

Worldwide the more animal protein consumed, the more osteoporosis:

Abelow, B. Cross-cultural association between dietary animal protein and hip fracture: a hypothesis. *Calcif Tissue Int* 50:14, 1992.

Scientific research has shown that an intake of 150 to 200 mg of calcium per day is adequate:

Paterson, C. Calcium requirements in man: a critical review. *Postgrad Med J* 54:244, 1978.

Plants provide an excellent balanced source of protein for people:

Young, V. Plant proteins in relation to human protein and amino acid nutrition. *Am J Clin Nutr* 59 (suppl):1203S, 1994.

People generally require about 2.5 percent of their calories from protein:

Rose, W. The amino acid requirements of adult man, XVI. The role of the nitrogen intake. *J Biol Chem* 217:997, 1955.

Hegsted, D. Minimum protein requirements of adults. *Am J Clin Nutr* 21:352, 1968.

Hoffman, W. Nitrogen requirement of normal men on a diet of protein hydrolysate enriched with limiting essential amino acids. *J Nutr* 44:123, 1951.

Dole, V. Dietary treatment of hypertension. Clinical and metabolic studies of people on the rice-fruit diet. *J Clin Invest* 29:1189, 1950.

Human breast milk at 5 percent protein supplies peak growth needs of infants:

Beaton, G. Protein requirements of infants: a reexamination of concepts and approaches. *Am J Clin Nutr* 48:1403, 1988.

Protein requirement established in 1974 by the World Health Organization:
 Passmore, Nicol, and Rao: *Handbook on human nutritional requirements.*
  Geneva, WHO Monogr Ser. No. 61, 1974.

Essential role of carbohydrates (energy for red blood, kidney, and brain cells):
 Jequier, E. Carbohydrates as a source of energy. *Am J Clin Nutr* 59(suppl):
  682S, 1994.

Our hunger drive is regulated primarily by carbohydrate consumption:
 Rolls, B. Satiety after preloads with different amounts of fat and carbohydrate: implications for obesity. *Am J Clin Nutr* 60:476, 1994.
 Blundell, J. Dietary fat and the control of energy intake: evaluating the effects of fat on meal size and postmeal satiety. *Am J Clin Nutr* 57 (suppl):
  772S, 1993.
 Tremblay, A. Impact of dietary fat content and fat oxidation on energy intake
  in humans. *Am J Clin Nutr* 49:799, 1989.
 Flatt, J. Dietary fat, carbohydrate balance, and weight maintenance: effects of
  exercise. *Am J Clin Nutr* 45:296, 1987.
 Rosenbaum, M. Obesity. *N Engl J Med* 337:396, 1997.

Beneficial effects of dietary fiber:
 Connor, W. Dietary fiber—nostrum or critical nutrient? (editorial) *N Engl J
  Med* 322:193, 1990.
 LaMont, J. Why fibre is good for you (commentary). *Lancet* 343:372, 1994.
 Wasan, H. Fibre-supplemented foods may damage your health (viewpoint).
  Lancet 348:319, 1996.

Chapter 3. Improving Your Chances for a Successful Pregnancy and a Safe Delivery

Ever-changing recommendations for amount of weight to gain during pregnancy:
 Feig, D. Eating for two: are guidelines for weight gain during pregnancy too
  liberal? *Lancet* 351:1054, 1998.

*World Health Organization pronounced that nutrition was of no great importance in
pregnancy:*
 FAO/WHO Expert Committee on Nutrition. *Sixth report.* (Rome: Food and
  Agriculture Organization, 1962). Nutr Meet Rep Ser no. 32.

One-fourth of pregnant women require surgical removal of their baby:
 Clarke, S. Changes in cesarean delivery in the United States, 1988 and 1993.
  Birth 22:63, 1995.
 Taffel, S. M. 1989 U.S. cesarean section rate steadies—VBAC rate rises to
  nearly one in five. *Birth* 18:73, 1991.

*Many less developed countries have better infant mortality rates and lower cesarean sec-
tion rates:*
 Guyer, B. Annual summary of vital statistics—1996. *Pediatrics* 100:905, 1997.

Van Roosmalen, J. Caesarean birth rates worldwide. A search for determinants. *Trop Geogr Med* 47:19, 1995.

Rates of cesarean delivery—United States, 1991. *MMWR Morb Mortal Wkly Rep* 42:285, 1993.

Weight gain of pregnant women from developed and underdeveloped countries:

Abrams, B. Weight gain and energy intake during pregnancy. *Clin Obstet Gynecol* 37:515, 1994.

Dhawan, S. Birth weights of infants of first generation Asian women in Britain compared with second generation Asian women. *BMJ* 311:86, 1995.

Maternal weight gain in pregnancy (editorial). *Lancet* 338:415, 1991.

The more weight you gain during pregnancy, the more likely you will retain that weight:

Schauberger, C. Factors that influence weight loss in the puerperium. *Obstet Gynecol* 79:424, 1992.

More diabetes, high blood pressure, pregnancy-induced hypertension with obesity:

Wolfe, H. Obesity in pregnancy. *Clin Obstet Gynecol* 37:596, 1994.

Pi-Sunyer, F. Medical hazards of obesity. *Ann Intern Med* 119:655, 1993.

Seventeen percent develop preeclampsia:

Gross, T. Obesity in pregnancy: risks and outcome. *Obstet Gynecol* 56:446, 1980.

Hollingsworth, D. Caloric restriction in pregnant diabetic women: a review of maternal obesity, glucose, and insulin relationships as investigated at the University of California, San Diego. *J Am Coll Nutr* 11:251, 1992.

Gestational diabetes risk may be as high as 20 percent in severely obese women:

Ruge, S. Obstetric risks in obesity. An analysis of the literature. *Obstet Gynecol Surv* 40:57, 1985.

Southern Medical Journal *found vegans essentially free from preeclampsia:*

Carter, J. Preeclampsia and reproductive performance in a community of vegans. *South Med J* 80:692, 1987.

New England Journal of Medicine *finds diet "the first-line treatment for women with gestational diabetes":* Dornhorst, A. Management of gestational diabetes mellitus. *N Engl J Med* 333:1281, 1995.

Effects of six-month Dutch famine on pregnancy:

Smith, C. Effects of maternal undernutrition upon the newborn infant in Holland (1944–1945). *J Pediatr* 30:229, 1947.

Stein, Z. Nutrition and mental performance. Prenatal exposure to the Dutch famine of 1944–1945 seems not related to mental performance at age 19. *Science* 178:708, 1972.

Between 60,000 and 80,000 extra calories are needed to grow a healthy baby:

Hytten, F. *The physiology of human pregnancy* (Oxford: Blackwell Scientific Publications, 1971).

Glucose is the primary metabolic fuel for your baby:

Koski, K. Effect of low carbohydrate diets during pregnancy on parturition and postnatal survival of the newborn rat pup. *J Nutr* 116:1938, 1986.

Pregnant women from the Philippines and rural Africa who do hard physical labor take in no more food:
Tuazon, M. Energy requirements of pregnancy in the Philippines. *Lancet* 2:1129, 1987.
Lawrence, M. Maintenance energy cost of pregnancy in rural Gambian women and influence of dietary status. *Lancet* 2:363, 1984.
Durnin, J. Is nutritional status endangered by virtually no extra intake during pregnancy? *Lancet* 2:823, 1985.

Plant foods provide an excellent source for proteins during pregnancy:
Young, V. Plant proteins in relation to human protein and amino acid nutrition. *Am J Clin Nutr* 59(suppl):1203S, 1994.

Two pounds of extra protein needed to grow a baby:
Hytten, F. *The physiology of human pregnancy* (Oxford: Blackwell Scientific Publications, 1971).

Pregnancy-induced hypertension not prevented by high protein intake:
Zlatnik. Dietary protein and preeclampsia. *Am J Obstet Gynecol* 147:354, 1983.
Rush, D. A randomized controlled trial of prenatal nutrition supplementation in New York City. *Pediatrics* 65:683, 1980.

Supplementation of protein during pregnancy in Guatemala results in worse outcome:
Stein, Z. Prenatal nutrition and birth weight: experiments and quasi-experiments in the past decade. *J Reprod Med* 21:287, 1978.

Supplementation with protein may adversely affect infant:
Viegas, O. Dietary protein energy supplementation of pregnant Asian mothers at Sorrento, Birmingham. II: Selective during the third trimester only. *BMJ* 285:592, 1982.

Pregnancy requires approximately 30 grams (one ounce) of calcium:
Pitkin, R. Calcium metabolism in pregnancy and the perinatal period: a review. *Am J Obstet Gynecol* 151:99, 1985.

Body increases its ability to absorb calcium from food and reduces losses through kidneys:
Ritchie, L. A longitudinal study of calcium homeostasis during human pregnancy and lactation and after resumption of menses. *Am J Clin Nutr* 67:693, 1998.

Neither number of children nor the duration of breast-feeding affect loss of bone:
Cummings, S. Risk factors for hip fracture in white women: study of Osteoporotic Fractures Research Group. *N Engl J Med* 332:767, 1995.
Koetting, C. Wrist, spine, and hip bone density in women with variable histories of lactation. *Am J Clin Nutr* 48:1479, 1988.

U.S.-Canadian guidelines revised to recommend no increase in calcium intake:
Institute of Medicine. *Dietary reference intakes. Calcium, phosphorus, magnesium, vitamin D, and fluoride* (Washington, D.C.: National Academy Press, 1998).

Iron absorption increases 9.1 times during pregnancy:
Barrett, J. Absorption of non-haem iron from food during normal pregnancy. *BMJ* 309:79, 1994.

Ascorbic acid enhances iron absorption, while other foods inhibit absorption:
Cook, J. Food iron availability: back to the basics (editorial). *Am J Clin Nutr* 67:593, 1998.

Iron intake of vegetarians higher than that of nonvegetarians:
Calkins, B. Diet, nutrition intake, and metabolism in populations at high and low risk for colon cancer. Nutrient intake. *Am J Clin Nutr* 40:896, 1984.
Carlson, E. A comparative evaluation of vegan, vegetarian, and omnivore diets. *J Plant Foods* 6:89, 1985.
Sanders, T. Blood pressure, plasma renin activity, and aldosterone concentrations in vegans and omnivore controls. *Hum Nutr: Appl Nutr* 41A:204, 1987.

Iron supplements offer no benefit and may be harmful to some women:
U.S. Preventive Services Task Force. Routine iron supplementation during pregnancy. *JAMA* 270:2846, 1993.

Iron inhibits absorption of zinc:
Dawson, E. Serum zinc changes due to iron supplementation in teen-age pregnancy. *Am J Clin Nutr* 50:848, 1989.
Crofton, R. Inorganic zinc and the intestinal absorption of ferrous iron. *Am J Clin Nutr* 50:141, 1989.

Blood B$_{12}$ levels below normal in babies with macrobiotic mothers:
Dagnelie, P. Increased risk of vitamin B-12 and iron deficiency in infants on macrobiotic diets. *Am J Clin Nutr* 50:818, 1989.

Birth defects increase by 480 percent with more than 10,000 IU of vitamin A daily:
Rothman, K. Teratogenicity of high vitamin A intake. *N Engl J Med* 333:1369, 1995.

Insufficient folic acid is the most frequently encountered vitamin deficiency in the Western world:
Kaminetzky, H. Nutritional needs in pregnancy. In *Principles and Practice of Obstetrics and Perinatology* (John Wiley & Sons, USA/Canada, 1981).

Folic acid deficiency leads to birth defects:
Rose, N. Periconceptional folate supplement and neural tube defects. *Clin Obstet Gynecol* 37:605, 1994.
Wald, N. Folic acid and the prevention of neural tube defects. *BMJ* 310:1019, 1995.
Shaw, G. Risks of orofacial clefts in children born to women using multivitamins containing folic acid periconceptionally. *Lancet* 345:393, 1995.

Even with adequate folic acid, obese women have children with more birth defects:
Werler, M. Prepregnant weight in relation to risk of neural tube defects. *JAMA* 275:1089, 1996.
Shaw, G. Risk of neural tube defect—affected pregnancies among obese women. *JAMA* 275:1093, 1996.

Mexican women have healthier babies than white Americans or Mexican-Americans:
Guendelman, S. Mexican women in the United States (commentary). *Lancet* 344:352, 1994.

Supplementation will not prevent about 30 percent of birth defects:
Goldenberg, R. Prepregnancy weight and pregnancy outcome (editorial). *JAMA* 275:1127, 1996.

Michigan children have 6.2 point decrease in IQ scores due to PCB exposure:
Jacobson, J. Intellectual impairment in children exposed to polychlorinated biphenyls in utero. *N Engl J Med* 335:783, 1996.

Disorders of the male reproductive tract have more than doubled in the past thirty to fifty years from environmental estrogens:
Sharpe, R. Are oestrogens involved in falling sperm counts and disorders of the male reproductive tract? *Lancet* 341:1392, 1993.

Brain cancer in young children linked to cured meats:
Bunin, G. Maternal diet and risk of astrocytic glioma in children: a report from the Children's Cancer Group (United States and Canada). *Cancer Causes Control* 5:177, 1994.

Vegetables, fruits, and fruit juices protect against brain cancers:
Bunin, G. Relation between maternal diet and subsequent primitive neuroectodermal brain tumors in young children. *N Engl J Med* 329:536, 1993.

Alcohol causes birth defects; one-third of children have fetal alcohol syndrome:
Olegard, R. Effects on the child of alcohol abuse during pregnancy. Retrospective and prospective studies. *Acta Paediatr Scand Suppl* 275:112, 1979.
Hanson, J. The effects of moderate alcohol consumption during pregnancy on fetal growth and morphogenesis. *J Pediatr* 92:457, 1978.

Caffeine and smoking reduce fertility:
Straton, C. Effects of caffeine consumption on delayed conception. *Am J Epidemiol* 142:1322, 1995.
Bolumar, F. Smoking reduces fecundity: a European multicenter study of infertility and subfecundity. *Am J Epidemiol* 143:578, 1996.

Caffeine increases miscarriage:
Infante-Rivard, C. Fetal loss associated with caffeine intake before and during pregnancy. *JAMA* 270:2940, 1993.

Caffeine may cause intrauterine growth retardation:
Golding, J. Reproduction and caffeine consumption—a literature review. *Early Hum Dev* 43:1, 1995.

The effects of cigarette smoking on the fetus:
> Lambers, D. The maternal and fetal physiologic effects of nicotine. *Semin Perinatol* 20:115, 1996.

Less risk of growth retardation on a healthy, high-vegetable diet:
> Cosgrove, M. Nucleotide supplementation and the growth of term small for gestational age infants. *Arch Dis Child Fetal Neonatal Ed* 74:F122, 1996.

Chapter 4. Giving Your Child a Healthful Head Start

Breast-feeding protects baby against blood-borne, brain, intestinal, chest, ear, and urinary tract infections:
> Xanthou, M. Human milk and intestinal host defense in newborns: an update. *Adv Pediatr* 42:171, 1995.
> Newburg, D. Role of human-milk lactadherin in protection against symptomatic rotavirus infection. *Lancet* 351:1160, 1998.

Breast milk contains sugars that prevent the attachment of unwelcome bacteria:
> Kunz, C. Biological functions of oligosaccharides in human milk. *Acta Paediatr* 82:903, 1993.
> Coppa, G. Preliminary study of breastfeeding and bacterial adhesion to uroepithelial cells. *Lancet* 335:569, 1990.

Breast-fed infants have one-fourth the risk of developing serious respiratory and intestinal diseases, and one-tenth the risk of being hospitalized:
> Howie, P. Protective effect of breast feeding against infection. *BMJ* 300:11, 1990.

Protects children from serious inflammatory bowel diseases (ulcerative colitis and Crohn's disease):
> Whorwell, P. Bottle feeding, early gastroenteritis, and inflammatory bowel disease. *BMJ* 1:382, 1979.
> Koletzko, S. Role of infant feeding practices in development of Crohn's disease in childhood. *BMJ* 298:1617, 1989.

In developing countries, bottle-fed infants are at least fourteen times more likely to die of diarrhea and four times more likely to die of pneumonia:
> Victoria, C. Evidence for protection by breast-feeding against infant deaths from infectious disease in Brazil. *Lancet* 2:319, 1987.

Breast-feeding reduces the risk of allergic diseases like eczema, asthma, and other food allergies later in life:
> Saarinen, U. Breastfeeding as prophylaxis against atopic disease: prospective follow-up study until 17 years old. *Lancet* 346:1065, 1995.
> Cant, A. Egg and cow's milk hypersensitivity in exclusively breast fed infants with eczema, and detection of egg protein in breast milk. *BMJ* 291:932, 1985.

Cancer risks, especially of lymphomas and acute leukemia, reduced by mother's milk:
> Davis, M. Infant feeding and childhood cancer. *Lancet* 2:365, 1988.
> McKinney, P. The inter-regional epidemiological study of childhood cancer

(IRESCC): a case control study of aetiological factors in leukaemia and lymphoma. *Arch Dis Child* 62:279, 1987.

Breast-feeding reduces risks of other health problems:
Pisacane, A. Breast feeding and hypertrophic pyloric stenosis: population based case-control study. *BMJ* 312:745, 1996.
A warm chain for breastfeeding (editorial). *Lancet* 344:1239, 1994.
Lucas, A. Breast milk and neonatal necrotising enterocolitis. *Lancet* 336:1519, 1990.
Standing Committee on Nutrition of the British Paediatric Association. Is breast feeding beneficial in the United Kingdom? *Arch Dis Child* 71:376, 1994.
Wilson, A. Relation of infant diet to childhood health: seven-year follow-up of cohort of children in Dundee infant feeding study. *BMJ* 316:21, 1998.
Paradise, J. Evidence in infants with cleft palate that breast milk protects against otitis media. *Pediatrics* 94:853, 1994.

The 1997 position statement on breast-feeding from the American Academy of Pediatrics:
Work Group on Breastfeeding. Breastfeeding and the use of human milk. *Pediatrics* 100:1035, 1997.

Behavioral abnormalities in bottle-fed infants noted more than sixty-five years ago:
Hoefer, C. Later development of breast fed and artificially fed infants. *JAMA* 92:615, 1929.

Children have demonstrated fewer speech difficulties:
Broad, F. Further studies of the effects of infant feeding on speech quality. *N Z Med J* 82:373, 1975.

Children who were breast-fed regularly produce higher scores on intelligence tests:
Fergusson, D. Breast-feeding and cognitive development in the first seven years of life. *Soc Sci Med* 16:1705, 1982.
Taylor, B. Breast feeding and child development at five years. *Dev Med Child Neurol* 26:73, 1984.
Morrow-Tlucak, M. Breast feeding and cognitive development in the first 2 years of life. *Soc Sci Med* 26:635, 1988.
Rogan, J. Breast-feeding and cognitive development. *Early Hum Dev* 31:181, 1993.
Temboury, M. Influence of breast-feeding on infants' intellectual development. *J Pediatr Gastroenterol Nutr* 18:32, 1994.
Greene, L. Relationship between early diet and subsequent cognitive performance during adolescence. *Biochem Soc Trans* 23:376S, 1995.
C du V Florey. Infant feeding and mental and motor development at 18 months of age in first born singletons. *Int J Epidemiol* 24:S21, 1995.
Morley, R. Nutrition and cognitive development. *Br Med Bull* 53:123, 1997.

IQ measured 8.3 points higher for premature infants who were breast-fed:
Lucas, A. Breast milk and subsequent intelligence quotient in children born premature. *Lancet* 339:261, 1992.
Cockburn, F. Neonatal brain and dietary lipids. *Arch Dis Child* 70:F1, 1994.

The more breast milk a child consumes, the higher that child's IQ will be later in life:
Pollack, J. Long term associations with infant feeding in clinically advantaged population of babies. *Dev Med Child Neurol* 36:429, 1994.

Breast milk provides a rich supply of essential fats and sugars for brain development:
Foreman–van Drongelen, M. Long-chain polyunsaturated fatty acids in preterm infants: status at birth and its influence on postnatal levels. *J Pediatr* 126:611, 1995.
Lanting, C. Neurological differences between 9-year-old children fed breast-milk or formula-milk as babies. *Lancet* 344:1319, 1994.
Jackson, K. Weaning foods cannot replace breast milk as sources of long-chain polyunsaturated fatty acids. *Am J Clin Nutr* 50:980, 1989.
Tram, T. Sialic acid content of infant saliva: comparison of breast with formula fed infants. *Arch Dis Child* 77:315, 1997.

Breast-feeding protects the nervous system from later damage that may lead to multiple sclerosis:
Pisacane, A. Breast feeding and multiple sclerosis. *BMJ* 308:1411, 1994.
Ben-Shlomo, Y. Dietary fat in the epidemiology of multiple sclerosis: has the situation been adequately assessed? *Neuroepidemiology* 11:214, 1992.

Dr. Yitzhak Koch and his colleagues have shown in animal studies:
Palmon, A. The gene for the neuropeptide gonadotropin-releasing hormone is expressed in the mammary gland of lactating rats. *Proc Natl Acad Sci USA* 91:4994, 1994.
Koch, Y. Hypothalamic hormones in milk. *Endocr Regul* 25:128, 1991.

Dr. Koch (New York Times). "Its activity is much more complex than people had thought":
Angier, N. Mother's milk found to be potent cocktail of hormones. *New York Times,* May 24, 1994.

Lower incidences of child abuse and of what is called "failure to thrive":
Kennell, J. Evidence for a sensitive period in the human mother. *Ciba Found Symp* 33:87, 1975.

Lactation was 99 percent effective in preventing pregnancy for up to six months:
Ramos, R. Effectiveness of lactation amenorrhoea in the prevention of pregnancy in Manila, the Philippines: non-comparative prospective trial. *BMJ* 313:909, 1996.

Breast-feeding promotes weight loss for mother:
Dewey, K. Maternal weight-loss patterns during prolonged lactation. *Am J Clin Nutr* 58:162, 1993.

Risk of breast cancer in premenopausal women is lower:
Newcomb, P. Lactation and a reduced risk of premenopausal breast cancer. *N Engl J Med* 330:81, 1994.
McTiernan, A. Evidence of a protective effect of lactation on risk of breast cancer in young women. *Am J Epidemiol* 124:353, 1986.

Risk of ovarian cancer in premenopausal women is lower:
  Whittemore, A. Personal characteristics relating to risk of invasive epithelial ovarian cancer in older women in the United States. *Cancer* 71 (2 Suppl): 558, 1993.
  Rosenblatt, K. WHO collaborative study of neoplasia and steroid contraceptives. *Int J Epidemiol* 22:192, 1993.

Lower risk of osteoporosis:
  Aloia, J. Risk factors for postmenopausal osteoporosis. *Am J Med* 78:95, 1985.

Cow's milk and infant formulas enhance attachment of bad bacteria to the cells:
  Andersson, B. Inhibition of attachment of Streptococcus pneumoniae and Haemophilus influenzae by human milk and receptor oligosaccharides. *J Infect Dis* 153:232, 1986.

Aluminum contamination of infant formulas:
  Hawkins, N. Potential aluminum toxicity in infants fed special infant formula. *J Pediatr Gastroenterol Nutr* 19:377, 1994.

Fifty percent of all newborns and 87 percent of three-month-old infants are fed a commercial formula:
  Hyams, J. Effects of infant formula on stool characteristics of young infants. *Pediatrics* 95:50, 1995.

Breast-fed infants have half the risk for developing diabetes:
  Mayer, E. Reduced risk of IDDM among breast-fed children. The Colorado IDDM Registry. *Diabetes* 37:1625, 1988.

The longer an infant is breast-fed, the lower his or her risk of diabetes:
  Scott, F. Cow's milk and insulin-dependent diabetes mellitus: is there a relationship? *Am J Clin Nutr* 51:489, 1990.
  Virtanen, S. Infant feeding in Finnish children less than 7 yrs of age with newly diagnosed IDDM. Childhood Diabetes in Finland Study Group. *Diabetes Care* 14:415, 1991.

In some susceptible young children, insulin-dependent diabetes is caused by cow's milk:
  Fava, D. Relationship between dairy product consumption and incidence of IDDM in childhood in Italy. *Diabetes Care* 17:1488, 1994.
  Work Group on Cow's Milk Protein and Diabetes Mellitus. Infant feeding practices and their possible relationship to the etiology of diabetes mellitus. *Pediatrics* 94:752, 1994.
  Cavallo, M. Cell-mediated immune response to β casein in recent-onset insulin-dependent diabetes: implications for disease pathogenesis. *Lancet* 348:926, 1996.
  Karjalainen, J. A bovine albumin peptide as a possible trigger of insulin-dependent diabetes. *N Engl J Med* 327:302, 1992.

Twelve of nineteen studies found an increased risk for SIDS with bottle-feeding:
Gilbert, R. Bottle feeding and the sudden infant death syndrome. *BMJ* 310:88, 1995.
Brooke, H. Case-control study of sudden infant death syndrome in Scotland, 1992–5. *BMJ* 314:1516, 1997.

Risk of SIDS increases two- to fourfold with bottle-feeding:
Mitchell, E. Bottle feeding and sudden infant death syndrome (letter). *BMJ* 311:122, 1995.
Cunningham, A. Breast-feeding and health in the 1980s: a global epidemiologic review. *J Pediatr* 118:659, 1991.
Bernshaw, N. Does breastfeeding protect against sudden infant death syndrome? *J Hum Lact* 7:73, 1991.
Ford, R. Breastfeeding and the risk of sudden infant death syndrome. *Int J Epidemiol* 22:885, 1993.

Bottle-fed infants regurgitate their stomach contents and inhale the cow's milk (or soy) protein:
Addy, D. Infant feeding: a current view. *BMJ* 1:1268, 1976.
Coombs, R. Allergy and cot death: with special focus on allergic sensitivity to cows' milk and anaphylaxis. *Clin Exp Allergy* 20:359, 1990.
Coombs, R. The enigma of cot death: is the modified-anaphylaxis hypothesis an explanation of some cases? *Lancet* 1:1388, 1982.
Parish, W. Hypersensitivity to milk and sudden death in infancy. *Lancet* 2:1106, 1960.

Many professional organizations recommend breast-feeding:
Lawrence, P. Breast milk: best source of nutrition for term and preterm infants. *Pediatr Clin N Am* 41:925, 1994.

Some doctors, nurses, hospitals, and drug companies discourage breast-feeding:
Anand, R. Health workers and the baby food industry. World Health Organization acts to end conflict of interest and promote breast feeding. *BMJ* 312:1556, 1996.
Freed, G. Breast-feeding. Time to teach what we preach. *JAMA* 269:243, 1993.
Losch, M. Impact of attitudes on maternal decisions regarding infant feeding. *J Pediatr* 126:507, 1995.
Waterston, T. Could hospitals do more to encourage breast feeding? Becoming a "baby friendly hospital" would help. *BMJ* 307:1437, 1993.
Costello, A. Protecting breast feeding from milk substitutes. The WHO code is widely violated and needs monitoring and supporting. *BMJ* 316:1103, 1998.

Dr. Carole A. Stashwick points out that doctors and nurses discourage mothers to breast-feed:
Brody, J. With all the reasons to breastfeed, too few do so. *New York Times*, April 6, 1994.

In 1992, 53.9 percent of women nursed their babies in the hospital:
 Brody, J. With all the reasons to breastfeed, too few do so. *New York Times,*
 April 6, 1994.

Contamination of breast milk with environmental chemicals:
 Wise, J. High amounts of chemicals found in breast milk. *BMJ* 314:1505,
 1997.
 Grandjean, P. Relation of a seafood diet to mercury, selenium, arsenic, and
 polychlorinated biphenyl and other organochlorine concentrations in
 milk. *Environ Res* 71:29, 1995.

Adding dairy products to a mother's diet will result in colic:
 Jakobsson, I. Cow's milk proteins cause infantile colic in breast-fed infants: A
 double-blind crossover study. *Pediatrics* 71:268, 1983.
 Clyne, P. Human breast milk contains bovine IgG. Relationship to infant
 colic? *Pediatrics* 87:439, 1991.

No increase in calcium intake is required by the nursing mother:
 Kalkwarf, H. The effect of calcium supplementation on the bone density dur-
 ing lactation and after weaning. *N Engl J Med* 337:523, 1997.
 Sowers, M. Changes in bone density with lactation. *JAMA* 269:3130, 1993.
 Prentice, A. Maternal calcium requirements during pregnancy and lactation.
 Am J Clin Nutr 59(suppl):477S, 1994.
 Laskey, M. Bone changes after 3 mo of lactation: influence of calcium intake,
 breast-milk output, and vitamin D-receptor genotype. *Am J Clin Nutr*
 67:685, 1998.
 Ritchie, L. A longitudinal study of calcium homeostasis during human pregnancy and lactation and after resumption of menses. *Am J Clin Nutr* 67:693,
 1998.

*The American Academy of Pediatrics recommends breast-feeding exclusively for the first
six months:*
 Work Group on Breastfeeding. Breastfeeding and the use of human milk.
 Pediatrics 100:1035, 1997.

Too early introduction of solids and liquids is harmful:
 Cohen, R. Effects of age of introduction of complementary foods on infant
 breast milk intake, total energy intake, and growth: a randomised intervention study in Honduras. *Lancet* 343:288, 1994.
 Charlton, J. Giving early solids to infants. May be harmful (letter). *BMJ*
 307:444, 1993.
 Forsyth, J. Relation between early introduction of solid food to infants and
 their weight and illnesses during the first two years of life. *BMJ* 306:572,
 1993.
 Smith, R. Breast feeding in the first six months. No need for extra fluids. *BMJ*
 304:1068, 1992.

Any additional liquids should be given by cup:
Lang, S. Cup feeding: an alternative method of infant feeding. *Arch Dis Child* 71:365, 1994.

Chapter 5. Preventing Premature Sexual Development in Children

Study in Pediatrics from the University of North Carolina at Chapel Hill:
Herman-Giddens, M. Secondary sexual characteristics and menses in young girls seen in office practice: a study from Pediatrics Research in Office Settings Network. *Pediatrics* 99:505, 1997.

Every ten years, the age at which girls experience puberty drops two to six months.
Tanner, J. Menarcheal age (letter). *Science* 214:604, 1981.
Wyshak, G. Secular changes in age in a sample of US women. *Ann Hum Biol* 10:75, 1983.
Manniche, E. Age at menarche: Nicolai Edvard Ravn's data on 3385 women in mid-19th century Denmark. *Ann Hum Biol* 10:79, 1983.

Many nations show progressive decrease in onset of maturity over last 150 years:
Beaton, G. Annex 3. Practical population indicators of health and nutrition. *WHO Monograph* 62:500, 1976.

In Britain, the average age of menarche has fallen from 16.5 years to 12.8 in 150 years:
Rees, M. Menarche when and why? *Lancet* 342:1375, 1993.

In the United States, age of menarche was 14 years in 1900 and 12.7 by 1960:
Beaton, G. Annex 3. Practical population indicators of health and nutrition. *WHO Monograph* 62:500, 1976.

In Japan, menarche was 16.5 years of age in 1875; by 1970 it fell to 12.5:
Kagawa, Y. Impact of westernization on the nutrition of Japanese: changes in physique, cancer, longevity, and centenarians. *Prev Med* 7:205, 1978.

The oldest onset of sexual maturity, between 18 and 19 years, was observed in Papua New Guinea:
Malcolm, L. Growth and development in New Guinea: a study of the Bundi people of the Madang District. Madang, Papua New Guinea, Institute of Human Biology, 1970. *Monograph Series*, no. 1.

Studies showing a correlation between diet and early onset of menstruation:
Kralj-Cereck, L. The influence of food, body build, and social origin on age of menarche. *Hum Biol* 28:393, 1956.
Lubin, J. Dietary factors and breast cancer risk. *Int J Cancer* 28:685, 1981.
Hughes, R. Intake of dietary fiber and the age of menarche. *Ann Hum Biol* 12:325, 1985.
de Ridder, C. Dietary habits, sexual maturation, and plasma hormones in pubertal girls: a longitudinal study. *Am J Clin Nutr* 54:805, 1991.

Menarche occurs later in vegetarians:

Sanchez, A. A hypothesis on the etiological role of diet on age of menarche. *Med Hypotheses* 7:1339, 1981.

Kissinger, D. The association of dietary factors with the age of menarche. *Nutr Res* 7:471, 1987.

Maclure, M. A prospective cohort study of nutrient intake and age at menarche. *Am J Clin Nutr* 54:649, 1991.

Vigorous physical activity delays menarche:

Frisch, R. Body fat, puberty, and fertility. *Biol Rev* 59:161, 1984.

Bernstein, L. The effects of moderate physical activity on menstrual cycle patterns in adolescence: implications for breast cancer prevention. *Br J Cancer* 55:681, 1987.

Merzenich, H. Dietary fat and sports activity as determinants for age of menarche. *Am J Epidemiol* 138:217, 1993.

Early onset of menarche is associated with more breast cancer:

Paffenbarger, R. Characteristics that predict risk of breast cancer before and after menopause. *Am J Epidemiol* 112:258, 1980.

Staszewski, J. Age at menarche and breast cancer. *J Natl Cancer Inst* 47:935, 1971.

Pike, M. Hormonal risk factors, breast tissue age, and the age-incidence of breast cancer. *Nature* 303:767, 1983.

Early onset of menarche is associated with more heart disease:

Colditz, G. A prospective study of age at menarche, parity, age at first birth, and coronary heart disease in women. *Am J Epidemiol* 126:861, 1987.

Eating rich foods increases the production of female hormones:

Woods, M. Hormone levels during dietary changes in premenopausal African-American women. *J Natl Cancer Inst* 88:1369, 1996.

Goldin, B. The effect of dietary fat and fiber on serum estrogen concentrations in premenopausal women under controlled dietary conditions. *Cancer* 74:1125, 1994.

Body fat makes more female hormones from androstenedione:

McDonald, P. Effect of obesity on conversion of plasma androstenedione to estrone in postmenopausal women with and without endometrial cancer. *Am J Obstet Gynecol* 130:448, 1978.

Bacteria convert bile acids into sex hormones:

Hill, P. Gut bacteria and the aetiology of cancer of the breast. *Lancet* 2:472, 1971.

Recirculating estrogens repeatedly stimulate hormone-sensitive tissue:

Gorbach, S. Estrogens, breast cancer, and intestinal flora. *Rev Infect Dis* 6 (suppl 1):S85, 1984.

Goldin, B. Estrogen excretion patterns and plasma levels in vegetarian and omnivorous women. *N Engl J Med* 307:1542, 1982.

Adlercreutz, H. Estrogen metabolism and excretion in Oriental and Caucasian women. *J Natl Cancer Inst* 86:1076, 1994.

Environmental chemicals have strong estrogenic activity:
Wolff, M.S.M. Blood levels of organochlorine residues and risk of breast cancer. *J Natl Cancer Inst* 85:648, 1993.
Vom Saal, F. Organochlorine residues and breast cancer (letter). *N Engl J Med* 338:988, 1998.

Combination estrogenic activity shot up 160- to 1,600-fold:
Kaiser, J. New yeast study finds strength in numbers. *Science* 272:1418, 1996.

Americans used record quantities of pesticides, insecticides, and herbicides in 1995:
Roberts, J. US pesticide use reaches new record. *BMJ* 312:1498, 1996.

Milk produced by pregnant cows contains high levels of estrogen:
Sharpe, R. Are oestrogens involved in falling sperm counts and disorders of the male reproductive tract? *Lancet* 341:1392, 1993.

Three million teenagers suffer from sexually transmitted diseases annually:
CDC National Center for Prevention Services, Surveillance, and Information Systems Branch, April 1994.

Early sexual maturation means sexual activity at a younger age and an earlier age of first pregnancy:
Soefer, E. Menarche: target age for reinforcing sex education for adolescents. *J Early Adolesc Health Care* 6:383, 1985.
Sandler, D. Age at menarche and subsequent reproductive events. *Am J Epidemiol* 119:765, 1984.

Teenage pregnancy statistics:
NCHS. *Monthly statistics report.* September 9, 1993.

Children who reach sexual maturity later in life eventually grow taller:
De Ridder, C. Dietary habits, sexual maturation, and plasma hormones in pubertal girls: a longitudinal study. *Am J Clin Nutr* 54:805, 1991.
Shangold, M. Relationship between menarcheal age and adult height. *West J Med* 82:443, 1989.

Higher estrogens cause shorter stature:
MacGillivray, M. Pediatric endocrinology update: an overview. The essential roles of estrogens in pubertal growth, epiphyseal fusion, and bone turnover: lessons from mutations in the genes for aromatase and the estrogen receptor. *Horm Res* 49 (suppl 1):2, 1998.

Chapter 6. Protecting Yourself Against Breast Cancer

Chances of developing breast cancer have become more common:
Feuer, E. The lifetime risk of developing breast cancer. *J Natl Cancer Inst* 85:892, 1993.

Cancer statistics:
   Landis, S. Cancer statistics, 1998. *CA Cancer J Clin* 48:6, 1998.

BRCA-1 gene only accounts for at most 5 percent of all breast cancers:
   Newman, B. Frequency of breast cancer attributable to BRCA1 in a population-based series of American women. *JAMA* 279:915, 1998.
   Eeles, R. Testing for the breast cancer predisposition gene, BRCA1. Documenting the outcome in gene carriers is essential (editorial). *BMJ* 313:572, 1996.

Cancer researcher Rolo Russell knew of cancer and meat association:
   Modan, B. Diet and cancer: causal relation or just wishful thinking? *Lancet* 340:162, 1992.

American Cancer Society recommends that Americans reduce their consumption of red meat:
   Burros, M. Risk seen in alcohol, red meat. Even modest amounts concern Cancer Society. *San Francisco Chronicle*, September 17, 1996.
   The American Cancer Society 1996 Advisory Committee on Diet, Nutrition, and Cancer Prevention. Guidelines on diet, nutrition, and cancer prevention: reducing the risk of cancer with healthy food choices and physical activity. *CA Cancer J Clin* 46:325, 1996.

Harvard School of Public Health concludes cancers caused by diet and lifestyle:
   Harvard report on cancer prevention. Causes of human cancer. Dietary factors. *Cancer Causes Control* 7 (suppl 1):S7, 1996.

Japanese women eating a traditional diet have one-sixth the risk of breast cancer as women in the United States:
   Ziegler, R. Relative weight, weight change, height, and breast cancer risk in Asian-American women. *J Natl Cancer Inst* 88:650, 1996.

Rural African women have one-seventeenth the risk of breast cancer as women in the United States:
   Walker, A. Is breast cancer avoidable? Could dietary changes help? *Int J Food Sci Nutr* 46:373, 1995.

Breast cancer is increasing as women worldwide change to a rich diet:
   Eng-Hen, N. Risk factors for breast carcinoma in Singaporean Chinese women. The central role of obesity. *Cancer* 80:725, 1997.

Two studies from Harvard University found no relationship between fat and breast cancer:
   Hunter, D. Cohort studies of fat intake and the risk of breast cancer—a pooled analysis. *N Engl J Med* 334:356, 1996.
   Willet, W. Dietary fat and the risk of breast cancer. *N Engl J Med* 316:22, 1987.
   Willet, W. Dietary fat and fiber in relation to risk of breast cancer. An 8-year follow-up. *JAMA* 268:2037, 1992.

Diet, lifestyle, hormone connection to breast cancer:
   Hulka, B. Breast cancer: cause and prevention. *Lancet* 346:883, 1995.

Free radicals are highly reactive substances that damage DNA and cause human diseases:
   Halliwell, B. Reactive oxygen species in living systems: source, biochemistry, and role in human disease. *Am J Med* 91 (suppl 3C):14S, 1991.
   Grisham, M. Oxidants and free radicals in inflammatory bowel disease. *Lancet* 344:859, 1994.

Bruce N. Ames, Ph.D., estimates that a rat experiences 100,000 oxidant hits each day:
   Ames, B. Oxidants, antioxidants, and the degenerative diseases of aging. *Proc Natl Acad Sci USA* 90:7915, 1993.

Breast cancer is a hormone-dependent disease:
   Lobo, R. Hormone replacement therapy. Oestrogen replacement after treatment for breast cancer? *Lancet* 341:1313, 1993.
   Toniolo, P. A prospective study of endogenous estrogens and breast cancer in postmenopausal women. *J Natl Cancer Inst* 87:190, 1995.

Research has shown that cancer cells require high levels of cholesterol to proliferate:
   Buchwald, H. Cholesterol inhibition, cancer, and chemotherapy. *Lancet* 339:1154, 1992.

Excess consumption of fats and oils promotes the growth of cancer:
   Wynder, E. Breast cancer: weighing the evidence for a promoting role of dietary fat. *J Natl Cancer Inst* 89:766, 1997.
   Kohlmeier, L. Adipose tissue trans fatty acids and breast cancer in the European Community Multicenter Study on Antioxidants, Myocardial Infarction, and Breast Cancer. *Cancer Epidemiol Biomarkers Prev* 6:705, 1997.
   Ip, C. Review of the effects of trans fatty acids, oleic acid, n-3 polyunsaturated fatty acids, and conjugated linoleic acid on mammary carcinogenesis in animals. *Am J Clin Nutr* 66 (6 suppl):1523S, 1997.
   Welsch, C. Relationship between dietary fat and experimental mammary tumorigenesis: a review and critique. *Cancer Res* 52 (7 suppl):2040S, 1992.

Canola oil caused blood levels of beta carotene and vitamin E to drop:
   Bierenbaum, M. Effects of canola oil on serum lipids in humans. *J Am Coll Nutr* 10:228, 1991.
   Wolff, M.S. M. Blood levels of organochlorine residues and risk of breast cancer. *J Natl Cancer Inst* 85:648, 1993.
   Vom Saal, F. Organochlorine residues and breast cancer (letter). *N Engl J Med* 338:988, 1998.

British girls start their first period at the age of thirteen, while Chinese girls start at seventeen:
   Key, T. Sex hormones in women in rural China and Britain. *Br J Cancer* 62:631, 1990.
   Armstrong, B. The role of diet in human carcinogenesis with special reference to endometrial cancer. In Hiatt, H. *Origins of human cancer. Cold Spring Harbor conferences on cell proliferation.* Vol. 4 (Cold Spring Harbor, N.Y.: Cold Spring Harbor Laboratory, 1977), 557.

Early onset of menarche is associated with more breast cancer:
Paffenbarger, R. Characteristics that predict risk of breast cancer before and after menopause. *Am J Epidemiol* 112:258, 1980.
Staszewski, J. Age at menarche and breast cancer. *J Natl Cancer Inst* 47:935, 1971.
Pike, M. Hormonal risk factors, breast tissue age, and the age-incidence of breast cancer. *Nature* 303:767, 1983.

Menopause occurs later in life in women with high estrogen levels from diet:
Key, T. Sex hormones in women in rural China and Britain. *Br J Cancer* 62:631, 1990.
Baird, D. Do vegetarians have earlier menopause? Proceedings of the Society of Epidemiology Research. *Am J Epidemiol,* 107, 1988.

Late menopause is associated with higher rates of breast cancer:
MacMahon, B. Etiology of human breast cancer: a review. *J Natl Cancer Inst* 50:21, 1973.

Growth of breast cancer from sex hormones:
Kuller, L. The etiology of breast cancer—from epidemiology to prevention. *Public Health Rev* 23:157, 1995.
Sharpe, R. Are estrogens involved in falling sperm counts and disorders of the male reproductive tract? *Lancet* 341:1392, 1993.

Women with fibrocystic breast disease are at greater risk of developing breast cancer:
Dupont, W. Long-term risk of breast cancer in women with fibroadenoma. *N Engl J Med* 331:10, 1994.
Bruzzi, P. Cohort study of association of risk of breast cancer with cyst type in women with gross cystic disease of the breast. *BMJ* 314:925, 1997.

Some studies show that women with breast cancer have higher-than-normal levels of prolactin and that dietary fat promotes higher levels of prolactin:
Baghurst, P. Diet, prolactin, and breast cancer. *Am J Clin Nutr* 56:943, 1992.
Ingram, D. Prolactin and breast cancer risk. *Med J Aust* 153:469, 1990.

Fats encourage the reabsorption of estrogens:
Gorbach, S. Estrogens, breast cancer, and intestinal flora. *Rev Infect Dis* 6 (suppl 1):S85, 1984.
Goldin, B. Estrogen excretion patterns and plasma levels in vegetarian and omnivorous women. *N Engl J Med* 307:1542, 1982.

Both animal and vegetable fats depress immune response and promote metastasis:
Giovannucci, E. A prospective study of dietary fat and risk of prostate cancer. *J Natl Cancer Inst* 85:1571, 1993.
Purasiri, P. Modulation in vitro of human natural cytotoxicity, lymphocyte proliferative response to mitogens, and cytokine production by essential fatty acids. *Immunology* 92:166, 1997.
Welsch, C. Relationship between dietary fat and experimental mammary tumorigenesis: a review and critique. *Cancer Res* 52 (7 suppl):2040S, 1992.

Karmali, R. Eicosanoids in neoplasia. *Prev Med* 16:493, 1987.

Ip, C. Review of the effects of trans fatty acids, oleic acid, n-3 polyunsaturated fatty acids, and conjugated linoleic acid on mammary carcinogenesis in animals. *Am J Clin Nutr* 66 (6 suppl):1523S, 1997.

Linoleic acid (corn, sunflower, and safflower oils) increases breast cancer in animals:

Ip, C. Requirement of essential fatty acid for mammary tumorigenesis in the rat. *Cancer Res* 45:1997, 1985.

Crevel, R. High-fat diets and the immune response of C57 B1 mice. *Br J Nutr* 67:17, 1992.

Linolenic acid (canola and linseed oils) seem to inhibit cancer growth:

Fernandes, G. Possible mechanisms through which dietary lipids, calorie restriction, and exercise modulate breast cancer. *Adv Exp Med Biol* 322:185, 1992.

Linolenic acids lose ability to block tumor growth with addition of linoleic acid:

Ip, C. Review of the effects of trans fatty acids, oleic acid, n-3 polyunsaturated fatty acids, and conjugated linoleic acid on mammary carcinogenesis in animals. *Am J Clin Nutr* 66 (6 suppl):1523S, 1997.

Olive oil can be cancer promoting or not, depending on varying amounts of linoleic acid:

Ip, C. Review of the effects of trans fatty acids, oleic acid, n-3 polyunsaturated fatty acids, and conjugated linoleic acid on mammary carcinogenesis in animals. *Am J Clin Nutr* 66 (6 suppl):1523S, 1997.

Fats coat the macrophage cell membrane and thus prevent it from recognizing cancer cells:

Fowler, K. Effects of purified dietary n-3 ethyl esters on murine T lymphocyte function. *J Immunol* 151:5186, 1993.

Jenski, L. Omega-3 fatty acid modification of membrane structure and function. I. Dietary manipulation of tumor cell susceptibility to cell- and complement-mediated lysis. *Nutr Cancer* 19:135, 1993.

Kelley, D. Essential nutrients and immunologic functions. *Am J Clin Nutr* 63:994S, 1996.

Oth, D. Modulation of CD4 expression on lymphoma cells transplanted to mice fed (n-3) polyunsaturated fatty acids. *Biochim Biophys Acta* 1027:47, 1990.

Kelley, D. Concentration of dietary N-6 polyunsaturated fatty acids and the human immune status. *Clin Immunol Immunopathol* 62:240, 1992.

Endres, S. Dietary supplementation with n-3 fatty acids suppresses interleukin-2 production and mononuclear cell proliferation. *J Leukoc Biol* 54:599, 1993.

Cholesterol-lowering diet and drugs have been shown to inhibit the growth of tumors in animals:

Buchwald, H. Cholesterol inhibition, cancer, and chemotherapy. *Lancet* 339:1154, 1992.

Littman, M. Effect of cholesterol-free, fat-free diet and hypocholesteremic agents on growth of transplantable animal tumors. *Cancer Chemother Rep* 50:25, 1966.

Cancer-causing cholesterol epoxides in a woman's breast fluids:
> Petrakis, N. Cholesterol and cholesterol epoxides in nipple aspirates of human breast fluid. *Cancer Res* 41:2563, 1981.

Grilling or frying all forms of meat releases at least ten known cancer-causing substances:
> Nagao, M. Dietary carcinogens and mammary carcinogenesis. Induction of rat mammary carcinomas by administration of heterocyclic amines in cooked foods. *Cancer* 74:1063, 1994.
>
> Snyderwine, E. Some perspectives on the nutritional aspects of breast cancer research. Food-derived heterocyclic amines as etiologic agents in human mammary cancer. *Cancer* 74:1070, 1994.

Pesticides, herbicides, and industrial chemicals are found in rich foods, specifically meat, fish, and dairy products:
> Schecter, A. Congener-specific levels of dioxins and dibenzofurans in US food and estimated daily toxic equivalent intake. *Environ Health Perspect* 102:962, 1994.
>
> Startin, J. Dioxins in food. In Schecter, A. ed. *Dioxins and health* (New York: Plenum Publishing Corp, 1994), 115–37.

Pesticide residues in produce imports 5,000 percent higher than current U.S. standards of DDT:
> Perlmutter, D. Organochlorines, breast cancer, and GATT. *JAMA* 271:1160, 1994.

Fourfold increase in relative risk of breast cancer with high DDT exposure:
> Wolff, M.S.M. Blood levels of organochlorine residues and risk of breast cancer. *J Natl Cancer Inst* 85:648, 1993.
>
> Milne, D. Small study implicates PCBs in breast cancer. *J Natl Cancer Inst* 84:834, 1992.
>
> Mussalo-Rauhamaa, H. Occurrence of beta-hexachlorocyclohexane in breast cancer patients. *Cancer* 66:2124, 1990.
>
> Dewailly, E. High organochlorine body burden in women with estrogen receptor-positive breast cancer. *J Natl Cancer Inst* 86:232, 1994.

Women with breast cancer have 50 to 60 percent higher concentration of DDE in breast specimens:
> Falck, F. Pesticides and polychlorinated biphenyl residues in human breast lipids and their relation to breast cancer. *Arch Environ Health* 47:143, 1992.

The National Research Council confirms chemicals cause cancer, but their importance is minimal:
> Brody, J. Calories, fat called major cancer risks. Chemicals in food less hazardous panel concludes. *San Francisco Chronicle,* February 16, 1996.

Chlorine forms compounds (trihalomethanes) known to cause cancers in humans:
> Doyle, T. The association of drinking water source and chlorination by-products with cancer incidence among postmenopausal women in Iowa: a prospective cohort study. *Am J Public Health* 87:1168, 1997.

Excess iron increases production of free radicals, which leads to cancer:
Bhasin, D. Dietary effects on breast cancer (letter). *Lancet* 338:186, 1991.

Phytates bind with iron, preventing it from producing free radicals:
Thompson, L. Phytic acid and minerals: effect on early markers of risk of mammary and colon carcinogenesis. *Carcinogenesis* 12:2041, 1991.
Graf, E. Antioxidant functions of phytic acid. *Free Radic Biol Med* 8:61, 1990.

Vegetarian women eliminate two to three times more estrogen in their feces:
Goldin, B. Estrogen excretion patterns and plasma levels in vegetarian and omnivorous women. *N Engl J Med* 307:1542, 1982.
Rose, D. Dietary fiber and breast cancer. *Nutr Cancer* 13:1, 1990.

Postmenopausal women who adopted a high-fiber, low-fat diet experienced an average drop in their estrogen levels of 50 percent:
Heber, D. Reduction of serum estradiol in postmenopausal women given free access to low-fat high-carbohydrate diet. *Nutrition* 7:137, 1991.

A twofold variation in estradiol levels means a threefold variation in breast cancer risk:
Toniolo, P. G. A prospective study of endogenous estrogens and breast cancer in postmenopausal women. *J Natl Cancer Inst* 87:190, 1995.

The rich American diet and resulting obesity seem to act to elevate these estrogen levels:
Heber, D. Reduction of serum estradiol in postmenopausal women given free access to low-fat high-carbohydrate diet. *Nutrition* 7:137, 1991.

A study of 6,500 Chinese done by Cornell researchers found that daily consumption of foods high in antioxidants was associated with lower rates of cancer:
Chen, J. Antioxidant status and cancer mortality in China. *Int J Epidemiol* 21:625, 1992.
Brody, J. Huge study of diet indicts fat and meat. *New York Times,* May 8, 1990.

Beta carotene supplements can compete with the other fifty dietary carotenoids:
Woodall, A. Caution with β-carotene supplements (letter). *Lancet* 347:967, 1996.
Pietrzik, K. Antioxidant vitamins, cancer, and cardiovascular disease (letter). *New Engl J Med* 335:1065, 1996.

Recent studies show increase in lung cancer with supplemental beta carotene:
Hennekens, C. Lack of effect of long-term supplementation with beta carotene on the incidence of malignant neoplasms and cardiovascular disease. *N Engl J Med* 334:1145, 1996.
Omenn, G. Effects of a combination of beta carotene and vitamin A on lung cancer and cardiovascular disease. *N Engl J Med* 334:1150, 1996.
The Alpha-Tocopherol, Beta Carotene Prevention Study Group. The effect of vitamin E and beta-carotene on the incidence of lung cancer and other cancers in male smokers. *N Engl J Med* 330:1029, 1994.

Phytoestrogens inhibit the growth of cancer by decreasing hormone stimulation:
Knight, D. A review of the clinical effects of phytoestrogens. *Obstetr Gynecol* 87:897, 1996.
Rose, D. Dietary fiber, phytoestrogens, and breast cancer. *Nutrition* 8:47, 1992.
Adlercreutz, H. Plasma concentrations of phyto-oestrogens in Japanese men. *Lancet* 342:1209, 1993.
Ingram, D. Case-control study of phytoestrogens and breast cancer. *Lancet* 350:990, 1997.
Adlercreutz, H. Phyto-oestrogens and Western diseases. *Ann Med* 29:95, 1997.

In the average Japanese woman who eats a plant-based diet, phytoestrogens are found to be one hundred to one thousand times higher than the estrogens made by her own body:
Adlercreutz, H. Dietary phyto-oestrogens and the menopause in Japan (letter). *Lancet* 339:1233, 1992.

More than fifteen phytoestrogens have so far been identified in human urine:
Ingram, D. Case-control study of phytoestrogens and breast cancer. *Lancet* 350:990, 1997.
Marwick, C. Learning how phytochemicals help fight disease. *JAMA* 274: 1328, 1995.

Genistein blocks blood vessels from growing to tumors:
Angier, N. Chemists learn why vegetables are good for you. *New York Times,* April 13, 1993.
Fotsis, T. Genistein, a dietary-derived inhibitor of in vitro angiogenesis. *Proc Natl Acad Sci USA* 90:2690, 1993.

Shiitake mushrooms may boost immune response:
Chang, R. Functional properties of edible mushrooms. *Nutr Rev* 54 (11 Pt 2): S91, 1996.

Progressive weight gain increases risk of breast cancer:
Huang, Z. Dual effects of weight and weight gain on breast cancer risk. *JAMA* 278:1407, 1997.
Kumar, N. Timing of weight gain and risk of breast cancer. *Cancer* 76:243, 1995.

Physical activity associated with lower risk of breast cancer:
Thune, I. Physical activity and the risk of breast cancer. *N Engl J Med* 336:1269, 1997.

Animals that are forced to exercise excessively have higher rates of breast cancer:
Thompson, H. Effect of amount and type of exercise on experimentally induced breast cancer. *Adv Exp Med Biol* 322:61, 1992.

Too much exercise increases risk of viral infections:
Nieman, D. Exercise, upper respiratory tract infection, and the immune system. *Med Sci Sports Exerc* 26:128, 1994.

Too much exercise and high-fat diets can suppress the immune system in humans:
Venkatraman, J. Influence of the level of dietary lipid intake and maximal exercise on the immune status in runners. *Med Sci Sports Exerc* 29:333, 1997.
Shephard, R. Exercise and the immune system. Natural killer cells, interleukins, and related responses. *Sports Med* 18:340, 1994.

Alcohol consumption increases the risk of breast cancer.
Ginsburg, E. Effects of alcohol ingestion on estrogens in postmenopausal women. *JAMA* 276:1747, 1996.
Fuchs, C. Alcohol consumption and mortality among women. *N Engl J Med* 332:1245, 1995.
Smith-Warner, S. Alcohol and breast cancer in women. A pooled analysis of cohort studies. *JAMA* 279:535, 1998.
Schatzkin, A. Alcohol and breast cancer. Where are we now and where do we go from here? *Cancer* 74:1101, 1994.

The more a woman smokes, the greater her risk of breast cancer:
Morabia, A. Relation of breast cancer with passive and active exposure to tobacco smoke. *Am J Epidemiol* 143:918, 1996.

Cancer-causing substances from cigarette smoke are found in breast fluids:
Petrakis, N. Mutagenic activity in nipple aspirates of human breast fluid. *Cancer Res* 40:188, 1980.
Hiatt, R. Smoking, menopause, and breast cancer. *J Natl Cancer Inst* 76:833, 1986.

Approximately 60 percent of women slowly detoxify the chemicals found in cigarette smoke:
Ambrosone, C. Cigarette smoking, N-acetyltransferase 2 genetic polymorphism, and breast cancer risk. *JAMA* 276:1494, 1996.

Women exposed to DES have a 35 percent higher risk of breast cancer:
Colton, T. Breast cancer in mothers prescribed stilbestrol in pregnancy: further follow-up. *JAMA* 269:2096, 1993.

A 50 percent increase in breast cancer for women who use hormone replacement therapy for more than 5 years:
McPherson, K. Breast cancer and hormone supplement in postmenopausal women. Among current users of combined supplements the risk rises with five or more years' treatment. *BMJ* 311:699, 1995.

Women who started using the birth-control pill before age thirty-six and used it for four years or more have 2.2 times greater risk for breast cancer than women who never used the pill:
Rookus, M. Oral contraceptives and risk of breast cancer in women aged 20–54 years. *Lancet* 344:844, 1994.

Calcium channel blockers increase breast cancer risk:
Fitzpatrick, A. Use of calcium channel blockers and breast carcinoma risk in postmenopausal women. *Cancer* 80:1438, 1997.

Pahor, M. Calcium channel blockers and incidence of cancer in aged populations. *Lancet* 348:493, 1996.

Jick, H. Calcium-channel blockers and risk of cancer. *Lancet* 349:525, 1997.

Cholesterol-lowering medications are suspected of increasing cancer risk:
Newman, T. Carcinogenicity of lipid-lowering drugs. *JAMA* 275:55, 1996.

Female flight attendants have an excess of breast cancer related to solar radiation:
Pukkala, E. Incidence of cancer among Finnish airline cabin attendants, 1967–92. *BMJ* 311:649, 1995.

Use of electric blankets has been tied to a small increase in breast cancer:
Vena, J. Risk of premenopausal breast cancer and use of electric blankets. *Am J Epidemiol* 140:974, 1994.

High-intensity magnetic fields decrease levels of melatonin:
Harland, J. Environmental magnetic fields inhibit the antiproliferative action of tamoxifen and melatonin in a human breast cancer cell line. *Bioelectromagnetics* 18:555, 1997.

Study of 383,700 people in Finland found no association between radiation and breast cancer:
Verkasalo, P. Magnetic fields of high voltage power lines and risk of cancer in Finnish adults: nationwide cohort study. *BMJ* 313:1047, 1996.

The long-term effect of full-term pregnancy is a reduction in your risk of breast cancer:
Kelsey, J. Reproductive factors and breast cancer. *Epidemiol Rev* 15:36, 1993.

Breast-feeding reduces the risk of breast cancer:
United Kingdom National Case-Control Study Group. Breast feeding and risk of breast cancer in young women. *BMJ* 307:17, 1993.

Newcomb, P. Lactation and a reduced risk of premenopausal breast cancer. *N Engl J Med* 330:81, 1994.

Women with a history of low secretion of milk and those who breast-feed from only one breast have an increased risk of breast cancer:
Michels, K. Prospective assessment of breastfeeding and breast cancer incidence among 89,887 women. *Lancet* 347:431, 1996.

Breast-feeding reduces the number of ovulations and surges of hormones:
Henderson, B. Do regular ovulatory cycles increase breast cancer risk? *Cancer* 56:1206, 1985.

Breast-feeding may eliminate carcinogens (organochlorines) through breast milk secretion:
McTiernan, A. Evidence for a protective effect of lactation on risk of breast cancer in young women. Results from a case-control study. *Am J Epidemiol* 124:353, 1986.

Adverse life events depress the immune system by production of adrenal hormones:
Chen, C. Adverse life events and breast cancer: case-control study. *BMJ* 311:1527, 1995.

A review of eighteen studies found emotional suppression is a risk factor for cancer:
Gross, J. Emotional expression in cancer onset and progression. *Soc Sci Med* 28:1239, 1989.

Divorce and widowhood show no relation to the onset or outcome of breast cancer:
Jones, D. Bereavement and cancer: some data on the deaths of spouses from the longitudinal study of the Office of Population Census and Surveys. *BMJ* 289:461, 1984.
Ewertz, M. Bereavement and breast cancer. *Br J Cancer* 53:701, 1986.
Kvikstad, A. Death of a husband or marital divorce related to risk of breast cancer in middle-aged women. A nested case-control study among Norwegian women born 1935–1954. *Eur J Cancer* 30A:473, 1994.

Early age of onset is to date the strongest indicator of genetic susceptibility:
Slattery, M. A comprehensive evaluation of family history and breast cancer risk. The Utah Population Database *JAMA* 270:1563, 1993.

Women with BRCA-1 gene have more breast cancer, but tests and treatment not shown to help:
Eeles, R. Testing for.the breast cancer predisposition gene, BRCA1. Documenting the outcome in gene carriers is essential (editorial). *BMJ* 313:572, 1996.
Collins, F. BRCA1—Lots of mutations, lots of dilemmas (editorial). *N Engl J Med* 334:186, 1996.
King, M. Inherited breast and ovarian cancer. What are the risks? What are the choices? *JAMA* 269:1975, 1993.

Thirty-five years ago, some scientists argued that lung cancer was not caused by smoking:
Breast Cancer Prevention Collaborative Group. Breast cancer: environmental factors. *Lancet* 340:904, 1992.

Chapter 7. Evaluating the Benefits of Mammography

Quote from Dr. Barbara Rimer to the New York Times:
Kolata, G. Breast cancer screening under 50: experts disagree if benefit exists. Statisticians find no proof that screening saves lives. *New York Times,* December 14, 1993.

American Cancer Society statistics and recommendations:
Dodd, G. Breast cancer detection and community practice. Executive summary report of a workshop cosponsored by General Motors Cancer Research Foundation and the American Cancer Society. *Cancer* 64:2639, 1989.

Positive findings on mammogram may lead to anguish and suicide:
Devitt, J. False alarms of breast cancer. *Lancet* 2:1257, 1989.
Weil, J. Positive findings of mammography may lead to suicide (letter). *BMJ* 314:754, 1997.

Dr. Edward Sondik told the New York Times:
> Kolata, G. Breast cancer screening under 50: experts disagree if benefit exists. Statisticians find no proof that screening saves lives. *New York Times,* December 14, 1997.

Chances of a false positive are more than 56 percent for women having a total of ten mammograms:
> Elmore, J. Ten-year risk of false positive screening mammograms and clinical breast examination. *N Engl J Med* 338:1089, 1998.

After false positive exam 26 percent of women still worried three months later:
> Lerman, C. Psychological and behavioral implications of abnormal mammograms. *Ann Intern Med* 114:657, 1991.

A significant percentage of breast cancers missed by mammography:
> Seidman, H. Survival experience in Breast Cancer Detection Demonstration Project. *CA Cancer J Clin* 37:258, 1987.
> Shapiro, S. Ten- to fourteen-year effect of screening on breast cancer mortality. *J Natl Cancer Inst* 69:349, 1992.
> Elmore, J. Variability in radiologists' interpretations of mammograms. *N Engl J Med* 331:1493, 1994.

One in twenty women screened have a mammographic abnormality:
> Wright, C. Breast cancer screening: a different look at the evidence. *Surgery* 100:594, 1986.

Up to 44 percent of women under fifty have a false negative mammogram:
> Edeiken, S. Mammography and palpable cancer of the breast. *Cancer* 61:263, 1988.

Between 10 and 15 percent of women are given clean bills of health by a mammogram:
> Baker, L. Breast cancer detection demonstration project: five-year summary report. *CA Cancer J Clin* 32:194–5, 1982.

Forty percent of women in their forties have DCIS on autopsy:
> Nielson, M. Breast cancer and atypia among young and middle-aged women: a study of 110 medicolegal autopsies. *Br J Cancer* 56:814, 1987.
> Welch, H. Using autopsy series to estimate the disease "reservoir" for ductal carcinoma in situ of the breast: how much more breast cancer can we find? *Ann Intern Med* 127:1023, 1997.

Dramatic increases in DCIS due to mammography—more than half of cancers now DCIS:
> Morrow, M. Preoperative evaluation of abnormal mammographic findings to avoid unnecessary breast biopsy. *Arch Surg* 129:1091, 1994.
> Alexander, H. Needle localized mammographic lesions: results and evolving treatment strategy. *Arch Surg* 125:1441, 1990.
> Silverstein, M. Non-palpable breast lesions: diagnosis with slightly overpenetrated screen-film mammography and hook wire–directed biopsy in 1014 cases. *Radiology* 171:633, 1989.

Ernster, V. Incidence of and treatment for ductal carcinoma in situ of the breast. *JAMA* 275:913, 1996.

Eight randomized controlled screening trials for mammography:

Fletcher, S. Report of the International Workshop on Screening for Breast Cancer. *J Natl Cancer Inst* 85:1644, 1993.

Shapiro, S. Determining the efficacy of breast cancer screening. *Cancer* 63:1873, 1989.

Shapiro, S. Ten- to fourteen-year effect of screening on breast cancer mortality. *J Natl Cancer Inst* 69:349, 1982.

Tabar, L. Reduction in mortality from breast cancer after mass screening with mammography. Randomised trial from the Breast Cancer Screening Working Group of the Swedish National Board of Health and Welfare. *Lancet* 1:829, 1985.

Tabar, L. Update of the Swedish two-county program for mammographic screening for cancer. *Radiol Clin North Am* 30:187, 1992.

Andersson, I. Mammographic screening and mortality from breast cancer: the Malmo mammographic screening trial. *BMJ* 297:943, 1988.

Verbeek, A. Reduction of breast cancer mortality through screening with modern mammography. *Lancet* 2:1222, 1984.

Roberts, M. Edinburgh trials of screening for breast cancer: Mortality at seven years. *Lancet* 335:241, 1990.

UK Trial of Early Detection of Breast Cancer Group. First results on mortality reduction in the UK trial of early detection of breast cancer. *Lancet* 2:411, 1988.

Rutqvist, L. Reduced breast-cancer mortality with mammography screening—an assessment of currently available date. *Int J Cancer Suppl* 5:76, 1990.

Miller, A. Canadian National Breast Screening Study 2: breast cancer detection and death rates among women ages 50 to 59. *Can Med Assoc J* 147:1477, 1992.

Miller, A. Canadian National Breast Screening Study 1: breast cancer detection and death rates among women ages 40 to 49. *Can Med Assoc J* 147:1459, 1992.

Bjurstam, N. The Gothenburg Breast Screening Trial: first results on mortality, incidence, and mode of detection for women ages 39–49 years at randomization. *Cancer* 80:2091, 1997.

Five meta-analyses show no significant benefit of mammography for women under fifty:

Nystrom, L. Breast cancer screening with mammography: overview of Swedish randomised trials. *Lancet* 341:973, 1993.

Glasziou, P. Mammographic screening trials for women aged under 50. A quality assessment and meta-analysis. *Med J Aust* 162:625, 1995.

Kerlikowske, K. Efficacy of screening mammography: a meta-analysis. *JAMA* 273:149, 1995.

Report of the Organizing Committee and Collaborators. Falun meeting.

Breast-cancer screening with mammography in women aged 40–49 years. *Int J Cancer* 68:693, 1996.

Fletcher, S. Report of the International workshop on Screening for Breast Cancer. *J Natl Cancer Inst* 85:1644, 1993.

Mammography's glowing results are disputed:

Schmidt, J. The epidemiology of mass breast cancer screening—a plea for a valid measure of benefit. *J Clin Epidemiol* 43:215, 1990.

Wright, C. Screening mammography and public health policy: the need for perspective. *Lancet* 346:29, 1995.

Dilhuydy, M. The debate over mass mammography: is it beneficial for women? *Eur J Radiol* 24:86, 1997.

Narod, S. On being the right size: a reappraisal of mammography trials in Canada and Sweden (letter). *Lancet* 349:1846, 1997.

Roberts, M. Breast screening: time for a rethink? *BMJ* 299:1153, 1989.

Skrabanek, P. False premises and false promises of breast cancer screening. *Lancet* 2:316, 1985.

One less death per year is achieved when a total of 7,086 women undergo a mammogram:

Wright, C. Screening mammography and public health policy: the need for prospective. *Lancet* 346:29–32, 1995.

In Finland, 200,000 women were screened to prevent twenty deaths:

Adab, P. Harm resulting from screening is likely to be high where prevalence of breast cancer is low (letter). *BMJ* 315:190, 1997.

Public funding for breast cancer screening in any age group is not justifiable:

Wright, C. Screening mammography and public health policy: the need for perspective. *Lancet* 346:29–32, 1995.

Only one study in its original analysis shows benefit for women under fifty:

Margolese, R. Screening mammography in young women: a different perspective. *Lancet* 347:881, 1996.

Bjurstam, N. The Gothenburg Breast Screening Trial: First results on mortality, incidence, and mode of detection for women ages 39–49 years at randomization. *Cancer* 80:2091, 1997.

Wright, C. Screening mammography and public health policy: the need for perspective. *Lancet* 346:29, 1995.

M. Maureen Roberts, clinical director of the Edinburgh Breast Cancer Screening Project, stated:

Roberts, M. Breast screening: time for a rethink? *BMJ* 299:1153, 1989.

The United States, Australia, Iceland, and the Canadian province of British Columbia recommend mammography for women under fifty:

Kolata, G. Breast cancer screening under 50: experts disagree if benefit exists. Statisticians find no proof that screening saves lives. *New York Times,* December 14, 1993.

The National Institutes of Health Consensus Development Conference statement:
National Institutes of Health Consensus Development Panel. National Institutes of Health Consensus Conference Statement: Breast cancer screening for women ages 40–49, January 21–23, 1997. *J Natl Cancer Inst* 89:1015, 1997.

Groups recommending and not recommending mammography for women under fifty:
Fletcher, S. Why question screening mammography for women in their forties? *Radiol Clin North Am* 33:1259, 1995.

For every one thousand women under fifty who had mammograms, no fewer than seven hundred would require further testing:
Fletcher, S. Report of the International Workshop on Screening for Breast Cancer. *J Natl Cancer Inst* 85:1644, 1993.

Nine out of every ten biopsies done on women in their forties find no cancer:
Eddy, D. The value of mammography screening in women under age 50 years. *JAMA* 259:1512, 1988.

Ductile carcinoma in situ accounted for 63 percent of cancers found in women under fifty:
Kerlikowske, K. Positive predictive value of screening mammography by age and family history of breast cancer. *JAMA* 270:2444, 1993.

The Canadian trial showed a 36 percent higher risk of dying from breast cancer for women under fifty who had mammograms:
Miller, A. Canadian National Breast Screening Study 1: breast cancer detection and death rates among women ages 40 to 49. *Can Med Assoc J* 147:1459, 1992.

According to Lancet editorial surgery and radiation increase risk of dying in screened group:
Breast cancer screening in women under 50 (editorial). *Lancet* 337:1575, 1991.

Editorial contradicts AMA position on mammography in women under fifty:
Davis, D. Mammographic screening. *JAMA* 271:152, 1994.

Overall, 81 percent of women experience discomfort during mammography:
Watmough, D. X-ray mammography and breast compression (letter). *Lancet* 340:122, 1992.
Austoker, J. Screening and self-examination for breast cancer. *BMJ* 309:168, 1994.

Compression of the breast during the test may cause the cancer cells to spread:
Watmough, D. X-ray mammography and breast compression (letter). *Lancet* 340:122, 1992.
Van Netten, J. Physical trauma and breast cancer (letter). *Lancet* 343:978, 1994.
Van Netten, J. Physical trauma and breast cancer (letter). *Lancet* 343:1365, 1994.
Levallius, B. Screening mammography (letter). *Lancet* 343:793, 1994.
Van Netten, J. Mammographic controversies: time for informed consent? (letter). *J Natl Cancer Inst* 89:1164, 1997.

Approximately one cancer in every two hundred thousand mammograms is produced by the radiation:

Freig, S. Mammographic screening of women aged 40–49 years. *Cancer* 76:2097, 1995.

Mammography Quality Standards Act of 1992:

Dodd, G. Mammography Quality Assurance Programs. *Cancer* 74:239, 1994.

Mammogram recommendations for older women (over sixty-nine):

Harris, J. Breast cancer (1). *N Engl J Med* 327:319, 1992.

Fletcher, S. Report of the International Workshop on Screening for Breast Cancer. *J Natl Cancer Inst* 85:1644, 1993.

Nystrom, L. Breast cancer screening with mammography: overview of Swedish randomised trials. *Lancet* 341:973, 1993.

The natural history of breast cancer—ten years of growth to become visible:

Meyers, F. Screening for cancer. Is it worth it? *West J Med* 163:166, 1995.

Fisher, B. The evolution of paradigms for the management of breast cancer: a personal perspective. *Cancer Res* 52:2371, 1992.

Henderson, I. Paradigmatic shifts in the management of breast cancer (editorial). *N Engl J Med* 332:951, 1995.

Gullino, P. Natural history of breast cancer. Progression from hyperplasia to neoplasia as predicted by angiogenesis. *Cancer* 39:2697, 1977.

MacDonald, I. The natural history of mammary carcinoma. *Am J Surg* 3:435, 1966.

Spread of cancer by the time of diagnosis has usually occurred:

Ganz, P. Treatment options for breast cancer—beyond survival (editorial). *Lancet* 326:1147, 1992.

Cancers found on mammograms may have doubling times of over two hundred days and been growing for fifteen to twenty years before discovery:

Arnerlov, C. Breast carcinoma growth rate described by mammographic doubling time and S-phase fraction. Correlations to clinical and histopathologic factors in a screened population. *Cancer* 70:1928, 1992.

Galante, E. Prognostic significance of the growth rate of breast cancer: preliminary evaluation on the follow-up of 196 breast cancers. *Tumori* 67:333, 1981.

Fournier, D. von. Growth rate of 147 mammary carcinomas. *Cancer* 45:2198, 1980.

Heuser, L. Growth rates of primary breast cancers. *Cancer* 43:1888, 1979.

Lundgren, B. Observations on growth rate of breast carcinomas and its possible implications for lead time. *Cancer* 40:1722, 1977.

Tumors found by screening are less aggressive than those found without:

Klemi, P. Aggressiveness of breast cancer found with and without screening. *BMJ* 304:467, 1992.

Mammography cannot detect a mass until twenty-five to thirty doublings have already occurred:
> Wright, C. Screening mammography and public health policy: the need for perspective. *Lancet* 346:29, 1995.

"We are not going to win the race by backing a loser":
> Wright, C. Screening for breast cancer, time to think—and stop? (letter) *Lancet* 346:439, 1995.

"We all know that mammography is an unsuitable screening test":
> Roberts, M. Breast screening: time for a rethink? *BMJ* 299:1153, 1989.

Mammography is big business:
> Brown, M. Is the supply of mammography machines outstripping need and demand? An economic analysis. *Ann Intern Med* 113:547, 1990.

Seventy-four percent of U.S. women have had at least one mammogram:
> Romans, M. Report from the Jacobs Institute—American Cancer Society workshop on mammography screening and primary care providers: current issues. *Women Health Issues* 2:169, 1992.

"Public imagination has been captured by mammography":
> Wright, C. Screening mammography and public health policy: the need for perspective. *Lancet* 346:29, 1995.

Quotation from Suzanne Fletcher, M.D., of the Harvard Medical School:
> Fletcher, S. Whither scientific deliberation in health policy recommendations? Alice in the Wonderland of breast cancer screening. *N Engl J Med* 336:1180, 1997.

"When medical scientists disagree . . . it means that whatever effect may be present is small":
> Pauker, S. Contentious Screening Decisions. Does the choice matter? (editorial) *N Engl J Med* 336:1243, 1997.

Advantage of mammography—treatment with more conservative surgery:
> Solin, L. The importance of mammographic screening relative to the treatment of women with carcinoma of the breast. *Arch Intern Med* 154:745, 1994.

Death rate from breast cancer has remained essentially unchanged for the past fifty years:
> Landis, S. Cancer statistics, 1998. *CA Cancer J Clin* 48:6, 1998.

High-fat diets are associated with a more suspicious mammographic pattern:
> Nordevang, E. Dietary habits and mammographic patterns in patients with breast cancer. *Breast Cancer Res Treat* 26:207, 1993.

A low-fat diet will improve the appearance of the breast on mammogram:
> Boyd, N. Effects at two years of a low-fat, high-carbohydrate diet on radiologic features of the breast: results from a randomized trial. Canadian Diet and Breast Cancer Prevention Study Group. *J Natl Cancer Inst* 89:488, 1997.

Chapter 8. Treating Breast Cancer with Surgery, Radiation, Chemotherapy, and Drugs

If the margins are free of cancer an excisional biopsy may be all the treatment you need:

Fisher, B. Lumpectomy margins and much more (editorial). *Cancer* 79:1453, 1997.

Page, D. Pathologic analysis of the National Surgical Adjuvant Breast Project (NSABP) B-17 trial. Unanswered questions remaining unanswered considering current concepts of ductal carcinoma in situ. *Cancer* 75:1219, 1995.

The breast tumor has been growing on the average for ten years before it was discovered:

Meyers, F. Screening for cancer. Is it worth it? *West J Med* 163:166, 1995.

Fisher, B. The evolution of paradigms for the management of breast cancer: a personal perspective. *Cancer Res* 52:2371, 1992.

Henderson, I. Paradigmatic shifts in the management of breast cancer (editorial). *N Engl J Med* 332:951, 1995.

Gullino, P. Natural history of breast cancer. Progression from hyperplasia to neoplasia as predicted by angiogenesis. *Cancer* 39:2697, 1977.

MacDonald, I. The natural history of mammary carcinoma. *Am J Surg* 3:435, 1966.

Routine laboratory, bone scans, liver scans, and chest X rays are no longer recommended:

Sacks, N. Primary management of carcinoma of the breast. *Lancet* 342:1402, 1993.

Incidence of ductal carcinoma in situ (or DCIS) has risen dramatically:

Silverstein, M. Ductal carcinoma in situ of the breast. *Br J Surg* 84:145, 1997.

The problem with DCIS are all the unknowns associated with the disease:

Fonseca, R. Ductal carcinoma in situ of the breast. *Ann Intern Med* 127:1013, 1997.

In 1983, 71 percent of DCIS cases were treated with mastectomy; today only 44 percent:

Ernster, V. Incidence of and treatment for ductal carcinoma of the breast. *JAMA* 275:913, 1996.

DCIS effectively treated with wide excision and no radiation:

Lagios, M. Ductal carcinoma in situ. The success of breast conservation therapy: a shared experience of two single institutional nonrandomized prospective studies. *Surg Oncol Clin N Am* 6:385, 1997.

Lagios, M. Widely excised DCIS rarely needs radiation. *Intern Med News*, February 1, 1998.

Page, D. Ductal carcinoma in situ of the breast. Understanding the misunderstood stepchild (editorial). *JAMA* 275:948, 1996.

In the state of Hawaii, during the years 1960 and 1961, 78 percent of women with breast cancer were given radical mastectomies:

Sieburg, V. Unpublished data from the Hawaii Tumor Registry.

No form of mastectomy offers a better survival benefit than that of a lumpectomy:

Fisher, B. Significance of ipsilateral breast tumor recurrence after lumpectomy. *Lancet* 338:327, 1991.

Veronesi, U. Radiotherapy after breast-preserving surgery in women with localized cancer of the breast. *N Engl J Med* 328:1587, 1993.

Liljegren, G. Sector resection with or without postoperative radiotherapy for stage I breast cancer: five-year results of a randomized trial. *J Natl Cancer Inst* 86:717, 1994.

The death rate from breast cancer has not changed during the last fifty years:

Landis, S. Cancer statistics, 1998. *CA Cancer J Clin* 48:6, 1998.

Negative surgical margins predict risk of a recurrence of cancer within the breast:

Smitt, M. The importance of the lumpectomy surgical margin status in long term results of breast conservation. *Cancer* 76:259, 1995.

Treatment of recurrence can be as successful as the first lumpectomy:

Smitt, M. The importance of the lumpectomy surgical margin status in long-term results of breast conservation. *Cancer* 76:259, 1995.

Timing your surgery according to your hormonal cycles may extend your life:

Hrushesky, W. Menstrual influence on surgical cure of breast cancer. *Lancet* 2:949, 1989.

Fentiman, I. Effect of menstrual phase on surgical treatment of breast cancer (letter). *Lancet* 344:402, 1994.

The follicular phase may support the aggressiveness of the cancer, weakening the immune system:

Astrow, A. Timing of breast cancer surgery: nodes, hormones, and retrospectoscopy (commentary). *Lancet* 343:1517, 1994.

Veronesi, U. Effect of menstrual phase on surgical treatment of breast cancer. *Lancet* 343:1545, 1994.

Spread of cancer by the time of diagnosis has usually occurred:

Ganz, P. Treatment options for breast cancer—beyond survival (editorial). *Lancet* 326:1147, 1992.

Recurrence of disease in the breast does not affect length of survival:

Fisher, B. Significance of ipsilateral breast tumor recurrence after lumpectomy. *Lancet* 338:327, 1991.

Crile, G. Factors influencing local recurrence of cancer after partial mastectomy. *Cleve Clin J Med* 57:143, 1990.

Nemoto, T. Factors affecting recurrence in lumpectomy without radiation for breast cancer. *Cancer* 67:2079, 1991.

Use of additional surgery or radiation for recurrence is just as effective:

McCready, D. Characteristics of local recurrence following lumpectomy for breast cancer. *Cancer Invest* 12:568, 1994.

Haffty, B. Conservative surgery and radiation therapy in breast carcinoma:

local recurrence and prognostic implications. *Int J Radiat Oncol Biol Phys* 17:727, 1989.

DCIS with lumpectomy alone has a 16 percent chance of local recurrence in forty-three months:

Fisher, B. Lumpectomy compared with lumpectomy and radiation therapy for the treatment of intraductal breast cancer. *N Engl J Med* 328:1581, 1993.

For invasive cancer, local recurrence after lumpectomy is about 25 percent within forty-three months:

Forrest, A. Randomised controlled trial of conservative therapy for breast cancer: 6-year analysis of the Scottish trial. *Lancet* 348:708, 1996.

At nine years the local relapse rate is about 43 percent with lumpectomy alone:

Fisher, B. Significance of ipsilateral breast tumor recurrence after lumpectomy. *Lancet* 338:327, 1991.

Survival benefits not improved with the addition of radiation to treatment with lumpectomy:

Fisher, B. Eight-year results of a randomized clinical trial comparing total mastectomy with lumpectomy with or without irradiation in the treatment of breast cancer. *N Engl J Med* 320:822, 1989.

Fisher, B. Reanalysis and results after 12 years of follow-up in a randomized clinical trial comparing total mastectomy with lumpectomy with or without radiation in the treatment of breast cancer. *N Engl J Med* 333:1456, 1995.

Early Breast Cancer Trialists' Collaborative Group. Effects of radiotherapy and surgery in early breast cancer. An overview of the randomised trials. *N Engl J Med* 333:1444, 1995.

Forrest, A. Randomised controlled trial of conservative therapy for breast cancer: 6-year analysis of the Scottish trial. *Lancet* 348:708, 1996.

The Uppsala-Orebro Breast Cancer Study Group. Sector resection with or without postoperative radiotherapy for stage I breast cancer: a randomized trial. *J Natl Cancer Inst* 82:277, 1990.

Clark, R. A randomized trial to assess the effectiveness of breast irradiation following lumpectomy and axillary dissection for node negative breast cancer. *J Natl Cancer Inst* 84:683, 1992.

Fisher, B. Significance of ipsilateral breast tumor recurrence after lumpectomy. *Lancet* 338:327, 1991.

At Cleveland Clinic, local recurrence rate is 11 percent at five years and 15 percent at ten years:

Hermann, R. Partial mastectomy without radiation is adequate treatment for patients with stages 0 and I carcinoma of the breast. *Surg Gynecol Obstet* 177:247, 1993.

Hermann, R. Early breast cancer: the Cleveland Clinic experience. *Primary Care & Cancer,* March 1989.

Hermann, R. The changing treatment of breast cancer (letter). *JAMA* 260:2834, 1988.

According to a 1995 overview of 17,273 women, radiation does not improve survival:
Early Breast Cancer Trialists' Collaborative Group. Effects of radiotherapy and surgery in early breast cancer. An overview of the randomized trials. *N Engl J Med* 333:1444, 1995.

Two recently published studies show small survival improvement with radiation:
Overgaard, M. Postoperative radiotherapy in high-risk pre-menopausal women with breast cancer who receive adjuvant chemotherapy. *N Engl J Med* 337:949, 1997.
Ragaz, J. Adjuvant radiotherapy and chemotherapy in node-positive premenopausal women with breast cancer. *N Engl J Med* 337:956, 1997.

Warnings about addition of radiotherapy:
Rogers, P. Regional node radiotherapy for breast cancer (letter). *Lancet* 351:374, 1998.

Side effects of radiation:
Rutqvist, L. Radiation therapies for breast cancer: current knowledge on advantages and disadvantages. *Recent Results Cancer Res* 127:119, 1993.

Radiation increases risk of dying from heart disease and other cancers:
Haybittle, J. Postoperative radiotherapy and late mortality: evidence from the Cancer Research Campaign trial for early breast cancer. *BMJ* 298:1611, 1989.
Cuzick, J. Overview of randomised trials of postoperative adjuvant radiotherapy in breast cancer. *Cancer Treatment Rep* 71:15, 1987.
Cuzick, J. Cause specific mortality in long-term survivors of breast cancer who participated in trials in radiotherapy. *J Clin Oncol* 12:447, 1994.
Gyenes, G. Evaluation of irradiated heart volumes in stage I breast cancer patients treated with postoperative adjuvant radiotherapy. *J Clin Oncol* 15:1348, 1997.
Houghton, J. Role of radiotherapy following total mastectomy in patients with early breast cancer. *World J Surg* 18:117, 1994.

Radiation increases the risk of cancer of the esophagus by about fivefold:
Ahsan, H. Radiation therapy for breast cancer and increased risk for esophageal carcinoma. *Ann Intern Med* 128:114, 1998.

Doctors recommending chemotherapy with negative lymph nodes:
Wyss-Desserich, M. Premenopausal node-negative breast cancer: may adjuvant chemotherapy be indicated by the analysis of nuclear DNA dynamics? *Breast Cancer Res Treat* 42:253, 1997.
Lee, K. Adjuvant therapy for node-negative breast cancer (letter). *N Engl J Med* 321:469, 1989.

Removing the lymph nodes does not increase your chance of surviving:
Fisher, B. Ten-year results of a randomized clinical trial comparing radical mastectomy and total mastectomy with or without radiation. *N Engl J Med* 312:674, 1985.
Cancer Research Campaign Working Party. Cancer Research Campaign

(Kings/Cambridge) trial for early breast cancer: a detailed update and the tenth year. *Lancet* 2:55, 1980.

Thirty-five percent of the women alive more than twenty years after diagnosis had positive lymph nodes:
   Fentiman, I. Which patients are cured of breast cancer? *BMJ* 289:1108, 1984.

Chemotherapy results are disappointing:
   Kearsley, J. Cytotoxic chemotherapy for common adult malignancies: "the emperor's new clothes" revisited? *BMJ* 293:871, 1986.
   GAO Report: The survival of breast cancer patients. GAO/PEMD-89-9. February 1989.
   Mueller, C. Adjuvant chemotherapy in stage I breast cancer. More harm than benefit. *Can Fam Physician* 39:2185, 1993.

Chemotherapy reduces the risk of recurrence of cancer by 28 percent and the risk of death by 16 percent:
   Early Breast Cancer Trialists' Collaborative Group. Systemic treatment of early breast cancer by hormonal, cytotoxic, or immune therapy. 133 randomised trials involving 31,000 recurrences and 24,000 deaths among 75,000 women. *Lancet* 339:1, 1992.
   Early Breast Cancer Trialists' Collaborative Group. Systemic treatment of early breast cancer by hormonal, cytotoxic, or immune therapy. 133 randomised trials involving 31,000 recurrences and 24,000 deaths among 75,000 women. *Lancet* 339:72, 1992.

Chemotherapy increased survival for patients with positive lymph nodes by 6.8 percent over ten years:
   Early Breast Cancer Trialists' Collaborative Group. Systemic treatment of early breast cancer by hormonal, cytotoxic, or immune therapy. 133 randomised trials involving 31,000 recurrences and 24,000 deaths among 75,000 women. *Lancet* 339:1, 1992.
   Early Breast Cancer Trialists' Collaborative Group. Systemic treatment of early breast cancer by hormonal, cytotoxic, or immune therapy. 133 randomised trials involving 31,000 recurrences and 24,000 deaths among 75,000 women. *Lancet* 339:72, 1992.

As few as 6 percent of women have their lives prolonged by fourteen months by chemotherapy:
   Mueller, C. The case against the use of adjuvant chemotherapy in breast cancer. *Am Coll Surg Bull* 78:25, 1993.

Chemotherapy impairs concentration, memory, thinking, and language:
   van Dam, F. Impairment of cognitive function in women receiving treatment for high-risk breast cancer: high-dose versus standard dose chemotherapy. *J Natl Cancer Inst* 90:210, 1998.

Chemotherapy causes sexual dysfunction, poor body image, and psychological distress:
   Schover, L. Partial mastectomy and breast reconstruction: a comparison of

their effects on psychosocial adjustment, body image, and sexuality. *Cancer* 75:54, 1995.

Weight gains of five to fifteen pounds are common with chemotherapy:
Faber-Langendeon, K. Weight gain in women receiving adjuvant chemotherapy for breast cancer. *JAMA* 276:855, 1996.

Viral infections are twice as common in women while they undergo chemotherapy:
Lenders, J. Viral infections during chemotherapy for breast cancer. *BMJ* 290:1626, 1985.

Twenty-nine percent reported, given the chance, they would never undergo chemotherapy again:
Palmer, B. Adjuvant chemotherapy for breast cancer: side effects and quality of life. *BMJ* 281:1594, 1980.

High-dose chemotherapy followed by bone marrow transplants:
Zujewski, J. Much ado about not . . . enough data: high dose chemotherapy with autologous stem cell rescue for breast cancer. Review. *J Natl Cancer Inst* 90:200, 1998.
Basade, M. High dose chemotherapy in metastatic breast cancer. *Lancet* 351:386, 1998.
Gradishar, W. High-dose chemotherapy for breast cancer. *Ann Intern Med* 125:599, 1996.

Effects of chemotherapy and those of surgery to remove the ovaries are similar:
Adjuvant systemic therapy for early breast cancer (editorial). *Lancet* 339: 27, 1992.

Improvements from chemotherapy come exclusively from the destruction of the ovaries:
Del Mastro, L. Adjuvant chemotherapy in breast cancer (letter). *N Engl J Med* 333:596, 1995.
Bianco, A. Prognostic role of amenorrhea induced by adjuvant chemotherapy in premenopausal patients with early breast cancer. *Br J Cancer* 63:799, 1991.
Adjuvant systemic therapy for early breast cancer (editorial). *Lancet* 339:27, 1992.
Padmanabhan, N. Mechanisms of action of adjuvant chemotherapy in early breast cancer. *Lancet* 2:411, 1986.

A review of 133 trials found chemotherapy, removal of the ovaries, and hormonal therapy equal in terms of survival:
Early Breast Cancer Trialists' Collaborative Group. Systemic treatment of early breast cancer by hormonal, cytotoxic, or immune therapy. 133 randomised trials involving 31,000 recurrences and 24,000 deaths among 75,000 women. *Lancet* 339:1, 1992.
Early Breast Cancer Trialists' Collaborative Group. Systemic treatment of early breast cancer by hormonal, cytotoxic, or immune therapy. 133 randomised trials involving 31,000 recurrences and 24,000 deaths among 75,000 women. *Lancet* 339:72, 1992.

Removal of ovaries improves survival 6.3 percent in fifteen years:
Barley, V. Time for reappraisal of ovarian ablation in early breast cancer (editorial). *Lancet* 348:1184, 1996.
Early Breast Cancer Trialists' Collaborative Group. Ovarian ablation in early breast cancer: overview of the randomised trials. *Lancet* 348:1189, 1996.

Removal of the ovaries by laparoscopy is the most economical, simple, and safe method:
Kwon, A. Prophylactic laparoscopic ovarian ablation for premenopausal breast cancer: medical and economic efficacy. *Surg Laparosc Endosc* 7:223, 1997.

Tamoxifen prolongs survival and delays recurrence when taken up to five years after surgery:
Early Breast Cancer Trialists' Collaborative Group. Tamoxifen for early breast cancer: an overview of the randomised trials. *Lancet* 351:1451, 1998.
Swedish Breast Cancer Cooperative Group. Randomized trial of two versus five years of adjuvant tamoxifen for postmenopausal early stage breast cancer. *J Natl Cancer Inst* 88:1543, 1996.
Fisher, B. Five versus more than five years of tamoxifen therapy for breast cancer patients with negative lymph nodes and estrogen receptor-positive tumors. *J Natl Cancer Inst* 88:1529, 1996.
Rea, D. Adjuvant tamoxifen: how long before we know how long? *BMJ* 316:1518, 1998.

Only 2 percent of women stop taking the tamoxifen because of menopausal side effects:
Controlled trial of tamoxifen as adjuvant therapy in management of early breast cancer. Analysis at four years by Nolvadex Trial Organisation. *Lancet* 1:257, 1983.

Tamoxifen reduced the risk of recurrence by 25 percent and the risk of death by 17 percent:
Controlled trial of tamoxifen as adjuvant therapy in management of early breast cancer. Analysis at four years by Nolvadex Trial Organisation. *Lancet* 1:257, 1983.

Combining chemotherapy and tamoxifen results in no further benefits:
Gelber, R. Adjuvant chemotherapy plus tamoxifen compared with tamoxifen alone for postmenopausal breast cancer: meta-analysis of quality-adjusted survival. *Lancet* 347:1066, 1996.

One serious drawback to tamoxifen therapy: an increase in risk of cancer of the uterus:
Neven, P. Tamoxifen and the uterus. Women given this drug need careful assessment. *BMJ* 309:1313, 1994.
van Leeuwen, F. Risk of endometrial cancer after tamoxifen treatment of breast cancer. *Lancet* 343:448, 1994.

"The war against cancer is far from over":
Bailar, J. Cancer undefeated. *N Engl J Med* 336:1569, 1997.

Ninety percent of cancers are caused by diet and lifestyle:
Doll, R. Nature and nurture: possibilities for cancer control. *Carcinogenesis* 17:177, 1996.

Wynder, E. Contribution of the environment to cancer incidence: an epidemiologic exercise. *J Natl Cancer Inst* 58:825, 1977.

Report by Dr. John C. Bailar in 1986 shows little or no progress against cancer:
Bailar, J. Progress against cancer? *New Engl J Med* 314:1226, 1986.

Chapter 9. Strengthening Your Cancer-Fighting Forces

In the 1920s, Otto Warburg began showing that normal cells can become cancerous:
Warburg, O. On the origin of cancer cells. *Science* 123:309, 1956.

The U.S. Senate Select Committee on Nutrition and Human Needs (1977), The National Cancer Institute (1979), the National Academy of Sciences (1982), the American Cancer Society (1984), and the U.S. Surgeon General (1988):
Statement by Arthur C. Upton, M.D., Director, National Cancer Institute: Status of the diet, nutrition, and cancer program before the subcommittee on nutrition. State Committee of Agriculture, Nutrition and Forestry, October 2, 1972.

U.S. Senate Report. *Dietary goals for the United States.* GPO Stock Number 052-070-03913-2, 1977.

Committee on Diet, Nutrition, and Cancer: Assembly of Life Sciences, National Research Council. *Diet, nutrition, and cancer* (Washington, D.C.: National Academy Press, 1982).

Nutrition and cancer: cause and prevention. An American Cancer Society Special Report. *Cancer* 34:121, 1984.

The Surgeon General's report on nutrition and health. U.S. Department of Health and Human Services. Public Health Service. DHHS (PHS) Publication Number 88-50210.

Fat triggers the oxidation process that deforms the DNA in cells:
Ames, B. Oxidants, antioxidants, and the degenerative diseases of aging. *Proc Natl Acad Sci USA* 90:7915, 1993.

Fat infiltrates the cell membranes of macrophages:
Yaqoob, P. The effect of dietary lipid manipulation on rat lymphocyte subsets and proliferation. *Immunology* 82:603, 1994.

Fowler, K. Effects of purified dietary n-3 ethyl esters on murine T lymphocyte function. *J Immunol* 151:5186, 1993.

Jenski, L. Omega-3 fatty acid modification of membrane structure and function. I. Dietary manipulation of tumor cell susceptibility to cell- and complement-mediated lysis. *Nutr Cancer* 19:135, 1993.

Kelley, D. Essential nutrients and immunologic functions. *Am J Clin Nutr* 63:994S, 1996.

Oth, D. Modulation of CD4 expression on lymphoma cells transplanted to mice fed (n-3) polyunsaturated fatty acids. *Biochim Biophys Acta* 1027:47, 1990.

Kelley, D. Concentration of dietary N-6 polyunsaturated fatty acids and the human immune status. *Clin Immunol Immunopathol* 62:240, 1992.

Endres, S. Dietary supplementation with n-3 fatty acids suppresses interleukin-2 production and mononuclear cell proliferation. *J Leukoc Biol* 54:599, 1993.

Evidence suggests a "dose-relationship" between fat intake and the incidence of breast cancer:
Wang, Y. Decreased growth of established human prostate LNCaP tumors in nude mice fed a low-fat diet. *J Natl Cancer Inst* 87:1456, 1993.

A very-low-fat, no-cholesterol diet retards the growth of cancer in animals:
Littman, M. Effect of cholesterol-free, fat-free diet and hypocholesteremic agents on growth of transplantable animal tumors. *Cancer Chemother Rep* 50:25, 1966.

Laval University found high intakes of saturated fat meant more cancerous involvement of the lymph nodes:
Verreault, R. Dietary fat in relation to prognostic indicators in breast cancer. *J Natl Cancer Inst* 80:81, 1988.

Hawaiian women with breast cancer who follow high-fat diets have three times the risk of dying:
Nomura, A. The effect of dietary fat on breast cancer survival among Caucasian and Japanese women in Hawaii. *Br Cancer Res Treat* 18:S135, 1991.

Vegetable fats promote cancer growth and death in women with breast cancer:
Rohan, T. Dietary factors and survival from breast cancer. *Nutr Cancer* 20:167, 1993.

Women with lower intake of total fat had tumors with more favorable DNA patterns:
Furst, C. DNA pattern and dietary habits in patients with breast cancer. *Eur J Cancer* 29A:1285, 1993.

Every 5 percent increase in intake of saturated fat increases the risk of dying by 50 percent:
Jain, M. Premorbid diet and the prognosis of women with breast cancer. *J Natl Cancer Inst* 86:1390, 1994.

Japanese women in Japan with breast cancer live longer than American women with breast cancer do:
Chlebowski, R. Adjuvant dietary fat intake reduction in postmenopausal breast cancer management. *Breast Cancer Res Treat* 20:73, 1991.

The risk of death increased by 40 percent for each kilogram (2.2 pounds) increase in fat intake per month:
Gregorio, D. Dietary fat consumption and survival among women with breast cancer. *J Natl Cancer Inst* 75:37, 1985.

Women following diets higher in total fat had much greater rates of cancer recurrence:
Holm, L. Treatment failure and dietary habits in women with breast cancer. *J Natl Cancer Inst* 85:32, 1993.

Reducing estrogen and prolactin by drugs or surgery retards breast cancer:
Weisburger, J. Dietary fat and risk of chronic disease: mechanistic insights from experimental studies. *J Am Diet Assoc* 97 (7 Suppl):S16, 1997.

Adams, J. Human breast cancer: concerted role of diet, prolactin and adrenal C19-delta 5-steroids in tumorigenesis. *Int J Cancer* 50:854, 1992.

Zumoff, B. Hormonal profiles in women with breast cancer. *Obstet Gynecol Clin North Am* 21:751, 1994.

Smithline, F. Prolactin and breast carcinoma. *N Engl J Med* 292:784, 1975.

Iowa Women's Health Study found that overweight women are almost twice as likely to die from breast cancer:

Zhang, S. Better breast cancer survival for postmenopausal women who are less overweight and eat less fat. The Iowa Women's Health Study. *Cancer* 76:275, 1995.

Women in their fifties who gained eleven pounds in ten years had twice the risk of breast cancer:

Ziegler, R. Relative weight, weight change, height, and breast cancer risk in Asian-American women. *J Natl Cancer Inst* 88:650, 1996.

The fat and cholesterol content of your diet, your weight, and your hormone levels encourage the growth of cancer:

McDougall, J. Preliminary study of diet as an adjunct therapy for breast cancer. *Breast* 10:18, 1984.

Bastarrachea, J. Obesity as an adverse prognostic factor for patients receiving adjuvant chemotherapy for breast cancer. *Ann Intern Med* 119:18, 1993.

Senie, R. Obesity at diagnosis of breast carcinoma influences duration of disease-free survival. *Ann Intern Med* 116:26, 1992.

Tartter, P. Cholesterol and obesity as prognostic factors in breast cancer. *Cancer* 47:2222, 1981.

There are hundreds of health-enhancing chemicals in a single plant such as broccoli:

Nestle, M. Broccoli sprouts as inducers of carcinogen-detoxifying enzyme systems: clinical, dietary, and policy implications. *Proc Natl Acad Sci USA* 94:11149, 1997.

Fahey, J. Broccoli sprouts: an exceptionally rich source of inducers of enzymes that protect against chemical carcinogens. *Proc Natl Acad Sci USA* 94:10367, 1997.

Verhoeven, D. A review of mechanisms underlying anticarcinogenicity by brassica vegetables. *Chem Biol Interact* 103:79, 1997.

Verhoeven, D. Epidemiological studies on brassica vegetables and cancer risk. *Cancer Epidemiol Biomarkers Prev* 5:733, 1996.

Beecher, C. Cancer preventive properties of varieties of *Brassica oleaceae*: a review. *Am J Clin Nutr* 59 (5 Suppl):1166S, 1994.

Women who ate more than five servings of vegetables had half the risk of breast cancer:

Freudenheim, J. Premenopausal breast cancer risk and intake of vegetables, fruits, and related nutrients. *J Natl Cancer Inst* 88:340, 1996.

"A variety of produce works like a soup filled with weak anticarcinogens":

The ultra-diet for healthy breasts. Experts say it is the key to staying breast cancer free. *Prevention*, September 1996, 68.

Breast cancer research from Queen Elizabeth II Medical Center in Australia:
Ingram, D. Diet and subsequent survival in women with breast cancer. *Br J Cancer* 69:592, 1994.

Beta carotene encourages macrophages to consume, or phagocytize, cancer cells:
Bendich, A. Beta-carotene and the immune response. *Proc Nutr Soc* 50:263, 1991.

Beta carotene increased lymphocytes and natural killer (NK) cells in men with cancer:
Prabhala, R. The effects of 13-cis-retinoic acid and beta-carotene on cellular immunity in humans. *Cancer* 67:1556, 1991.

A large population study of 6,500 Chinese done by Cornell University researchers on the effects of beta carotene:
Chen, J. Antioxidant status and cancer mortality in China. *Int J Epidemiol* 21:625, 1992.

A substance in soybeans and soybean products blocks blood flow to tumors:
Fotsis, T. Genistein, a dietary-derived inhibitor of in vitro angiogenesis. *Proc Natl Acad Sci USA* 90:2690, 1993.

The New York Times reported that genistein could help in the prevention and treatment of cancers:
Angier, N. Chemists learn why vegetables are good for you. *New York Times,* April 13, 1993.

A substantial reduction in breast cancer risk with a high intake of phytoestrogens:
Ingram, D. Case-control study of phyto-estrogens and breast cancer. *Lancet* 350:990, 1997.

Broccoli, cabbage, kale, Brussels sprouts, collards, and mustard greens contain indoles and sulforanphane:
Verhoeven, D. A review of mechanisms underlying anticarcinogenicity by brassica vegetables. *Chem Biol Interact* 103:79, 1997.
Preobrazhenskaya, M. Ascorbigen and other indole-derived compounds from brassica vegetables and their analogs as anticarcinogenic and immunomodulating agents. *Pharmacol Ther* 60:301, 1993.

Daily consumption of 30 grams of fiber will lower your estrogen levels by 20 percent:
Rose, D. High-fiber diet reduces serum estrogen concentrations in premenopausal women. *Am J Clin Nutr* 54:520, 1991.

Chances of having a small tumor instead of a large mass are greater with a high-fiber diet:
Holm, L. Dietary habits and prognostic factors in breast cancer. *J Natl Cancer Inst* 81:1218, 1989.

Regular exercise independently lowers estrogen levels, while alcohol consumption raises it:
Thune, I. Physical activity and the risk of breast cancer. *N Engl J Med* 336:1269, 1997.
Smith-Warner, S. Alcohol and breast cancer in women. A pooled analysis of cohort studies. *JAMA* 279:535, 1998.

Cancer-causing chemicals produced by the combustion of tobacco are found in the breast fluids:
> Petrakis, N. Mutagenic activity in nipple aspirates of human breast fluid. *Cancer Res* 40:188, 1980.

Women who participated in a support group lived twice as long:
> Spiegel, D. Effect of psychological treatment on survival of patients with metastatic breast cancer. *Lancet* 2:888, 1989.

Social support predicted both higher natural killer cell activity and recurrence:
> Levy, S. Immunological and psychosocial predictors of disease recurrence in patients with early-stage breast cancer. *Behav Med* 17:67, 1991.

Intensive follow-up programs don't help improve survival:
> The GIVIO Investigators. Impact of follow-up testing on survival and health-related quality of life in breast cancer patients. A multicenter randomized controlled trial. *JAMA* 271:1587, 1994.
> Del Turco, M. Intensive diagnostic follow-up after treatment of primary breast cancer. A randomized trial. *JAMA* 271:1593, 1994.
> Kattlove, H. A benefits package for breast cancer includes selective screening, choice of surgery, adjuvant therapy, and no routine follow-up. *JAMA* 273:142, 1995.
> Dewar, J. Follow up in breast cancer. A suitable case for reappraisal. *BMJ* 310:685, 1995.

A large-scale study of two thousand women is being conducted by the National Cancer Institute:
> Henderson, M. Nutritional aspects of breast cancer. *Cancer* 76:2053, 1995.

Chapter 10. Safeguarding Your Uterus

Statistics on hysterectomies:
> Graves E. *National hospital discharge survey: annual summary, 1990. Vital and health statistics.* Series 13, No. 112 (Washington, D.C.: Government Printing Office, 1987). DHHS (PHS) Publication Number 92-1773.
> Ravnikar, V. Hysterectomies. Where are the indications? *Obstet Gynecol Clin N Am* 21:405, 1994.
> Bachmann, G. Hysterectomy: a critical review. *J Reprod Med* 35:839, 1990.

By age sixty, one-third of women will have had a hysterectomy:
> Pokras, R. National Center for Health Statistics. *Hysterectomies in the United States, 1965–84. Vital and health statistics.* Series 13, No. 92 (Washington, D.C.: Government Printing Office, 1987). DHHS (PHS) Publication Number 88-1753.

Barely half of the women in California will carry their uterus to the grave:
> Lilford, R. Hysterectomy: will it pay the bills in 2007? The treatment of choice for cancer, but a choice of treatment for menorrhagia. *BMJ* 314:160, 1997.

Five recent studies suggest that retaining the uterus protects premenopausal women from heart disease:

Grimes, D. Shifting indications for hysterectomy: nature, nurture, or neither? (commentary) *Lancet* 344:1652, 1994.

After a hysterectomy premenopausal women experience a threefold increase in heart disease:

Centerwell, B. Premenopausal hysterectomy and cardiovascular disease. *Am J Obstet Gynecol* 139:58, 1981.

Gordon, T. Menopause and coronary heart disease: The Framingham Study. *Ann Intern Med* 89:157, 1978.

The risk of hypertension is increased after a hysterectomy:

Luoto, R. Cardiovascular morbidity in relation to ovarian function after hysterectomy. *Obstet Gynecol* 85:515, 1995.

Women report a general loss of sexual desire and response following a hysterectomy:

Poad, D. Sexual function after pelvic surgery in women. *Aust NZ J Obstet Gynaecol* 34:471, 1994.

Richards, D. A post-hysterectomy syndrome. *Lancet* 2:983, 1974.

Sloan, D. The emotional and psychosexual aspects of hysterectomy. *Am J Obstet Gynecol* 131:598, 1978.

Utian, W. Effect of hysterectomy, oophorectomy, and estrogen therapy on libido. *Int J Gynaecol Obstet* 13:97, 1975.

Kilkku, P. Supravaginal uterine amputation vs. hysterectomy. Effects on libido and orgasm. *Acta Obstet Gynecol Scand* 62:147, 1983.

Mental depression, anxiety, and difficult sexual relations may follow hysterectomy:

Carranza-Lira, S. Changes in symptomatology, hormones, lipids, and bone density after hysterectomy. *Int J Fertil Womens Med* 42:43, 1997.

Wright, J. Psychological aspects of heavy periods, does endometrial ablation provide the answer? *Br J Hosp Med* 55:289, 1996.

Complications after surgery occur in 25 to 50 percent of cases, though most are minor:

Bachmann, G. Hysterectomy: a critical review. *J Reprod Med* 35:839, 1990.

Constipation is reported by about one-third of women after a hysterectomy:

Van Dam, J. Changes in bowel function after hysterectomy. *Dis Colon Rectum* 40:1342, 1997.

Even when ovaries remain, hysterectomy can cause premature menopausal symptoms:

Siddle, N. The effect of hysterectomy on the age of ovarian failure: identification of a subgroup of women with premature loss of ovarian function and literature review. *Fertil Steril* 47:94, 1987.

Watson, N. Bone loss after hysterectomy with ovarian conservation. *Obstet Gynecol* 86:72, 1995.

Reidel, H. Ovarian failure phenomena after hysterectomy. *J Reprod Med* 31:597, 1986.

A survey of 6,622 women showed more symptoms of menopause after hysterectomy:
Oldenhave, A. Hysterectomized women with ovarian conservation report more severe climacteric complaints than do normal climacteric women of similar age. *Am J Obstet Gynecol* 168:765, 1993.

After a hysterectomy, women are often told by their doctors to "see a psychiatrist":
Oldenhave, A. Indications for hysterectomy (letter). *Lancet* 329:275, 1993.

Appropriate use of the operation—cancer:
Rose, P. Endometrial carcinoma. *N Engl J Med* 335:640, 1996.

Cervical cancer is believed to be caused by a virus:
Elkas, J. Cancer of the uterine cervix. *Curr Opin Obstet Gynecol* 10:47, 1998.

Evidence suggests that a plant-based diet confers some protection from cervical cancer:
Buckley, D. Dietary micronutrients and cervical dysplasia in Southwestern Indian women. *Nutr Cancer* 17:179, 1992.
Potishman, N. A case-control study of nutrient status and invasive cervical cancer. *Am J Epidemiol* 134:1347, 1991.
Brock, K. Nutrients in diet and plasma and risk of in situ cancer. *J Natl Cancer Inst* 80:580, 1988.
Butterworth, C. Folate deficiency and cervical dysplasia. *JAMA* 267:528, 1992.

After two consecutive negative Pap tests, have this test done every three years until age fifty:
Wijngaarden, W. Rationale for stopping cervical screening in women over 50. *BMJ* 306:967, 1993.

Obstetrical indications for a hysterectomy:
Carlson, K. Indications for hysterectomy. *N Engl J Med* 328:856, 1993.
Bachmann, G. Hysterectomy: a critical review. *J Reprod Med* 35:839, 1990.

Hysterectomy undertaken to prevent cancer, however, cannot be justified:
Bachmann, G. Hysterectomy: a critical review. *J Reprod Med* 35:839, 1990.
Cole, P. Elective hysterectomy. *Am J Obstet Gynecol* 129:117, 1977.

Hysterectomies are most commonly performed on premenopausal women:
Pokras, R. Hysterectomies in the United States, 1965–84. *Am J Public Health* 78:852, 1988.

Twice as many hysterectomies are performed in the United States than in England and Sweden:
McPherson, K. Small-area variations in the use of common surgical procedures: an international comparison of New England, England, and Norway. *N Engl J Med* 307:1310, 1982.

Hysterectomy is more common in Southern states than in the Northeast:
Graves, E. *National hospital discharge survey: annual summary, 1990. Vital and health statistics.* Series 13, No. 112 (Washington, D.C.: Government Printing Office, 1987). DHHS (PHS) Publication Number 92-1773.

Having a male doctor substantially increases the risk of having a hysterectomy:
   Domenighetti, G. Hysterectomy and sex of the gynecologist (letter). *N Engl J Med* 313:1482, 1985.
   Coulter, A. Influence of sex of general practitioner on management of menorrhagia. *Br J Gen Pract* 45:471, 1995.
   Bachmann, G. Hysterectomy: a critical review. *J Reprod Med* 35:839, 1990.
   Bickell, N. Gynecologists' sex, clinical beliefs, and hysterectomy rates. *Am J Public Health* 84:1649, 1994.

The older your doctor is, the greater your chances of having the operation:
   Bachmann, G. Hysterectomy: a critical review. *J Reprod Med* 35:839, 1990.

The number of hysterectomies peaked in 1975, when 725,000 were performed:
   Pokras, R. Hysterectomies in the United States, 1965–84. *Am J Public Health* 78:852, 1988.

Having a gynecologist as your primary care physician increases the likelihood of hysterectomy:
   Roos, N. Hysterectomy: variations in rates across small areas and across physicians' practices. *Am J Public Health* 74:327, 1984.

Having health insurance increases the chance of having a hysterectomy to 40 percent:
   Selwood, T. Incidence of hysterectomy in Australia. *Med J Aust* 2:201, 1978.

"A cooperative patient with a uterus and good health insurance":
   Patton, W. Indications for hysterectomy (letter). *Lancet* 329:276, 1993.

The older you get, the greater your chances of undergoing a hysterectomy:
   Van Keep, P. Hysterectomy in six European countries. *Maturitas* 5:69, 1983.

The less you know about the pros and cons of hysterectomy, the more likely it is that you will have one:
   Domenighetti, G. Effect of information campaign by mass media on hysterectomy rates. *Lancet* 2:1470, 1988.

A second opinion may reduce hysterectomy by as much as 28 percent:
   McSherry, C. Second surgical opinion programs: dead or alive? *J Am Coll Surg* 185:451, 1997.

Many doctors do not really know when this operation is truly necessary:
   Carlson, K. Indications for hysterectomy. *N Engl J Med* 328:856, 1993.

Excess estrogen causes dysfunctional uterine bleeding or abnormal uterine bleeding:
   Deligeoroglou, E. Dysfunctional uterine bleeding. *Ann NY Acad Sci* 816:158, 1997.

Excess estrogen causes cancer of the endometrium of the uterus:
   Mack, T. Estrogen and endometrial cancer in a retirement community. *N Engl J Med* 294:1262, 1976.
   Food and Drug Administration. Estrogens and endometrial cancer. *FDA Bull* 6:18, 1976.

Armstrong, B. Environmental factors and cancer incidence and mortality in different countries, with special reference to dietary practices. *Int J Cancer* 15:61, 1975.

Haenszel, W. Studies of Japanese migrants. I. Mortality from cancer and other disease among Japanese in the United States. *J Natl Cancer Inst* 40:43, 1968.

Excess estrogen causes fibroids:
Ross, R. Risk factors for uterine fibroids: reduced risk associated with oral contraceptives. *BMJ* 293:359, 1986.

Fibroids are uncommon in African women who remain in Africa:
Oram, R. The management of uterine fibroids in the Rhodesian African. *Cent Afr J Med* 16:143, 1970.

Gibney, E. Hysterectomy in the rural tropics. *Cent Afr J Med* 38:72, 1992.

Ross, R. Risk factors for uterine fibroids: reduced risk associated with oral contraceptives. *BMJ* 293:359, 1986.

Fibroids are caused by high levels of estrogens from high-fat diets and obesity:
Shikora, S. Relationship between obesity and uterine leiomyomata. *Nutrition* 7:251, 1991.

Fibroids shrink away during menopause:
Carlson, K. Indications for hysterectomy. *N Engl J Med* 328:856, 1993.

Appropriate reasons for hysterectomy to remove fibroids:
Bachmann, G. Hysterectomy: a critical review. *J Reprod Med* 35:839, 1990.

Carlson, K. Indications for hysterectomy. *N Engl J Med* 328:856, 1993.

Ravnikar, V. Hysterectomies. Where are the indications? *Obstet Gynecol Clin North Am* 21:405, 1994.

Six refutable reasons to remove fibroids:
Carlson, K. Indications for hysterectomy. *N Engl J Med* 328:856, 1993.

Ravnikar, V. Hysterectomies. Where are the indications? *Obstet Gynecol Clin North Am* 21:405, 1994.

Freidman, A. Should uterine size be an indication for surgical intervention in women with myomas? *Am J Obstet Gynecol* 168:751, 1993.

Alternatives to hysterectomy for fibroid treatment:
Healy, D. Toward removing uterine fibroids without surgery: subcutaneous infusion of luteinizing hormone–releasing hormone agonist commencing in the luteal phase. *J Clin Endocrinol Metab* 63:619, 1986.

West, C. Shrinkage of uterine fibroids during therapy with goserelin (Zoladex®): a luteinizing hormone–releasing hormone agonist administered as a monthly subcutaneous depot. *Fertil Steril* 48:45, 1987.

Friedman, A. Treatment of leiomyomata uteri with leuprolide acetate depot: a double-blind, placebo-controlled, multicenter study. *Obstet Gynecol* 77:720, 1991.

Fibroids will likely regress as the function of the ovaries decreases, and estrogen levels fall:
Novak, E. *Novak's gynecologic and obstetric pathology,* 8th ed. (Philadelphia, London: WB Saunders, 1979), 260–69.
Carlson, K. Indications for hysterectomy. *N Engl J Med* 328:856, 1993.

Alternatives to hysterectomy for AUB:
Parkin, D. Prognostic factors for success of endometrial ablation and resection. *Lancet* 351:1147, 1998.
Sharp, N. Microwaves for menorrhagia: a new fast technique for endometrial ablation. *Lancet* 346:1003, 1995.
Alexander, D. Randomised trial comparing hysterectomy with endometrial ablation for dysfunctional uterine bleeding: psychiatric and psychosocial aspects. *BMJ* 312:280, 1996.
O'Connor, H. Medical Research Council randomised trial of endometrial resection versus hysterectomy in management of menorrhagia. *Lancet* 349:897, 1997.
Carlson, K. Alternatives to hysterectomy for menorrhagia (editorial). *N Engl J Med* 335:198, 1996.
Andersson, J. Levonorgestrel-releasing intrauterine device in the treatment of menorrhagia. *Br J Obstet Gynaecol* 97:690, 1990.

Alternatives to hysterectomy for carcinoma in situ:
Jones, H. Treatment of cervical intraepithelial neoplasia. *Clin Obstet Gynecol* 33:826, 1990.
Wright T. Treatment of cervical intraepithelial neoplasia with loop electrosurgical excision procedure. *Obstet Gynecol* 79:173, 1992.

Alternatives to hysterectomy for endometrial hyperplasia, genital prolapse, endometriosis, chronic pelvic pain:
Carlson, K. Indications for hysterectomy. *N Engl J Med* 328:856, 1993.
Ravnikar, V. Hysterectomies. Where are the indications? *Obstet Gynecol Clin North Am* 21:405, 1994.
Grimes, D. Shifting indications for hysterectomy: nature, nurture, or neither? (commentary) *Lancet* 344:1652, 1994.
Bachmann, G. Hysterectomy: a critical review. *J Reprod Med* 35:839, 1990.
Peters, A. A randomized clinical trial to compare two different approaches in women with chronic pelvic pain. *Obstet Gynecol* 77:740, 1991.

Vaginal hysterectomy is associated with fewer complications:
Casey, M. A critical analysis of laparoscopic assisted vaginal hysterectomies compared with vaginal hysterectomies. *J Gynaecol Surg* 10:7, 1994.
Dicker, R. Complications of abdominal and vaginal hysterectomy among women of reproductive age in the United States: the Collaborative Review of Sterilization. *Am J Obstet Gynecol* 144:841, 1982.

Removal of cervix causes reduction in orgasms:
Kilkku, P. Supravaginal uterine amputation vs hysterectomy: effects on libido and orgasm. *Acta Obstet Gynaecol Scand* 62:147, 1983.

Removal of cervix increases risk of complications:
Drife, J. Conserving the cervix at hysterectomy. *Br J Obstet Gynaecol* 101:563, 1994.
Grimes, D. Shifting indications for hysterectomy: nature, nurture, or nei-ther? *Lancet* 344:1652, 1994.
Nathorst-Boos, J. Consumer's attitude to hysterectomy: the experience of 678 women. *Acta Obstet Gynaecol Scand* 71:230, 1992.

In Sweden 21 percent of hysterectomies leave the cervix:
Nathorst-Boos, J. Consumer's attitude to hysterectomy: the experience of 678 women. *Acta Obstet Gynaecol Scand* 71:230, 1992.

Seven hundred women would have to have their healthy ovaries removed to prevent one case of cancer:
Schweppe, K. Prophylactic oophorectomy. *Geburtshilfe Frauenheilkunde* 39: 1024, 1979.

Chapter 11. Building Strong Bones

For the first five years after menopause, women lose 5 to 8 percent of their bone mass:
Ross, P. Osteoporosis. Frequency, consequences, and risk factors. *Arch Intern Med* 156:1399, 1996.

Estrogen reduces a woman's risk of heart attack and stroke:
Heckbert, S. Duration of estrogen replacement therapy in relation to the risk of incident myocardial infarction in postmenopausal women. *Arch Intern Med* 157:1330, 1997.
Lobo, R. Benefits and risks of estrogen replacement therapy. *Am J Obstet Gynecol* 173:982, 1995.

"Eating a high-protein diet is like pouring acid rain on your bones":
Personal communication from Robert Heaney, M.D., specialist in osteoporo-sis from Creighton University, Omaha, Nebraska, to Tom Monte.

Bone-depleting factors: sedentary lifestyle, cigarette smoking, excess consumption of salt and caffeine:
Kannus, P. Effect of starting age of physical activity on bone mass in the domi-nant arm of tennis and squash players. *Ann Intern Med* 123:27, 1995.
Hopper, J. The bone density of female twins discordant for tobacco use. *N Engl J Med* 330:387, 1994.
Law, M. A meta-analysis of cigarette smoking, bone mineral density, and risk of hip fracture: recognition of a major effect. *BMJ* 315:841, 1997.
Need, A. Effect of salt restriction on urinary hydroxyproline excretion in postmenopausal women. *Arch Intern Med* 151:757, 1991.
Harris, S. Caffeine and bone loss in healthy postmenopausal women. *Am J Clin Nutr* 60:573, 1994.
Hernandez-Avila, M. Caffeine, moderate alcohol intake, and risk of fractures of the hip and forearm in middle-aged women. *Am J Clin Nutr* 54:157, 1991.

Osteoporosis is big business:
  Silverman, S. Effect of bone density information on decisions about hormone replacement therapy: a randomized trial. *Obstet Gynecol* 89:321, 1997.
  Sheldon, T. Bone densitometry in clinical practice. Clinical uses of densitometry are not yet proved (letter). *BMJ* 311:686, 1995.
  Ettinger, B. Use of bone densitometry results for decisions about therapy for osteoporosis (letter). *Ann Intern Med* 125:623, 1996.

Statistics on osteoporosis:
  Ross, P. Osteoporosis. Frequency, consequences, and risk factors. *Arch Intern Med* 156:1399, 1996.
  Cummings, S. Risk factors for hip fracture in white women. *N Engl J Med* 332:767, 1995.

Each year, about 10 percent of your skeleton is broken down in a process called resorption:
  Heaney, R. Menopausal changes in bone remodeling. *J Lab Clin Med* 92:964, 1978.

"You only have the bones you need. The more demands you make of your body in the form of exercise, the more bone you produce"; Tufts' exercise recommendations:
  Personal communication from Roger Fielding, exercise physiologist, U.S. Department of Agriculture's Human Nutrition Research Center on Aging, Tufts University, Boston, to Tom Monte.

Osteoporosis is formally defined as loss of bone density and strength and is not caused by calcium deficiency:
  Consensus Development Conference. Prophylaxis and treatment of osteoporosis. *Am J Med* 90:107, 1991.

American women are big calcium consumers but have high levels of osteoporosis:
  Abelow, B. Cross-cultural association between dietary animal protein and hip fracture: a hypothesis. *Calcif Tissue Int* 50:14, 1992.

A fifty-year-old woman faces a 17.5 percent chance that she will fracture her hip:
  Donaldson, L. Incidence of fractures in a geographically defined population. *J Epidemiol Community Health* 44:241, 1990.
  Compston, J. Bone densitometry in clinical practice. *BMJ* 310:1507, 1995.

Actual calcium requirements of people are quite small:
  Heaney, R. Calcium nutrition and bone health in the elderly. *Am J Clin Nutr* 36:986, 1982.
  Paterson, C. Calcium requirements in man: a critical review. *Postgrad Med J* 54:244, 1978.

Worldwide the more animal protein consumed the more osteoporosis:
  Abelow, B. Cross-cultural association between dietary animal protein and hip fracture: a hypothesis. *Calcif Tissue Int* 50:14, 1992.

Acidification from animal protein dissolves the bones—plants are usually alkaline:
  Sebastian, A. Improved mineral balance and skeletal metabolism in post-

menopausal women treated with potassium bicarbonate. *N Engl J Med* 330:1776, 1994.

Sebastian, A. Improved mineral balance and skeletal metabolism in post-menopausal women treated with potassium bicarbonate (letter). *N Engl J Med* 331:279, 1994.

Excess consumption of animal protein causes calcium losses in people in natural living conditions:

Hu, J. Dietary intakes and urinary excretion of calcium and acids: a cross-sectional study of women in China. *Am J Clin Nutr* 58:398, 1993.

Itoh, R. Dietary protein intake and urinary excretion of calcium: a cross-sectional study in healthy Japanese population. *Am J Clin Nutr* 67:438, 1998.

Animal foods are rich sources of sulfa-containing amino acids.

Breslau, N. Relationship of animal protein-rich diet to kidney stone formation and calcium metabolism. *J Clin Endocrinol Metab* 66:140, 1988.

Trilok, G. Sources of protein-induced endogenous acid production and excretion by human adults. *Calcif Tissue Int* 44:335, 1989.

Methionine is twice as prevalent in meats as it is in grains; there is five times more methionine in beef as there is in beans:

Brockis, J. The effects of vegetable and animal protein diets on calcium, urate, and oxalate excretion. *Br J Urology* 54:590, 1982.

Doubling the protein increases calcium loss by 50 percent:

Hegsted, M. Urinary calcium and calcium balance in young men as affected by level of protein and phosphorus intake. *J Nutr* 111:553, 1981.

A study of thirty-eight women found protein intake associated with wrist bone density:

Metz, J. Intakes of calcium, phosphorus, and protein, and physical activity level are related to radial bone mass in young adult women. *Am J Clin Nutr* 58:537, 1993.

In five districts of China calcium loss was found to be associated with animal protein:

Hu, J. Dietary intakes and urinary excretion of calcium and acids: a cross-sectional study of women in China. *Am J Clin Nutr* 58:398, 1993.

A study of 886 men and women found the more protein consumed, the more calcium lost:

Itoh, R. Sodium excretion in relation to calcium and hydroxyproline excretion in Japanese population. *Am J Clin Nutr* 63:735, 1996.

The Nurse's Health Study recently found 22 percent greater risk of forearm fractures:

Feskanich, D. Protein consumption and bone fractures in women. *Am J Epidemiol* 143:472, 1996.

Worldwide, osteoporosis increases with the consumption of dairy products and calcium supplements:

Hu, J. Dietary intakes and urinary excretion of calcium and acids: a cross-sectional study of women in China. *Am J Clin Nutr* 58:398, 1993.

Abelow, B. Cross-cultural association between dietary animal protein and hip fracture: a hypothesis. *Calcif Tissue Int* 50:14, 1992.

Most of the world's population consumes only 300 to 500 milligrams of calcium each day:
Ho, S. Determinants of bone mass in the Chinese old-old population. *Osteoporos Int* 5:161, 1995.
Haines, C. Dietary calcium intake in postmenopausal Chinese women. *Eur J Clin Nutr* 48:591, 1994.

Dairy protein from skim milk causes calcium loss and a negative calcium balance:
Recker, R. The effect of milk supplements on calcium metabolism, bone metabolism, and calcium balance. *Am J Clin Nutr* 41:254, 1985.

A study of 84,484 nurses found drinking coffee increased the risk of hip fracture:
Hernandez-Avila, M. Caffeine, moderate alcohol intake, and risk of fractures of the hip and forearm in middle-aged women. *Am J Clin Nutr* 54:157, 1991.

Excess salt consumption has also been shown to promote calcium loss:
Need, A. Effect of salt restriction on urinary hydroxyproline excretion in postmenopausal women. *Arch Intern Med* 151:757, 1991.

Women who smoke lose an average of 5 to 10 percent more bone mass than nonsmokers:
Hopper, J. The bone density of female twins discordant for tobacco use. *N Engl J Med* 330:387, 1994.

The role of dietary calcium remains controversial:
Jones, G. Progressive loss of bone in the femoral neck in elderly people: longitudinal findings from Dubbo osteoporosis epidemiology. *BMJ* 309:691, 1994.

Calcium inhibits iron absorption:
Hallberg, L. Calcium: effect of different amounts of nonheme- and heme-iron absorption in humans. *Am J Clin Nutr* 53:112, 1991.
Cook, J. Calcium supplementation: effect on iron absorption. *Am J Clin Nutr* 53:106, 1991.

That same 300 mg calcium supplement will also increase your risk of kidney stones:
Curhan, G. Comparison of dietary calcium with supplemental calcium and other nutrients as factors affecting the risk of kidney stones in women. *Ann Intern Med* 126:497, 1997.

Many supplements are contaminated with significant amounts of lead and/or aluminum:
Whiting, S. Safety of some calcium supplements questioned. *Nutrition Reviews* 52:95, 1994.

Calcium citrate increase absorption of aluminum:
Nolan, C. Aluminum and lead absorption from dietary sources in women ingesting calcium citrate. *South Med J* 87:894, 1994.

Aluminum makes the bones more fragile by inhibiting mineralization:
Mjoberg, B. Aluminum, Alzheimer's disease, and bone fragility. *Acta Orthop Scand* 68:511, 1997.

Aluminum plays an important role in the cause of Alzheimer's disease:
  Shin, R. Interaction of aluminum with paired helical filament tau is involved in neurofibrillary pathology of Alzheimer's disease. *Gerontology* 43 (Suppl 1): 16, 1997.
  Armstrong, R. Aluminium and Alzheimer's disease: review of possible pathogenic mechanisms. *Dementia* 7(1):1, 1996.
  Shin, R. Neurofibrillary pathology and aluminum in Alzheimer's disease. *Histol Histopathol* 10:969, 1995.
  McLachlan, D. Aluminium and the pathogenesis of Alzheimer's disease: a summary of evidence. *Ciba Found Symp* 169:87, 1992.

Animal fat plays a role in the cause of Alzheimer's disease:
  Kalmijn, S. Dietary fat intake and the risk of incident dementia in the Rotterdam Study. *Ann Neurol* 42:776, 1997.

Chapter 12. Monitoring Bone Health and Choosing Treatment

Half of all spinal fractures are asymptomatic:
  Ross, P. Pain and disability associated with new vertebral fractures and other spine conditions. *J Clin Epidemiol* 47:231, 1994.

A single spinal fracture means three times the risk of a future fracture:
  Ross, P. Pre-existing fractures and bone mass predict vertebral fracture incidence in women. *Ann Intern Med* 114:919, 1991.

Bone mineral density testing techniques and interpretation:
  Miller, P. Clinical utility of bone mass measurements in adults: consensus of an international panel. *Semin Arthritis Rheum* 25:361, 1996.
  Hagiwara, S. Noninvasive bone mineral density measurement in the evaluation of osteoporosis. *Rheum Dis Clin N Am* 20:651, 1994.
  Johnston, C. Identification of patients with low bone mass by single photon absorptiometry and single-energy x-ray absorptiometry. *Am J Med* 98 (suppl 2A):37S, 1995.
  Rizzoli, R. The role of dual energy x-ray absorptiometry of lumbar spine and proximal femur in the diagnosis and follow-up of osteoporosis. *Am J Med* 98 (suppl 2A):33S, 1995.
  Baran, D. Quantitative ultrasound: a technique to target women with low bone mass for preventive therapy. *Am J Med* 98 (suppl 2A):48S, 1995.
  Hans, D. Ultrasonographic heel measurements to predict hip fracture in elderly women: the EPIDOS prospective study. *Lancet* 348:511, 1996.
  Kanis, J. The diagnosis of osteoporosis. *J Bone Min Res* 9:1137, 1994.

Lowest BMD group (those with scores of 22.5) have 8.5 times the risk of fracture:
  Cummings, S. Bone density at various sites for prediction of hip fracture. *Lancet* 341:72, 1993.

A low BMD and one previous fracture means twenty-five times higher risk of another fracture:
  Ross, P. Pre-existing fractures and bone mass predict vertebral fracture incidence in women. *Ann Intern Med* 114:919, 1991.

Best age for BMD is between sixty and sixty-five:
Tayler, E. Measurement of bone density in osteoporosis (letter). *BMJ* 311: 263, 1995.
Bone densitometry. *Med Lett Drugs Ther* 38:103, 1996.
Compston, J. Bone densitometry in clinical practice. *BMJ* 310:1507, 1995.
Ettinger, B. Use of bone densitometry results for decisions about therapy for osteoporosis (letter). *Ann Intern Med* 125:623, 1996.

No significant difference in bone strength when women start hormone replacement therapy at menopause or after age sixty:
Schneider, D. Timing of postmenopausal estrogen for optimal bone mineral density. The Rancho Bernardo Study. *JAMA* 277:543, 1997.

Any skeletal site is equally useful for making the diagnosis of osteoporosis:
Melton, L. Long-term fracture prediction by bone mineral assessed at different skeletal sites. *J Bone Min Res* 8:1227, 1993.

Bone turnover speeds up at menopause and peaks between one and three years after:
Stepan, J. Bone loss and biochemical indices of bone remodeling in surgically induced premenopausal women. *Bone* 8:279, 1987.

Crosslinks increase significantly after menopause, indicating increased resorption:
Delmas, P. Biochemical markers of bone turnover I: theoretical consideration and clinical use in osteoporosis. *Am J Med* 95 (suppl 5A): 11S, 1993.
Riis, B. Biochemical markers of bone turnover II: diagnosis, prophylaxis, and treatment of osteoporosis. *Am J Med* 95 (suppl 5A): 17S, 1993.

"Fast losers" of bone lost 50 percent more bone than slow losers:
Hansen, M. Role of peak bone mass and bone loss in postmenopausal osteoporosis: 12-year study. *BMJ* 303:961, 1991.

Combination of both tests, BMD and crosslinks, is best for determining treatment needs:
Riis, B. The role of bone loss. *Am J Med* 98 (suppl 2A):29S, 1995.
Raisz, L. The osteoporosis revolution. *Ann Intern Med* 126:458, 1997.

Crosslinks testing predicted which women would respond to calcitonin:
Civitelli, R. Bone turnover in postmenopausal osteoporosis. Effect of calcitonin treatment. *J Clin Invest* 82:1268, 1988.

Osteoporosis testing has become big business:
Silverman, S. Effect of bone density information on decisions about hormone replacement therapy: a randomized trial. *Obstet Gynecol* 89:321, 1997.
Sheldon, T. Bone densitometry in clinical practice. Clinical uses of densitometry are not yet proved (letter). *BMJ* 311:686, 1995.
Ettinger, B. Use of bone densitometry results for decisions about therapy for osteoporosis (letter). *Ann Intern Med* 125:623, 1996.

Of similar predictive value are a history of maternal hip fracture, weight loss since age twenty-five, and the habit of standing for less than four hours:
Cummings, S. Risk factors for hip fracture in white women. *N Engl J Med* 332:767, 1995.

Dr. Deborah Marshall can't justify screening programs:
   Marshall, D. Ability of bone mineral density to predict osteoporotic fractures (letter). *Lancet* 313:561, 1996.
   Marshall, D. Meta-analysis of how well measures of bone mineral density predict occurrence of osteoporotic fractures. *BMJ* 312:1254, 1996.

There is very little hard scientific evidence proving the effectiveness of HRT therapy:
   Cummings, R. Commentary on meta-analysis: bone mineral density measurement predicts risk for fractures in women. *ACP Journal Club* Sept/Oct 1996, 48.

Difference in BMD between patients with fractures and controls are too small for effective screening:
   Law, M. Strategies for prevention of osteoporosis and hip fracture. *BMJ* 303:453, 1991.

The effectiveness of preventing fractures has not been established by properly done prospective studies:
   Lange, S. Hormone replacement therapy. Be cautious about using HRT for women without symptoms of oestrogen deficiency. *BMJ* 314:1415, 1997.

Consensus view is that population-based screening cannot be justified at present:
   Compston, J. Bone densitometry in clinical practice. *BMJ* 310:1507, 1995.

It would cost $6 billion to "screen" every woman in the United States near menopause for BMD:
   Norris, R. Medical cost of osteoporosis. *Bone* 13:S11, 1992.

BMD test should be used to motivate women to accept or continue HRT:
   Johnston, C. Risk assessment: theoretical considerations. *Am J Med* 95 (suppl 5A): 2S, 1993.

Magnitude of force is actually more important than frequency of exercise:
   Taaffe, D. Differential effects of swimming versus weight bearing activity on bone mineral status of eumenorrheic athletes. *J Bone Miner Res* 10:586, 1995.
   Whalen, R. Influences of physical activity on the regulation of bone density. *J Biomech* 21:825, 1988.

The results of the Postmenopausal Estrogen/Progestin Interventions Trial:
   The Writing Group for the PEPI Trial. Effects of hormone therapy on bone mineral density. Results from the Postmenopausal Estrogen/Progestin Interventions (PEPI) Trial. *JAMA* 276:1389, 1996.

Estrogen replacement therapy for six years leads to BMD values 10 percent higher than those of untreated women and reduces fractures by about 50 percent:
   Cauley, J. Estrogen replacement therapy and fractures in older women. *Ann Intern Med* 122:9, 1995.

Designer Estrogens:
   Raloxifene for postmenopausal osteoporosis. *Med Lett Drugs Ther* 40:29, 1998.

El-Hajj Fuleihan, G. Tissue-specific estrogens—the promise for the future. *N Engl J Med* 337:1686, 1997.

Rifkind, B. Designer drugs, magic bullets, and gold standards. *JAMA* 279: 1483, 1998.

994 postmenopausal women with osteoporosis were treated with Fosamax or a placebo:

Liberman, U. Effect of oral alendronate on bone mineral density and incidence of fractures in postmenopausal osteoporosis. *N Engl J Med* 333: 1437, 1995.

Fosamax reduces hip fractures:

Karpf, D. Prevention of nonvertebral fractures by Alendronate. A meta-analysis. *JAMA* 277:1159, 1997.

Hosking, D. Prevention of bone loss with alendronate in postmenopausal women under 60 years of age. *N Engl J Med* 338:485, 1998.

Severe esophageal side effects of Fosamax:

Groen, P. Esophagitis associated with the use of alendronate. *N Engl J Med* 335:1016, 1996.

Long-term calcitonin treatment results in measurable increases in BMD:

Reginster, J. Calcitonin for prevention and treatment of osteoporosis. *Am J Med* 95 (suppl 5A):44S, 1993.

Benefits of calcium, vitamin D, and fluoride treatments not great:

Wood, A. Treatment of postmenopausal osteoporosis. *N Engl J Med* 338:736, 1998.

Eastell, R. Gains in bone mineral density with resolution of vitamin D intoxication. *Ann Intern Med* 127:203, 1997.

Lips, P. Vitamin D supplementation and fracture incidence in elderly persons. A randomized placebo-controlled clinical trial. *Ann Intern Med* 124:400, 1996.

Chapter 13. Balancing the Positives and Negatives of Hormone Replacement Therapy

Oral estrogen appears to slow the body's rate of fat burning and increase body fat:

Poehlman, E. Changes in energy balance and body composition at menopause: a controlled longitudinal study. *Ann Intern Med* 123:673, 1995.

O'Sullivan, A. Estrogen, lipid oxidation, and body fat (letter). *N Engl J Med* 333:669, 1995.

Many women actually enjoy sex more after menopause:

Butler, R. Love and sex after 60: how to evaluate and treat the sexually-active woman. *Geriatrics* 49:33, 1994.

Koster, A. Sexual desire and menopausal development. A prospective study of Danish women born in 1936. *Maturitas* 16:49, 1993.

Fibroids and fibrocystic breast disease naturally regress after menopause unless you use estrogen:

Sener, A. The effects of hormone replacement therapy on uterine fibroids in postmenopausal women. *Fertil Steril* 65:354, 1996.

Pastides, H. Estrogen replacement therapy and fibrocystic breast disease. *Am J Prev Med* 3:282, 1987.

Women who eat a low-fat, high-fiber diet experience menopause two years earlier:

Key, T. Sex hormones in women in rural China and Britain. *Br J Cancer* 62:631, 1990.

Armstrong, B. The role of diet in human carcinogenesis with special reference to endometrial cancer. In Hiatt, H. *Origins of human cancer. Cold Spring Harbor conferences on cell proliferation.* Vol 4 (Cold Spring Harbor, N.Y.: Cold Spring Harbor Laboratory, 1977), 557.

Baird, D. Do vegetarians have earlier menopause? Proceedings of the Society of Epidemiology Research. *Am J Epidemiol,* 107, 1988.

Alcohol consumption raises estrogen levels and delays menopause:

Ginsburg, E. Effects of alcohol ingestion on estrogens in postmenopausal women. *JAMA* 276:1747, 1996.

Stress and alcohol are factors in hot flashes:

Gannon, L. Correlates of menopausal hot flashes. *J Behav Med* 10:277, 1987.

Weight gain is the result of a decrease in physical activity and the amount of energy burned:

O'Sullivan, A. Estrogen, lipid oxidation, and body fat (letter). *N Engl J Med* 333:669, 1995.

Japanese women rarely complain of unpleasant menopausal symptoms:

Lock, M. Menopause in Japanese women (letter). *JAMA* 274:1265, 1995.

Adlercreutz, H. Dietary phyto-oestrogens and the menopause in Japan. *Lancet* 339:1233, 1992.

Lock, M. Contested meanings of menopause. *Lancet* 337:1270, 1991.

"There appears to be no 'midlife crisis' for the majority of Japanese women":

Lock, M. Menopause in Japanese women (letter). *JAMA* 274:1265, 1995.

There is no word for hot flashes in the Japanese language:

Lock, M. Contested meanings of menopause. *Lancet* 337:1270, 1991.

Avis, N. The evolution of menopausal symptoms. *Bailliere's Clin Endo Metab* 7:17, 1993.

Phytoestrogens mitigate menopausal symptoms and reduce cancer risk:

Peterson, G. Genistein inhibition of the growth of human cancer cells: independence from estrogens and the multi-drug resistance gene. *Biochem Biophys Res Com* 179:661, 1991.

Sixty grams of soy protein changes balance of hormones to inhibit breast cancer:

Cassidy, A. Biological effects of a diet of soy protein rich in isoflavones on the menstrual cycle of premenopausal women. *Am J Clin Nutr* 60:333, 1994.

Vegetarians have much higher levels of phytoestrogens than meat eaters:

Adlercreutz, H. Quantitative determination of lignans and isoflavonoids in plasma of omnivorous and vegetarian women by isotope dilution gas chromatography-mass spectrometry. *Scan J Clin Lab Invest Suppl* 215:5, 1993.

Levels of phytoestrogen in women on a macrobiotic diet, lacto-ovo-vegetarians, and meat eaters:

Adlercreutz, H. Determination of urinary lignans and phytoestrogen metabolites, potential antiestrogens, and anticarcinogens, in urine of women on various diets. *J Steroid Biochem* 25:791, 1986.

Japanese women have sixty to one hundred times higher levels of phytoestrogens in their urine than Finnish women do:

Adlercreutz, H. Dietary phyto-oestrogens and the menopause in Japan. *Lancet* 339:1233, 1992.

Benefits of HRT:

Quigley, M. Estrogen therapy arrests bone loss in elderly women. *Am J Obstet Gynecol* 156:1516, 1987.

Naessen, T. Hormone replacement therapy and risk for first hip fracture. A prospective, population-based cohort study. *Ann Intern Med* 113:95, 1990.

Jacobs, H. Postmenopausal hormone replacement therapy. *BMJ* 305:1403, 1992.

Belchetz, P. Hormonal treatment of postmenopausal women. *N Engl J Med* 330:1062, 1994.

Tang, M. Effect of oestrogen during menopause on risk and age at onset of Alzheimer's disease. *Lancet* 348:429, 1996.

Raz, R. A controlled trial of intravaginal estriol in postmenopausal women with recurrent urinary tract infections. *N Engl J Med* 329:753, 1993.

A significant amount of the reduction seen in heart disease is due to healthier lifestyles, not HRT:

Cauley, J. Estrogen replacement therapy and mortality among older women. The study of osteoporotic fractures. *Arch Intern Med* 157:2181, 1997.

Whooley, M. Postmenopausal hormone therapy and mortality (letter). *N Engl J Med* 337:1389, 1997.

Green, J. Postmenopausal hormone therapy and mortality (letter). *N Engl J Med* 337:1390, 1997.

Hemminki, E. Impact of postmenopausal hormone therapy on cardiovascular events and cancer: pooled data from clinical trials. *BMJ* 315:149, 1997.

Barrett-Connor, E. Postmenopausal estrogen and prevention bias. *Ann Intern Med* 115:455, 1991.

No reduction in cardiovascular mortality from estrogens in these studies:

Sidney, S. Myocardial infarction and the use of estrogen and estrogen-progestogen in postmenopausal women. *Ann Intern Med* 127:501, 1997.

Barrett-Connor, E. Prospective study of endogenous sex hormones and fatal cardiovascular disease in postmenopausal women. *BMJ* 311:1193, 1995.

Wilson, P. Postmenopausal estrogen use, cigarette smoking, and cardiovascular mortality in women over 50. *N Engl J Med* 313:1038, 1985.

Hazards of HRT:
Collaborative Group on Hormonal Factors in Breast Cancer. Breast cancer and hormone replacement therapy: collaborative reanalysis of data from 51 epidemiological studies of 52,705 women with breast cancer and 108,411 women without breast cancer. *Lancet* 350:1047, 1997.
Jacobs, H. Postmenopausal hormone replacement therapy. *BMJ* 305:1403, 1992.
Colditz, G. The use of estrogens and progestins and the risk of breast cancer in postmenopausal women. *N Engl J Med* 332:1589, 1995.
Gutthann, S. Hormone replacement therapy and risk of venous thromboembolism: population based case-control study. *BMJ* 314:796, 1997.

Only 20 to 30 percent of all menopausal women actually begin HRT, and about half stop shortly after starting:
Silverman, S. Effect of bone density information on decisions about hormone replacement therapy: a randomized trial. *Obstet Gynecol* 89:321, 1997.

Improvements in symptoms are the most reliable indications that the treatment is correct:
Lange, S. Be cautious about using HRT for women without symptoms of oestrogen deficiency (letter). *BMJ* 314:1415, 1997.

Oral estrogen appears to slow the body's rate of fat burning and increases body fat:
Poehlman, E. Changes in energy balance and body composition at menopause: a controlled longitudinal study. *Ann Intern Med* 123:673, 1995.

Estrogen therapy increases the risk of gallbladder disease by 2.5 times:
A report from the Boston Collaborative Drug Surveillance Program, Boston University Medical Center: Surgically confirmed gallbladder disease, venous thrombosis, and breast tumors in relation to postmenopausal estrogen therapy. *N Engl J Med* 290:15, 1974.

Women who use estrogen with synthetic progestin for more than five years have an increased risk of uterine cancer:
Beresford, S. Risk of endometrial cancer in relation to use of oestrogen combined with cyclic progestagen therapy in postmenopausal women. *Lancet* 349:458, 1997.
Pike, M. Estrogen-progesterone therapy and endometrial cancer. *J Natl Cancer Inst* 89:1110, 1997.

Synthetic progestin (Provera) may actually increase the risk of breast cancer:
Bergkvist, L. The risk of breast cancer after estrogen and estrogen-progestin replacement. *N Engl J Med* 321:293, 1989.
Stanford, J. Exogenous progestins and breast cancer. *Epidemiol Rev* 15:98, 1993.

Unlike natural progesterone, Provera has an adverse effect on blood cholesterol and triglyceride levels:

Ottosson, U. Subfractions of high-density lipoprotein cholesterol during estrogen replacement therapy: a comparison between progestogens and natural progesterone. *Am J Obstet Gynecol* 151:746, 1985.

Burkman, R. Lipid and lipoprotein changes in relation to oral contraception and hormonal replacement therapy. *Fertil Steril* 49 (suppl):39S, 1988.

The Writing Group for the PEPI Trial. Effects of estrogen or estrogen/progestin regimens on heart disease risk factors in postmenopausal women. The Postmenopausal Estrogen/Progestin Interventions (PEPI) Trial. *JAMA* 273:199, 1995.

Adams, M. Medroxyprogesterone acetate antagonizes inhibitory effects of conjugated equine estrogens on coronary artery atherosclerosis. *Arterioscler Thromb Vasc Biol* 17:217, 1997.

The liver removes hormones taken by mouth:

Chetkowski, R. Biologic effects of transdermal estradiol. *N Engl J Med* 314: 1615, 1986.

Without the liver's involvement there is no improvement in blood cholesterol levels:

Walsh, B. Effects of postmenopausal estrogen replacement on the concentration and metabolism of plasma lipoproteins. *N Engl J Med* 325:1196, 1991.

Transdermal route minimizes adverse effects of HRT:

Whitehead, M. Transdermal administration of oestrogen/progestagen hormone replacement therapy. *Lancet* 335:310, 1990.

Transdermal estrogen effective at preventing osteoporosis:

Lufkin, E. Treatment of postmenopausal osteoporosis with transdermal estrogen. *Ann Intern Med* 117:1, 1992.

Skin patch does not elevate blood fats, or triglycerides:

O'Sullivan, A. Estrogen, lipid oxidation, and body fat (letter). *N Engl J Med* 333:669, 1995.

Women using the patch also avoid the weight gain associated with taking oral estrogen:

Linn, E. Clinical significance of the androgenicity of progestins in hormonal therapy in women. *Clin Ther* 12:447, 1990.

Estrogen relieves stress incontinence in about 50 percent of women and prevents urethra inflammation:

Samsioe, G. Occurrence, nature, and treatment of urinary incontinence in a 70-year-old female population. *Maturitas* 7:335, 1985.

Raz, R. A controlled trial of intravaginal estriol in postmenopausal women with recurrent urinary tract infections. *N Engl J Med* 329:753, 1993.

As little as 7.5 micrograms (mcg) of estradiol administered through vaginal tissues result in a 2.1 percent increase in forearm bone density:

Naessen, T. Bone loss in elderly women prevented by ultralow doses of parental 17β-estradiol. *Am J Obstet Gynecol* 177:115, 1997.

No significant difference in bone density when women start taking estrogen at menopause or after age sixty:

Schneider, D. Timing of postmenopausal estrogen for optimal bone mineral density. The Rancho Bernardo Study. *JAMA* 277:543, 1997.

Michaelsson, K. Hormone replacement therapy and risk of hip fracture: population based case-control study. *BMJ* 316:1858, 1998.

Progestins increase the risk of breast cancer, while natural progesterone lowers it:

Lewis, P. Risk factors for breast cancer (letter). *BMJ* 309:1662, 1994.

McPherson, K. Breast cancer and hormonal supplements in postmenopausal women. Among current users of combined supplements the risk rises with five or more years' treatment. *BMJ* 311:699, 1995.

Going, J. Proliferative and secretory activity in human breast during natural and artificial menstrual cycles. *Am J Pathol* 130:193, 1988.

Persson, I. Combined oestrogen-progestogen replacement and breast cancer risk (letter). *Lancet* 340:1044, 1992.

Colditz, G. The use of estrogens and progestins and the risk of breast cancer in postmenopausal women. *N Engl J Med* 332:1589, 1995.

Bergkvist, L. The risk of breast cancer after estrogen and estrogen-progestin replacement. *N Engl J Med* 321:293, 1989.

Bergkvist, L. Breast cancer and estrogen replacement (letter). *N Engl J Med* 322:204, 1990.

Pike, M. Estrogens, progestogens, normal breast cell proliferation, and breast cancer risk. *Epidemiol Rev* 15:17, 1993.

Stanford, J. Exogenous progestins and breast cancer. *Epidemiol Rev* 15:98, 1993.

Chang, K. Influences of percutaneous administration of estradiol and progesterone on human breast epithelial cell cycle in vivo. *Fertil Steril* 63:785, 1995.

Progesterone reverses the precancerous changes in the uterus caused by estrogen:

Paterson, M. Endometrial disease after treatment with oestrogens and progestogens in the climacteric. *BMJ* 1:822, 1980.

Clarke, C. Progestin regulation of cell proliferation. *Endocr Rev* 11:266, 1990.

Affinito, P. Endometrial hyperplasia: efficacy of a new treatment with a vaginal cream containing natural micronized progesterone. *Maturitas* 20:191, 1994.

Progesterone benefits PMS:

Dennerstein, L. Progesterone and the premenstrual syndrome: a double blind crossover trial. *BMJ* 290:1617, 1985.

Progesterone cream can reverse the precancerous changes in breast tissue:

Chang, K. Influences of percutaneous administration of estradiol and progesterone on human breast epithelial cell cycle in vivo. *Fertil Steril* 63:785, 1995.

Assessment of cancer protection from progesterone by ultrasound tests or endometrial biopsy:

Castelo-Branco, C. Transvaginal sonography of the endometrium in postmenopausal women: monitoring the effect of hormone replacement therapy. *Maturitas* 19:59, 1994.

Vaginal progesterone creams relieve breast pain in 65 percent of menstruating women:

Nappi, C. Double-blind controlled trial of progesterone vaginal cream treatment for cyclic mastodynia in women with benign breast disease. *J Endocrinol Invest* 15:801, 1992.

Progesterone has bone-building benefits:

Prior, J. Progesterone as a bone-tropic hormone. *Endocrine Rev* 11:386, 1990.

Lee, J. Osteoporosis reversal with transdermal progesterone (letter). *Lancet* 336:1327, 1990.

Lee, J. Osteoporosis reversal, the role of progesterone. *Int Clin Nutr Rev* 10:384, 1990.

Adverse side effects of testosterone include elevation of blood cholesterol and development of male cosmetic features; effects of testosterone:

Rosenberg, M. Estrogen-androgen for hormone replacement. A review. *J Reprod Med* 42:394, 1997.

Kaunitz, A. The role of androgens in menopausal hormonal replacement. *Endocrinol Metab Clin North Am* 26:391, 1997.

Sherwin, B. Effects of parenteral administration of estrogen and androgen on plasma hormone levels and hot flashes in the surgical menopause. *Am J Obstet Gynecol* 148:552, 1984.

Methyltestosterone is toxic to the liver:

Murray-Lyon, I. Hepatic complications of androgen therapy. *Gastroenterology* 73:1461, 1977.

Premarin consists of many horse estrogens:

Adams, W. Conjugated estrogens bioequivalence: comparison of four products in postmenopausal women. *J Pharmocol Sci* 68:986, 1979.

Ethical issues of animal abuse concerning the use of Premarin:

Minerva. *BMJ* 309:1382, 1994.

Cox, D. Should a doctor prescribe hormone replacement therapy which has been manufactured from mare's urine? *J Med Ethics* 22:199, 1996.

150 herbs traditionally used by herbalists for treating a variety of health problems:

Zava, D. Estrogen and progestin bioactivity of foods, herbs, and spices. *Proc Soc Exp Biol Med* 21:369, 1998.

For black cohosh, a recent study found no sign of estrogen activity on rats:

Einer-Jensen, N. Cimicifuga and Melbrosia lack oestrogenic effects in mice and rats. *Maturitas* 25:149, 1996.

When 110 women took black cohosh, luteinizing hormone was decreased 20 percent:
    Duker, E. Effects of extracts from Cimicifuga racemosa on gonadotropin release in menopausal women and ovariectomized rats. *Planta Med* 57:420, 1991.

Women in the black cohosh group had greater relief of menopausal symptoms, anxiety, and depression:
    Warnecke, G. Using phyto-treatment to influence menopausal symptoms. *Med Welt* 36:871, 1985.
    Stoll, W. Phytotherapy influences atrophic vaginal epithelium. *Theripeuticon* 1:23, 1987.

Black cohosh relieves hot flashes, profuse perspiration, headache, dizziness . . . :
    Lehmann, W. Clinical and endocrinologic examinations about therapy of climacteric symptoms following hysterectomy with remaining ovaries. *Zentralblatt Gynakol* 110:611, 1988.
    Stolze, H. The other way to treat symptoms of menopause. *Gyne* 1:14, 1982.

Ingestion of large doses of black cohosh may result in nausea, vomiting, and miscarriage:
    The Lawrence Review of Natural Products, September 1992.

Chaste berry extracts inhibit prolactin secretion of rat pituitary cells:
    Sliutz, G. Agnus castus extracts inhibit prolactin secretion of rat pituitary cells. *Horm Metab Res* 25:253, 1993.

After three months of chaste berry therapy prolactin release was reduced and estrogen increased:
    Milewicz, A. Vitex agnus castus in the treatment of luteal phase defects due to latent hyperprolactinemia. Results of a randomized placebo-controlled double-blind study. *Arzneimittelforschung* 43:752, 1993.

Licorice has estrogenic effects:
    Costello, C. Estrogenic substances from plants: I Glycyrrhiza. *J Am Pharm Soc* 39:177, 1950.
    Kumagai, A. Effect of glycyrrhizin on estrogen action. *Endocrinol Japan* 14:34, 1967.
    Tamaya, T. Inhibition by plant herb extracts of steroid binding in uterus, liver, and serum of the rabbit. *Acta Obstet Gynaecol Scand* 65:839, 1986.

Ginseng is known to have estrogenic activity:
    Carr, B. Oestrogen-like effect of ginseng. *BMJ* 281:1110, 1980.

Ginseng face cream caused vaginal bleeding in a postmenopausal woman:
    Hopkins, M. Ginseng face cream and unexplained vaginal bleeding. *Am J Obstet Gynecol* 159:1121, 1988.

Hops appear to have an estrogen effect and bind to estrogen receptors of human cells:
    Zava, D. Estrogen and progestin bioactivity of foods, herbs, and spices. *Proc Soc Exp Biol Med* 21:369, 1998.

Dong quai stimulates uterine tissue:

Harada, M. Effect of Japanese angelica root and peony root on uterine contraction in the rabbit in situ. *J Pharmacobiodyn* 7:304, 1984.

Chang, S. Stimulating action of Carthamus tinctorius L., Angelica sinensis (Oliv.) Diels, and Leonurus sibircus L. on the uterus. *Chung Kuo Chung Yao Tsa Chih* 20:173, 1995.

A study of seventy-one postmenopausal women found no differences between the dong quai and a placebo:

Hirata, J. Does dong quai have estrogenic effects in postmenopausal women? A double-blind, placebo-controlled trial. *Fertil Steril* 68:981, 1997.

St. John's wort extracts were found to be about as effective as standard antidepressants:

Linde, K. St John's wort for depression—an overview and meta-analysis of randomised clinical trials. *BMJ* 313:253, 1996.

The Medical Letter Inc., St John's wort. *Med Lett Drugs Ther* 39:107, 1997.

Benefits from gingko have been reported for poor circulation:

Kleinjnen, J. Gingko biloba. *Lancet* 340:1136, 1992.

Gingko has been shown to slow the progress of dementia:

LeBars, P. A placebo-controlled, double-blind, randomized trial of an extract of gingko biloba for dementia. *JAMA* 278:1327, 1997.

Kleinjnen, J. Gingko biloba. *Lancet* 340:1136, 1992.

Kava reduced menopausal complaints after one week:

Warnecke, G. Psychosomatic dysfunction in the female climacteric. Clinical effectiveness and tolerance of Kava Extract WS 1409. *Fortschr Med* 109:119, 1991.

Kava found to have superior benefits over antidepressants and tranquilizers:

Volz, H. Kava-kava extract WS 1490 versus placebo in anxiety disorders—a randomized placebo-controlled 25-week outpatient trial. *Pharmacopsychiatry* 30:1, 1997.

Other research supporting kava's benefits:

Kinzler, E. Effect of a special kava extract in patients with anxiety-tension, and excitation states of non-psychotic genesis. Double blind study with placebos over 4 weeks. *Arzneimittelforschung* 41:584, 1991.

Use of kava for treating alcohol abuse and some forms of psychosis:

Cawte, J. Parameters of kava used as a challenge to alcohol. *Aust NZ J Psychiatry* 20:70, 1986.

Heavy kava users complain of poor health, a "puffy" face, and underweight:

Mathews, J. Effects of the heavy use of kava on physical health: summary of a pilot survey in an aboriginal community. *Med J Aust* 148:548, 1988.

Focus on a healthy starch-based diet, exercise, stress reduction:

Taunton, J. Exercise for the older woman: choosing the right prescription. *Br J Sports Med* 31:5, 1997.

Lucerno, M. Alternatives to estrogen for the treatment of hot flashes. *Ann Pharmacother* 31:915, 1997.

Exercise relieves mild depression and anxiety:

Daniel, M. Opiate receptor blockade by naltrexone and mood state after acute physical activity. *Br J Sports Med* 26:111, 1992.

Raglin, J. Exercise and mental health. Beneficial and detrimental effects. *Sports Med* 9:323, 1990.

Folkins, C. Physical fitness training and mental health. *Am Psychol* 36:373, 1981.

Carr, D. Physical conditioning facilitates the exercise-induced secretion of beta-endorphins and beta-lipotropin in women. *N Engl J Med* 305:560, 1981.

Greist, J. Running through your mind. *J Psycho-Somatic Res* 22:259, 1978.

Mersey, D. Health benefits of aerobic exercise. *Postgrad Med* 90:103, 1991.

Keith, R. Alterations in dietary carbohydrate, protein, and fat intake and mood state in trained female cyclists. *Med Sci Sports Exercise* 23:212, 1991.

A healthy, low-animal-protein diet allows the production of neurochemicals:

Wurtman, J. Carbohydrate craving in obese people: suppression by treatments affecting serotoninergic transmission. *Int J Eating Disorders* 1:2, 1981.

Wurtman, J. Effect of nutrient intake on premenstrual depression. *Am J Obstet Gynecol* 161:1228, 1989.

Wurtman, J. Behavioral effects of nutrients. *Lancet* 1:1145, 1983.

Glaeser, B. Changes in brain levels of acidic, basic, and neutral amino acids after consumption of single meals containing various portions of protein. *J Neurochem* 41:1016, 1983.

Lieberman, H. The effects of dietary neurotransmitter precursors on human behavior. *Am J Clin Nutr* 42:366, 1985.

Avoiding too much sleep is one of the most powerful antidepressants:

Wehr, T. Improvement of depression and triggering of mania by sleep deprivation. *JAMA* 267:548, 1992.

Wu, J. The biological basis of an antidepressant response to sleep deprivation and relapse: review and hypothesis. *Am J Psychiatry* 147:14, 1990.

Leibenluft, E. Is sleep deprivation useful in treatment of depression? *Am J Psychiatry* 149:159, 1992.

Wu, J. Effect of sleep deprivation on brain metabolism of depressed patients. *Am J Psychiatry* 149:538, 1992.

Chapter 14. Breaking the Cycle of Cardiovascular Disease

Statistics on cardiovascular disease in women:

Newnham, H. Women's hearts are hard to break. *Lancet* 349 (suppl 1):SI3, 1997.

Writing Group. Cardiovascular disease in women. A statement for healthcare professionals from the American Heart Association. *Circulation* 96:2468, 1997.

Women do not get the same kinds of treatment that men do for heart disease:

Schrott, H. Adherence to National Cholesterol Education Program treatment goals in postmenopausal women with heart disease. *JAMA* 277:1281, 1997.

Malacrida, R. A comparison of the early outcome of acute myocardial infarction in men and women. *N Engl J Med* 338:8, 1998.

Thomas, J. Coronary artery disease in women. A historical perspective. *Arch Intern Med* 158:333, 1998.

Coronary artery disease and women. Justifies equal opportunity management. *BMJ* 309:555, 1994.

Clarke, K. Do women with acute myocardial infarction receive the same treatment as men? *BMJ* 309:563, 1994.

Wilkinson, P. Acute myocardial infarction in women: survival analysis in first six months. *BMJ* 309:566, 1994.

Becker, R. Comparison of clinical outcomes for men and women after acute myocardial infarction. *Ann Intern Med* 120:638, 1994.

Karlson, B. Prognosis in myocardial infarction in relation to gender. *Am Heart J* 128:477, 1994.

Atherosclerosis causes hearing loss:

Rosen, S. Epidemiologic hearing studies in the USSR. *Arch Otolaryng* 91:424, 1970.

Rosen, S. Dietary prevention of hearing loss. *Arch Otolaryng* 70:242, 1970.

Spencer, J. Hyperlipoproteinemias in the etiology of inner ear disease. *Laryngoscope* 85:639, 1973.

Gates, G. The relation of hearing loss in the elderly to the presence of cardiovascular disease and cardiovascular risk factors. *Arch Otolaryngol Head Neck Surg* 119:156, 1993.

Cruickshanks, K. Cigarette smoking and hearing loss. The Epidemiology of Hearing Loss Study. *JAMA* 279:1715, 1998.

Atherosclerosis leads to ruptured discs and back pain:

Kauppila, L. Can low-back pain be due to lumbar-artery disease? *Lancet* 346:888, 1995.

Heliovaara, M. Low back pain and subsequent cardiovascular mortality. *Spine* 20:2109, 1995.

Kauppila, L. Prevalence of stenotic changes in arteries supplying the lumbar spine. A postmortem angiographic study on 140 subjects. *Ann Rheum Dis* 56:591, 1997.

Atherosclerosis causes impotence:

Virag, R. Is impotence an arterial disorder? A study of arterial risk factors in 440 impotent men. *Lancet* 1:181, 1985.

Morley, J. Sexual function with advancing age. *Med Clin North Am* 73:1483, 1989.

Rosen, M. Cigarette smoking: an independent risk factor for atherosclerosis in the hypogastric-cavernous arterial bed of men with arteriogenic impotence. *J Urol* 145:759, 1991.

Azadzoi, K. Study of etiologic relationship of arterial atherosclerosis to corporal veno-occlusive dysfunction in the rabbit. *J Urol* 155:1795, 1996.

The processes of atherosclerosis and thrombosis:

Ambrose J. Thrombosis in ischemic heart disease. *Arch Intern Med* 156:1382, 1996.

Steinberg, D. Beyond cholesterol. Modifications of low-density lipoprotein that increase its atherogenicity. *N Engl J Med* 320:915, 1989.

Fuster, V. The pathogenesis of coronary artery disease and the acute coronary syndromes (first of two parts). *N Engl J Med* 326:242, 1992.

Ulbricht, T. Coronary heart disease: seven dietary factors. *Lancet* 338:985, 1991.

Constantinides, P. Plaque fissuring in human coronary thrombosis. *J Atheroscler Res* 6:1, 1966.

Oliva, P. Pathophysiology of acute myocardial infarction, 1981. *Ann Intern Med* 94:236, 1981.

Davies, M. Plaque fissuring—the cause of acute myocardial infarction, sudden ischemic death, and crescendo angina. *Br Heart J* 53:363, 1985.

Epstein, S. Sounding board: sudden cardiac death without warning. Possible mechanisms and implications for screening asymptomatic populations. *N Engl J Med* 321:320, 1989.

Richardson, P. Influence of plaque configuration and stress distribution on fissuring of coronary atherosclerotic plaques. *Lancet* 2:941, 1989.

Fuster, V. The pathogenesis of coronary artery disease and the acute coronary syndromes (second of two parts). *N Engl J Med* 326:310, 1992.

Patterson, D. The culprit coronary artery lesion. *Lancet* 338:1379, 1991.

Brown, B. Regression of atherosclerosis—an ounce of prevention. *West J Med* 159:208, 1993.

Brown, B. Atherosclerosis regression, plaque disruption, and cardiovascular events: a rationale for lipid lowering in coronary artery disease. *Ann Rev Med* 44:365, 1993.

Ideal cholesterol is less than 150 mg/dl:

Roberts, W. Atherosclerotic risk factors—are there ten or is there only one? *Am J Cardiol* 64:552, 1989.

Kannel, W. Is the serum total cholesterol an anachronism? *Lancet* 2:950, 1979.

Reversal of atherosclerosis:

Strom, A. Mortality from circulatory diseases in Norway 1940–1945. *Lancet* 1:126, 1951.

Wissler, R. Studies of regression of advanced atherosclerosis in experimental animals and man. *Ann NY Acad Sci* 275:363, 1976.

Armstrong, M. Regression of coronary atheromatosis in Rhesus monkeys. *Circ Res* 27:59, 1970.

Duffield, R. Treatment of hyperlipidaemia retards progression of symptomatic femoral atherosclerosis. *Lancet* 2:639, 1983.

Nikkila, E. Prevention of progression of coronary atherosclerosis by treatment of hyperlipidaemia: a seven-year prospective angiographic study. *Br Med J* 289:220, 1984.

Ost, C. Regression of peripheral atherosclerosis during therapy with high doses of nicotinic acid. *Scand J Clin Lab Invest* (suppl) 99:241, 1967.

Barndt, R. Regression and progression of early femoral atherosclerosis in treated hyperlipoproteinemic patients. *Ann Intern Med* 86:139, 1977.

Hennerici, M. Spontaneous progression and regression of small carotid atheroma. *Lancet* 1:1415, 1985.

Basta, L. Regression of atherosclerotic stenosing lesions of the renal arteries and spontaneous cure of systemic hypertension through control of hyperlipidemia. *Am J Med* 61:420, 1976.

Bassler, T. Regression of athroma. *West J Med* 132:474, 1980.

Roth, D. Noninvasive and invasive demonstration of spontaneous regression of coronary artery disease. *Circulation* 62:888, 1980.

Hubbard, J. Nathan Pritikin's heart. *N Engl J Med* 313:52, 1985.

Brensike, J. Effects of therapy with cholestyramine on progression of coronary atherosclerosis: results of the NHLBI Type II Coronary Intervention Study. *Circulation* 69:313, 1984.

Cashin-Hemphill, L. Beneficial effects of colestipol-niacin on coronary atherosclerosis: a 4-year follow-up. *JAMA* 264:3013, 1990.

Arntzenius, A. Diet, lipoproteins, and the progression of coronary atherosclerosis: the Leiden Intervention Trial. *N Engl J Med* 312:805, 1985.

Blankenhorn, D. Beneficial effects of combined colestipol-niacin therapy on coronary atherosclerosis and coronary venous bypass grafts. *JAMA* 257:3233, 1987.

Buchwald, H. Effect of partial ileal bypass surgery on mortality and morbidity from coronary heart disease in patients with hypercholesterolemia: Report of the Program on the Surgical Control of Hyperlipidemias (POSCH). *N Engl J Med* 323:946, 1990.

Brown, B. Regression of coronary artery disease as a result of intensive lipid-lowering therapy in men with high levels of apolipoprotein B. *N Engl J Med* 323:1289, 1990.

Kane, J. Regression of coronary atherosclerosis during treatment of familial hypercholesterolemia with combined drug regiments. *JAMA* 264:3007, 1990.

Watts, G. Effects on coronary artery disease of lipid-lowering diet, or diet plus cholestyramine in the St. Thomas' Atherosclerosis Regression Study (STARS). *Lancet* 339:563, 1992.

Schuler, G. Regular physical exercise and low-fat diet: effects on progression of coronary artery disease. *Circulation* 86:1, 1992.

Schuler, G. Myocardial perfusion and regression of coronary artery disease in patients on a regimen of physical exercise and low fat diet. *J Am Coll Cardiol* 19:34, 1992.

Brown, B. Regression of atherosclerosis—an ounce of prevention. *West J Med* 159:208, 1993.

Haskell, W. Effects of intensive multiple risk factor reduction on coronary atherosclerosis and clinical cardiac events in men and women with coronary artery disease: the Stanford Coronary Risk Intervention Project (SCRIP). *Circulation* 89:975, 1994.

Blankenhorn, D. The influence of diet on the appearance of new lesions in human coronary artery disease. *JAMA* 263:1646, 1990.

Blankenhorn, D. Coronary angiographic changes with lovastatin therapy. The Monitored Atherosclerosis Regression Study (MARS). *Ann Intern Med* 119:969, 1993.

Ornish, D. Can lifestyle changes reverse coronary heart disease? *Lancet* 336:129, 1990.

Levine, G. Cholesterol reduction in cardiovascular disease. *N Engl J Med* 332:512, 1995.

Superko, R. Coronary artery disease regression. Convincing evidence for the benefit of aggressive lipoprotein management. *Circulation* 90:1056, 1994.

Thompson, G. Familial Hypercholesterolaemia Regression Study: a randomised trial of low-density-lipoprotein apheresis. *Lancet* 345:811, 1995.

Treasure, C. Beneficial effects of cholesterol-lowering therapy on the coronary endothelium in patients with coronary artery disease. *N Engl J Med* 332:481, 1995.

There is a lot of confusion today about HDL cholesterol:

McMurray, M. Changes in lipid and lipoprotein levels and body weight in the Tarahumara Indians after consumption of an affluent diet. *N Engl J Med* 325:1704, 1991.

Brinton, E. A low-fat diet decreases high density lipoprotein (HDL) cholesterol levels by decreasing HDL apolipoprotein transport rates. *J Clin Invest* 85:144, 1990.

Published results of the McDougall Program:

McDougall, MD. Rapid reduction of serum cholesterol and blood pressure by a twelve-day, very low fat, strictly vegetarian diet. *J Am Coll Nutr* 14:491, 1995.

Worldwide people with the lowest HDL have the lowest heart disease:

Knuiman, J. HDL-cholesterol in men from thirteen countries (letter). *Lancet* 2:367, 1981.

Simple carbohydrates raise triglycerides, complex carbohydrates don't:

Hudgins, L. Human fatty acid synthesis is reduced after the substitution of dietary starch for sugar. *Am J Clin Nutr* 67:631, 1998.

Anderson, J. Metabolic effects of high-carbohydrate, high-fiber diets for insulin-dependent diabetic individuals. *Am J Clin Nutr* 1991 54:936, 1991.

Fruit (fructose) raises cholesterol and triglycerides in sensitive people:
  Hollenbeck, C. Dietary fructose effects on lipoprotein metabolism and risk
    for coronary artery disease. *Am J Clin Nutr* 58 (suppl):800S, 1993.
  Hallfrisch, J. Metabolic effects of fructose. *FASEB J* 4:2652, 1992.
  Swanson, J. Metabolic effects of dietary fructose in healthy subjects. *Am J Clin
    Nutr* 55:851, 1992.

Overfeeding subjects causes triglycerides to rise:
  Schaefer, E. Body weight and low-density lipoprotein cholesterol changes af-
    ter consumption of a low-fat ad libitum diet. *JAMA* 274:1450, 1995.

Slower introduction of a high-carbohydrate diet results in no increase in triglycerides:
  Ullmann, D. Will a high-carbohydrate, low-fat diet lower plasma lipids and
    lipoproteins without producing hypertriglyceridemia. *Atheroscler Thromb*
    11:1059, 1991.

Exercise lowers triglycerides:
  Tsetsonis, N. Reduction in postprandial lipemia after walking: influence of
    exercise intensity. *Med Sci Sports Exerc* 28:1235, 1996.

Elevated homocysteine levels are associated with increased risk of heart and other diseases:
  Nygard, O. Plasma homocysteine levels and mortality in patients with coro-
    nary artery disease. *N Engl J Med* 337:230, 1997.
  Graham, I. Elevated total homocysteine levels increased the risk for vascular
    disease. *JAMA* 277:1775, 1997.
  Nygard, O. Total homocysteine and cardiovascular risk profile. The Horda-
    land Homocysteine Study. *JAMA* 274:1526, 1995.
  Rimm, E. Folate and vitamin B6 from diet and supplements in relation to risk
    of coronary heart disease among women. *JAMA* 279:359, 1998.
  Heijer, M. Hyperhomocysteinemia as a risk factor for deep-vein thrombosis.
    N Engl J Med 334:759, 1996.
  Fermo, I. Prevalence of moderate hyperhomocysteinemia in patients with early-
    onset venous and arterial occlusive disease. *Ann Intern Med* 123:747, 1995.

A 12 percent rise in homocysteine increases the risk of artery disease by more than threefold:
  Selhub, J. Association between plasma homocysteine concentrations and
    extracranial carotid-artery stenosis. *N Engl J Med* 332:286, 1995.
  Selhub, J. Vitamin status and intake as primary determinants of homocys-
    teinemia in an elderly population. *JAMA* 270:2693, 1993.

Exercise improves circulation:
  McKirnan, M. Clinical significance of coronary vascular adaptions to exercise
    in training. *Med Sci Sports Exerc* 26:1262, 1994.
  Tomanek, R. Exercise-induced coronary angiogenesis: a review. *Med Sci Sports
    Exerc* 26:1245, 1994.

Garlic lowers cholesterol:
  Warshafsky, S. Effect of garlic on total serum cholesterol. A metaanalysis. *Ann
    Intern Med* 119:599, 1993.

Jain, A. Can garlic reduce levels of serum lipids? A controlled clinical study. *Am J Med* 94:632, 1993.

Mansell, P. Garlic. Effects on serum lipids, blood pressure, coagulation, platelet aggregation, and vasodilatation. *BMJ* 303:379, 1991.

Brosche, T. Garlic (letter). *BMJ* 303:785, 1991.

Odorless garlic also lowers cholesterol:

Steiner, M. A double-blind crossover study in moderately hypercholesterolemic men that compared the effect of aged garlic extract and placebo administration on blood lipids. *Am J Clin Nutr* 64:866, 1996.

Lau, B. Effect of odor-modified garlic preparation on blood lipids. *Nutr Res* 7:139, 1987.

Steiner, M. Cardiovascular and lipid changes in response to aged garlic extract ingestion. *J Am Coll Nutr* 13:524, 1994.

Vitamin C (2 grams) lowers cholesterol and platelet adhesiveness:

Bordia, A. The effect of vitamin C on blood lipids, fibrinolytic activity and platelet adhesiveness in patients with coronary artery disease. *Atherosclerosis* 35:181, 1980.

Turley, S. The role of ascorbic acid in the regulation of cholesterol metabolism and in the pathogenesis of atherosclerosis. *Atherosclerosis* 24:1, 1976.

Vitamin E supplements lower cholesterol:

Qureshi, A. Lowering of serum cholesterol in hypercholesterolemic humans by tocotrienols (palmvitee). *Am J Clin Nutr* 53:1021S, 1991.

Dietary fiber lowers cholesterol:

Salenius, J. Long term effects of guar gum on lipid metabolism after carotid endarterectomy. *BMJ* 310:95, 1995.

Ripsin, C. Oat products and lipid lowering: a meta-analysis. *JAMA* 267:3317, 1992.

Davidson, M. The hypocholesterolemic effects of B-glucan in oatmeal and oat bran. *JAMA* 265:1833, 1991.

Activated charcoal lowers cholesterol:

Neuvonen, P. The mechanism of the hypocholesterolaemic effect of activated charcoal. *Eur J Clin Invest* 19:251, 1989.

Kuusisto, P. Effect of activated charcoal on hypercholesterolaemia. *Lancet* 2:366, 1986.

Friedman, E. Reduction in hyperlipidemia in hemodialysis patients treated with charcoal and oxidized starch (oxystarch). *Am J Clin Nutr* 31:1903, 1978.

Neuvonen, P. Activated charcoal in the treatment of hypercholesterolaemia: dose-response relationship and comparison with cholestyramine. *Eur J Clin Pharmacol* 37:225, 1989.

Powerful cholesterol-lowering effects of gugulipid:
   Nityanand, S. Clinical trials with gugulipid. A new hyolipidaemic agent. *J Assoc Physicians India* 37:323, 1989.
   Satyavati, G. Gum guggul (Commiphora mukul)—the success story of an ancient insight leading to a modern discovery. *Indian J Med Res* 87:327, 1988.
   Verma, S. Effect of Commiphora mukul (gum guggulu) in patients of hyperlipidemia with special reference to HDL-cholesterol. *Indian J Med Res* 87:356, 1988.

Vitamin B_3 (niacin) supplements lower cholesterol, but long-acting forms cause hepatitis:
   McKenney, J. A comparison of the efficacy and toxic effects of sustained- vs immediate-release niacin in hypercholesterolemic patients. *JAMA* 271:672, 1994.
   Henkin, Y. Niacin revisited: clinical observations on an important underutilized drug. *Am J Med* 91:239, 1991.
   Gray, D. Efficacy and safety of controlled-release niacin in dyslipoproteinemic veterans. *Ann Intern Med* 121:252, 1994.

HRT lowers cholesterol and reduces risk of heart disease:
   Darling, G. Estrogen and progestin compared with simvastatin for hypercholesterolemia in postmenopausal women. *N Engl J Med* 337:595, 1997.
   Kessler, C. Estrogen replacement therapy and coagulation: relationship to lipid and lipoprotein changes. *Obstet Gynecol* 89:326, 1997.
   Also see chapter 13, "Balancing the Positives and Negatives of Hormone Replacement Therapy."

Incidence of hypertension varies around the world; the disease is rare among people living on starch-based, low-salt diets:
   Freis, E. Salt, volume and the prevention of hypertension. *Circulation* 53:589, 1976.
   Finn, R. Blood pressure and salt intake: an intra-population study. *Lancet* 1:1097, 1981.

A diet rich in fruits and vegetables lowers blood pressure:
   Appel, L. A clinical trial of the effects of dietary patterns on blood pressure. *N Engl J Med* 336:1117, 1997.

Serious side effects of calcium channel blockers:
   Pahor, M. Risk of gastrointestinal hemorrhage with calcium antagonists in hypertensive persons over 67 years old. *Lancet* 347:1061, 1996.
   Psaty, B. The risk of myocardial infarction with antihypertensive drug therapies. *JAMA* 274:620, 1995.
   Horton, R. Spinning the risks and benefits of calcium antagonists. *Lancet* 346:586, 1995.
   Furberg, C. Calcium antagonists: not appropriate as first line antihypertensive drugs. *Am J Hypertens* 9:122, 1996.
   Pahor, M. Calcium channel blockers and incidence of cancer in aged populations. *Lancet* 348:493, 1996.

Fitzpatrick, A. Use of calcium channel blockers and breast carcinoma risk in postmenopausal women. *Cancer* 80:1438, 1997.

Lindberg, G. Use of calcium channel blockers and risk of suicide: ecological findings confirmed in population cohort study. *BMJ* 316:741, 1998.

Adverse effects of diuretics:

Siscovick, D. Diuretic therapy for hypertension and the risk of cardiac arrest. *N Engl J Med* 330:1852, 1994.

Hoes, A. Diuretics, β-blockers, and the risk for sudden cardiac death in hypertensive patients. *Ann Intern Med* 123:481, 1995.

Ballantyne, D. Long-term effects of antihypertensives on blood lipids. *J Hum Hypertens* 4 (suppl 2):35, 1990.

Multiple Risk Factor Intervention Trial Research Group. Multiple Risk Factor Intervention Trial. Risk factor changes and mortality results. *JAMA* 248:1465, 1982.

Holme, I. Treatment of mild hypertension with diuretics. The importance of ECG abnormalities in the Oslo Study and in MRFIT. *JAMA* 251:1298, 1984.

Kannel, W. Sudden death: lessons from subsets in population studies. Lessons from epidemiology. *J Am Coll Cardiol* 5:141B, 1985.

Anti-HT therapy seems to add to sudden death risk in some. *Int Med News* 18:60, 1985.

Grimm, R. Effects of thiazide diuretics on plasma lipids and lipoproteins in mildly hypertensive patients. A double-blind controlled trial. *Ann Intern Med* 94:7, 1981.

Ames, R. Serum cholesterol during treatment of hypertension with diuretic drugs. *Arch Intern Med* 144:710, 1984.

Diuretics, hyperuricaemia, and tienilic acid (editorial). *Lancet* 2:681, 1980.

Murphy, M. Glucose intolerance in hypertensive patients treated with diuretics; a fourteen-year follow-up. *Lancet* 2:1293, 1982.

Holland, O. Diuretic-induced ventricular ectopic activity. *Am J Med* 70:762, 1981.

Intellectual performance in hypertensive patients (editorial). *Lancet* 1:87, 1984.

Effects of ACE inhibitors:

Armario, P. Adverse effects of direct-acting vasodilators. *Drug Safety* 11:80, 1994.

Schnaper, H. Angiotensin-converting enzyme inhibitors for systemic hypertension in young and elderly patients. *Am J Cardiol* 69:54C, 1992.

Parish, R. Adverse effects of angiotension-converting enzyme (ACE) inhibitors. An update. *Drug Safety* 7:14, 1992.

Adverse effects of β-blockers:

Hoes, A. Diuretics, β-blockers, and the risk for sudden cardiac death in hypertensive patients. *Ann Intern Med* 123:481, 1995.

Observe blood pressure for three to six months before treatment, because BP often drops without treatment:

WHO/ISH Mild Hypertension Liaison Committee. 1989 guidelines for the management of mild hypertension: memorandum from WHO/ISH meeting. *J Hypertens* 7:689, 1989.

Report by the Management Committee: the Australian therapeutic trial in mild hypertension. *Lancet* 1:1261, 1980.

Blood pressure at home more accurate than in the doctor's office:

White, W. Average daily blood pressure, not office blood pressure, determines cardiac function in patients with hypertension. *JAMA* 261:873, 1989.

Aggressive treatment of blood pressure kills—do not lower diastolic below 90 with drugs:

Alderman, M. Treatment-induced blood pressure reduction and the risk of myocardial infarction. *JAMA* 262:920, 1989.

Cruickshank, J. Benefits and potential harm of lowering blood pressure. *Lancet* 1:581, 1987.

Farnett, L. The J-curve phenomenon and the treatment of hypertension. Is there a point beyond which pressure reduction is dangerous? *JAMA* 265:489, 1991.

Cruickshank, J. Coronary flow reserve and the J curve relation between diastolic blood pressure and myocardial infarction. *BMJ* 297:1227, 1988.

Kuller, L. Unexpected effects of treating hypertension in men with electrocardiographic abnormalities: a critical analysis. *Circulation* 73:114, 1986.

Cooper, S. The relation between degree of blood pressure reduction and mortality among hypertensives in the Hypertensive Detection and Follow-up Program. *Am J Epidemiol* 127:387, 1988.

Berglund, G. Goals of antihypertensive therapy. Is there a point beyond which pressure reduction is dangerous? *Am J Hypertens* 2:586, 1989.

McCloskey, L. Level of blood pressure and risk of myocardial infarction among treated hypertensive patients. *Arch Intern Med* 152:513, 1992.

Smith, B. Do no harm. Antihypertensive therapy and the "J" curve (editorial). *Arch Intern Med* 152:473, 1992.

Samuelsson, O. The J-shaped relationship between coronary heart disease and achieved blood pressure level in treated hypertension: further analysis of 12 years of follow-up of treated hypertensives in Primary Prevention Trial in Gothenberg, Sweden. *J Hypertens* 8:547, 1990.

Lindblad, U. Control of blood pressure and risk of first acute myocardial infarction: Skaraborg hypertensive project. *BMJ* 308:681, 1994.

Caffeine raises blood pressure:

Sung, B. Prolonged increase in blood pressure by a single dose of caffeine in mildly hypertensive men. *Am J Hypertens* 7:755, 1994.

Superko, R. Effects of cessation of caffeinated-coffee consumption on ambulatory and resting blood pressure in men. *Am J Cardiol* 73:780, 1994.

Alcohol raises blood pressure:

Moore, R. Alcohol consumption and blood pressure in the 1982 Maryland hypertension survey. *Am J Hypertens* 3:1, 1990.

Potter, J. Pressor effect of alcohol in hypertension. *Lancet* 1:119, 1984.

Marmiot, M. Alcohol and blood pressure: the INTERSALT study. *BMJ* 308: 1263, 1994.

Patients experience a dramatic improvement in circulation with a low-fat diet—no more sludging:

Cullen, C. Intravascular aggregation and adhesiveness of the blood elements associated with alimentary lipemia and injections of large molecular substances. *Circulation* 9:335, 1954.

Friedman, M. Serum lipids and conjunctival circulation after fat ingestion in men exhibiting type-A behavior patterns. *Circulation* 29:874, 1964.

Friedman, M. Effect of unsaturated fats upon lipemia and conjunctival circulation. A study of coronary-prone (pattern A) men. *JAMA* 193:883, 1965.

Kuo, P. The effect of lipemia upon coronary and peripheral arterial circulation in patients with essential hyperlipidemia. *Am J Med* 26:68, 1959.

Exercise improves a woman's health and her heart:

Blair, S. Influences of cardiorespiratory fitness and other precursors on cardiovascular disease and all-cause mortality in men and women. *JAMA* 276:205, 1996.

Duncan, J. Women walking for health and fitness. How much is enough? *JAMA* 266:3295, 1991.

Lemaitre, R. Leisure-time physical activity and the risk of nonfatal myocardial infarction in postmenopausal women. *Arch Intern Med* 155:2302, 1995.

NIH Consensus Development Panel on Physical Activity and Cardiovascular Health. Physical activity and cardiovascular health. *JAMA* 276:241, 1996.

Stefanick, M. Effects of diet and exercise in men and women with low levels of HDL cholesterol and high levels of LDL cholesterol. *N Engl J Med* 339:12, 1998.

Pima Indians develop diabetes and other degenerative diseases on the Western diet:

Ringrose, H. Nutrient intakes in an urbanized Micronesian population with high diabetes prevalence. *Am J Clin Nutr* 32:1334, 1979.

In the 1920s, Dr. Shirley Sweeney found fat paralyzed insulin activity:

Sweeney, S. Dietary factors that influence the dextrose tolerance test: a preliminary study. *Arch Intern Med* 40:818, 1927.

University of Kentucky researchers found that two-thirds of adult diabetics no longer needed insulin after adopting a low-fat diet:

Kiehm, T. Beneficial effects of a high carbohydrate, high fiber diet on hyperglycemia in diabetic men. *Am J Clin Nutr* 29:895, 1976.

Anderson, J. Long-term effects of high-carbohydrate, high-fiber diets on glucose and lipid metabolism: a preliminary report on patients with diabetes. *Diabetes Care* 1:77, 1978.

Chapter 15. Surviving Is the Bottom Line

People who are not well insured do not get the same quality of care:
   Newacheck, P. Health insurance and access to primary care for children.
   N Engl J Med 338:513, 1998.
   Mort, E. Physician response to patient insurance status in ambulatory care
   clinical decision-making. Implications for quality of care. *Med Care* 34:783,
   1996.
   Bloom, B. Access to health care. Part 2: Working-age adults. *Vital Health Stat
   10* 197:1, 1997.
   Simpson, G. Access to health care. Part 1: Children. *Vital Health Stat 10* 196:1,
   1997.

Fee for services vs. managed care:
   Hillman, A. Health maintenance organizations, financial incentives, and
   physicians' judgments. *Ann Intern Med* 112:891, 1990.
   Angell, M. Quality and the medical marketplace—following elephants.
   N Engl J Med 335:883, 1996.
   Woolhandler, S. Extreme risk—the new corporate proposition for physicians.
   N Engl J Med 333:1706, 1995.
   Bodenheimer, T. How large employers are shaping the health market
   place. First of two parts. *N Engl J Med* 338:1003, 1998.

Forty-three percent of HMOs ask Medicare patients about their health prior to enrollment:
   Woolhandler, S. Extreme risk—the new corporate proposition for physicians.
   N Engl J Med 333:1706, 1995.

Total capitation for an internist is between $11 and $14 per member per month:
   Spong, F. What is in a reasonable capitation agreement. *ACP Observer,* January 1997, 7.

*An internist may take home more than $150,000 in bonuses and incentives for saving
money:*
   Woolhandler, S. Extreme risk—the new corporate proposition for physicians.
   N Engl J Med 333:1706, 1995.

*Contracts with doctors that prevent them from divulging their financial arrangements
with insurance companies:*
   Woolhandler, S. Extreme risk—the new corporate proposition for physicians.
   N Engl J Med 333:1706, 1995.

Appendix B. Early Detection Tests

*The National Cancer Institute estimates a 30 percent reduction in tobacco use would yield
a 10 percent reduction in cancer deaths:*
   McPhee, S. Screening for cancer. Useful despite its limitations. *West J Med*
   163:169, 1995.

American Cancer Society recommendations for breast cancer prevention:
  Cancer facts and figures—1996. American Cancer Society, 1996.

There is no evidence that a doctor's physical examination of your breasts, your own breast self-examination, or breast ultrasound will reduce your chance of dying of breast cancer:
  Austoker, J. Screening for ovarian, prostatic, and testicular cancers. *BMJ* 309:315, 1994.

Results of breast self-examination show no benefits and possible harm:
  Baines, C. Reflections on breast self-examination (editorial). *J Natl Cancer Inst* 89:339, 1997.
  Morrison, A. Is self-examination effective in screening for breast cancer? *J Natl Cancer Inst* 83:226, 1991.
  Mant, D. Breast self examination: should we discourage it? (editorial) *J R Coll Gen Pract* 39:180, 1989.
  Frank, J. Breast self-examination in young women: more harm than good? *Lancet* 2:654, 1985.

63,636 women between ages forty-five and sixty-four in England who were offered breast self-examination education had a higher death rate from breast cancer:
  UK Trial of Early Detection Cancer Group. First results on mortality reduction in the UK trial of early detection of breast cancer. *Lancet* 2:411, 1988.

Another study found a higher risk of developing advanced breast cancer in women who reported they performed breast self-examination than in those who did not:
  Newcomb, P. Breast self-examination in relation to occurrence of advanced breast cancer. *J Natl Cancer Inst* 83:260, 1991.

A study of Chinese women who worked in a textile factory found no benefit of breast self-examination:
  Thomas, D. Randomized trial of breast self-examination in Shanghai: methodology and preliminary results. *J Natl Cancer Inst* 89:355, 1997.

"Fecal blood appears to be a poor marker for colorectal neoplasia. Most cancers and the vast majority of polyps will be missed":
  Ahlquist, D. Accuracy of fecal occult blood screening for colon rectal neoplasia. A prospective study using Hemoccult and HemoQuant Tests. *JAMA* 269:1262, 1993.
  Simon, J. Should all people over the age of 50 have regular fecal occult-blood tests? Postpone population screening until problems are solved. *N Engl J Med* 338:1151, 1998.

More recent studies suggest fecal blood may be helpful:
  Fletcher, R. Should all people over the age of 50 have regular fecal occult-blood tests? If it works why not do it? *N Engl J Med* 338:1153, 1998.
  Ransohoff, D. Clinical guideline: part II. Screening for colorectal cancer with the fecal occult blood test: a background. *Ann Intern Med* 126:811, 1997.

In one often-cited study, sigmoidoscopy examination once every ten years reduced the risk of dying from colorectal cancer by 59 percent:

> Selby, J. A case-control study of screening sigmoidoscopy and mortality from colorectal cancer. *N Engl J Med* 326:653, 1992.

Cancer begins with a small symptomless polyp, or projecting growth, which takes ten to thirty-five years to become cancer:

> Bhattacharya, I. Screening colonoscopy: the cost of common sense. *Lancet* 347:1744, 1996.

> Morson, B. Genesis of colonrectal cancer. *Clin Gastroenterol* 5:505, 1976.

> Stryker, S. Natural history of untreated colonic polyps. *Gastroenterology* 93: 1009, 1987.

The National Polyp Study showed an incidence of colon cancer 76 to 90 percent lower than expected:

> Winawer, S. Prevention of colorectal cancer by colonoscopy polypectomy. The National Polyp Study Workgroup. *N Engl J Med* 329:1977, 1993.

An effective way to screen would be to do one exam between the ages of fifty-five and sixty:

> Atkin, W. Prevention of colorectal cancer by once-only sigmoidoscopy. *Lancet* 341:736, 1993.

> Lieberman, D. Cost-effectiveness model for colon cancer screening. *Gastroenterology* 109:1781, 1995.

> Selby, J. Screening sigmoidoscopy for colorectal cancer (commentary). *Lancet* 341:728, 1993.

My preferred method for colon cancer screening is a double-contrast barium enema and a flexible sigmoidoscope:

> Chapman, A. United States has recommended screening for colon cancer. Why has barium enema been suggested? (letter) *BMJ* 314:1624, 1997.

> Selby, J. A case-control study of screening sigmoidoscopy and mortality from colorectal cancer. *N Engl J Med* 326:653, 1992.

> Dodd, G. The role of the barium enema in the detection of colonic neoplasms. *Cancer* 70:1272, 1992.

Colonoscopy examinations miss 24 percent of polyps:

> Rex, D. Colonoscopic miss rates of adenomas determined by back-to-back colonoscopies. *Gastroenterology* 112:24, 1997.

Mass screening for cervical cancer may be doing more harm than good:

> McCormick, J. Cervical smears? A questionable practice? *Lancet* 2:207, 1989.

> Raffle, A. Cervical screening: what is the point? (letter) *Lancet* 346:246, 1995.

Death rates from cervical cancer were declining before screening began:

> Raffle, A. Cervical screening: what is the point? (letter) *Lancet* 346:246, 1995.

Study of screening in Bristol, England, of 225,974 women found 15,000 healthy women were being incorrectly told that they are "at risk":

Raffle, A. Detection rates for abnormal cervical smears: what are we screening for? *Lancet* 345:1469, 1995.

Raffle, A. Informed participation in screening is essential (letter). *BMJ* 314: 1762, 1997.

"Abnormal cells can be found in the smears of numerous women never destined to get cervical cancer":

Raffle, A. Detection rates for abnormal cervical smears: what are we screening for? *Lancet* 345:1469, 1995.

Many health organizations recommend discontinuation of smears after the ages of sixty to sixty-five:

Fahs, M. Cost effectiveness of cervical screening for the elderly. *Ann Intern Med* 117:520, 1992.

"All women over 50 . . . with negative results on smear testing every three years may be safely discharged from further screening":

Van Wijngaarden. Rationale for stopping cervical screening in women over 50. *BMJ* 306:967, 1993.

After a hysterectomy, Pap smears should be stopped:

Fetters, M. Effectiveness of vaginal Papanicolaou smear screening after total hysterectomy for benign disease. *JAMA* 275:940, 1996.

The Canadian Task Force was unable to recommend any screening techniques for endometrial cancer and the American College of Physicians agrees:

Pritchard, K. Screening for endometrial cancer: is it effective? (editorial) *Ann Intern Med* 110:177, 1989.

Pelvic examination for ovarian cancer is not effective and bimanual examination should not be performed as a routine screening in asymptomatic women:

Austoker, J. Screening for ovarian, prostatic, and testicular cancers. *BMJ* 309:315, 1994.

Testing for ovarian cancer is ineffective:

American College of Physicians. Screening for ovarian cancer: recommendations and rationale. *Ann Intern Med* 121:141, 1994.

Carlson, K. Screening for ovarian cancer. *Ann Intern Med* 121:124, 1994.

Austoker, J. Screening for ovarian, prostatic, and testicular cancers. *BMJ* 309:315, 1994.

NIH Consensus Development Panel on Ovarian Cancer. Ovarian cancer: screening, treatment, and follow-up. *JAMA* 273:491, 1995.

Schapira, M. The effectiveness of ovarian cancer screening. A decision analysis model. *Ann Intern Med* 118:838, 1993.

It is widely accepted that screening for lung cancer is not recommended:

Eddy, D. Screening for lung cancer. *Ann Intern Med* 111:232, 1989.

McDougall's recommendations:

Meyers, F. Screening for cancer. Is it worth it? *West J Med* 163:166, 1995.

General Index

RECIPE INDEX